Healing the Body Politic

Healing the Body Politic

El Salvador's Popular Struggle for Health Rights–From Civil War to Neoliberal Peace

SANDY SMITH-NONINI

RUTGERS UNIVERSITY PRESS

NEW BRUNSWICK, NEW JERSEY, AND LONDON

LIBRARY OF CONGRESS CATALOGING-IN-PUBLICATION DATA

Smith-Nonini, Sandra C.
    Healing the body politic : El Salvador's popular struggle for health rights from civil war to neoliberal peace / Sandy Smith-Nonini.
        p. cm. — (Studies in medical anthropology)
    Includes bibliographical references and index.
    ISBN 978–0–8135–4735–0 (hardcover : alk. paper) — ISBN 978–0–8135–4736–7 (pbk. : alk. paper)
    1. Public health—El Salvador.   2. Health policy—El Salvador.   3. Community health services—El Salvador.   4. Social conflict—Health aspects—El Salvador.
    I. Title.
    RA454.S2S65   2010
    362.1097284—dc22

                                                                              2009025348

A British Cataloging-in-Publication record for this book is available
from the British Library.

Visit our Web site: http://rutgerspress.rutgers.edu

Manufactured in the United States of America

Dedicated to
Marta Lidia "Tita" Guzmán
(1967–1989)
Spokesperson for UNADES, a union of
victims of the 1986 earthquake

Tita, a single mother of two young children
and a close friend,
is believed to have been captured and killed
by the National Police, on June 3, 1989,
after a series of police threats
and arrests of activists in the organization.
We never found her body.

There is no such thing as "disappeared."

CONTENTS

PART FOUR
War by Other Means

ACKNOWLEDGMENTS

This book evolved from over two decades of involvement in health rights issues in El Salvador, so the paltry list of mentors, supporters, friends, and co-conspirators here will surely fail to do justice to the many obligations I incurred. Generous financial support from a Richard Carley Hunt Postdoctoral Writing Fellowship, awarded by the Wenner Gren Foundation, made revision of the manuscript possible. The quality of my research during the postwar period was enhanced by a research grant from the Inter-American Foundation, and travel grants from the Tinker and Mellon Foundations, awarded by the Duke University—University of North Carolina Latin American Studies Program.

I am very grateful to Susan Greenblatt for excellent research assistance with interviews in San Salvador on the antiprivatization movement in 2000, 2002–2003, and 2007. I benefited greatly from Leigh Binford's reading and gentle editing of the entire manuscript, and from the skillful guidance of my editor, Adi Hovav, and the Studies in Medical Anthropology series editor Mac Marshall. I owe a special debt to Catherine Lutz, Orin Starn, and Donald Nonini, who believed in me before I believed in myself, offering encouraging feedback on early drafts, and helping to keep my small boat afloat through the shoals of the culture wars.

Other colleagues who encouraged this endeavor through shared insights or feedback on writings include Bernard Bloom, Jeff Boyer, Leo Chavez, Carole Crumley, Marisol de la Cadena, Arturo Escobar, Paul Farmer, John Gershman, Kris Heggenhougan, Dorothy Holland, Alex Irwin, Jim Yong Kim, Richard Lee, Bill Maurer, Tom May, Joyce Millen, Tommie Sue Montgomery, Carolyn Nordstrom, Jim Peacock, Jim Quesada, Peter Redfield, Michelle Rivkin-Fish, and the graduate students of the UNC Moral Economies of Medicine seminar.

Since my first visit to El Salvador on a small National Central America Health Rights task force in 1985, I benefited from the generosity of hundreds of Salvadorans who took time out of their busy lives to help me understand the complicated politics of their struggles over community health and basic human rights. I am grateful especially to Eduardo Espinoza, Violeta Menjivar, Margarita Posada, Ernesto Selva-Sutter, Hector Silva, and Miguel Saenz Varela. For reasons of privacy I cannot fully acknowledge all those whose patience and hospitality made my fieldwork enjoyable and productive, but I throw *besos especiales* to Delmy, Francisco, Victoria, Tina, Rene, Teófilo, Dagoberto, and Cece. Special thanks to David Bedell and Bob Bristow for all those rides to Chalate and to the wonderful *promotores de salud popular* in rural Chalatenango who have worked so professionally for long years with little recognition.

During the tumultuous years of 1987–1989 my life in San Salvador was enriched by shared experiences with many intrepid colleagues engaged in human rights work and journalism, including Leslie Toser, Robyn Braverman, Tom Long, Kathleen Lynch, and Corinne Dufka—all of whom also pitched in with childcare for my son, Roque, when his irresponsible mother was on deadline. I'm especially grateful to Davida Coady and the San Carlos Foundation for funding my investigative reporting on violations of medical neutrality, and to Flora Skelly, my editor at *American Medical News*, who continued to publish the reports despite their controversial reception by conservative readers. During my 1989 stint as a stringer for the *New York Times* I was grateful for the trust and confidence placed in me by San Salvador Bureau Chief Lindsey Gruson. The humor of Jeremy Bigwood helped keep us all sane, and I again thank Doug Mine, who intervened to spring me and a colleague from the Fourth Brigade headquarters after the incident described in the Prologue.

El Salvador's civil war had a way of minting extraordinary people whose courage and service under horrific circumstances became a beacon for the rest of us. I had the privilege of knowing several genuine heroes, including Lutheran bishop Medardo Gomez, Charles Clements, the late Sister Ann Manganaro, and Brenda Hubbard and Lanny Smith, of Doctors for Global Health. Many who I cannot name (because of lost records or protected identities) delivered health services behind the lines at enormous risk during the war, some losing their lives. Hundreds continued to volunteer throughout the long postwar period of neoliberal austerity. May this book serve to pay homage to your sacrifice.

Finally, nothing would have been possible without Roque, the amazing son I brought home from El Salvador, and my husband, Don, whose love and passion for justice is the wellspring of my energy.

PROLOGUE: TERROR AND HEALING IN EL SALVADOR

In the first spring of the new millennium, eight years after the civil war, residents of San Salvador found themselves caught in an eerie déjà vu. On March 6, 2000, hundreds of riot police, in an action reminiscent of the war years, fired tear gas into a hospital emergency room occupied by protesting health workers, then stormed the building. At least two patients died in the chaos and dozens were injured. The violence came during a prolonged health strike that had paralyzed hospitals across the country as two medical unions protested President Francisco Flores's plans to privatize social security health services.

Under pressure, Flores, of the right-wing National Republican Alliance (ARENA) party, backed off on his privatization plan only to unveil a new version of the plan months later. By fall 2002 the opposition, now joined by public hospital employees and a broad sector of the democratic left, struck again with health strikes, road closings, and a series of massive "White Marches" in which hundreds of thousands filled the streets dressed in white to show solidarity with striking doctors and nurses. Once again efforts by ARENA elites backed by multilateral lenders favoring privatization were set back. In June 2003 Flores agreed to a joint health reform commission that would include leaders of the social movement. After that, in a rare move, the World Bank agreed to remove privatization conditions from loan agreements.

The marches were the largest street mobilizations since the war ended, and to the surprise of many, they were not led by the leftist party of former guerrillas—the Farabundo Martí National Liberation Front (FMLN)—whose leaders had belatedly thrown their support behind the radicalized health workers after the protests gained popular momentum. In retrospect, given the frustrations of polarized party politics in El Salvador, many observers credit the credibility and legitimacy of the organized physicians for the success of the mobilizations. It is rare for medical professionals to leave the relative comfort of medical practice to lead political movements. However, health workers have played critical roles for many years in El Salvador's volatile politics. Three recent mayors of San Salvador have been doctors, including leftists Violeta Menjívar and Hector Silva, who are credited with initiating innovative community health strategies in urban barrios, and Norman Quijano, the ARENA candidate who narrowly defeated Menjívar in January 2009.

This ethnography tells the story of contemporary struggles over health rights in El Salvador and builds a theoretical argument for the role of the "body politic," a concept that seeks to restore materiality and practice in dialectical understandings of political power and social movements. Most of my fieldwork was carried out during the mid-1990s peace process that followed the twelve-year civil war, with a focus on a "popular" health system built by the FMLN, dissident peasants, and nongovernmental organizations (NGOs) in northeast Chalatenango, a mountainous region that served as a rearguard for guerrillas during the war. I studied efforts of the ARENA-led Ministry of Health to regain control over health in the former war zone during the 1990s, and conversely, the struggles of the popular health movement to reform the ministry's rural health policies.[1] More recent research from 2000 to 2007 focused on the social movement behind the White Marches as health workers led a national mobilization against privatization. My research has been shaped by previous experiences in El Salvador investigating military impacts on health work as a volunteer with health rights NGOs in 1985–1989 and reporting on the war for U.S. newspapers from 1987 through early 1990.

From a political "realist" perspective, it takes a certain moxie to insist on human health as any sort of criteria during a war, especially during the early 1980s when the political murder rate had soared to one thousand souls a month. The exercise becomes more macabre, stepping back a little more from the bloodbath, when one considers the statistics on agricultural modernization backed by military repression since the 1960s, which relegated hundreds of thousands of campesino small-holders to a marginalized existence as seasonal or surplus labor. In truth, hardly anyone in the privileged north had paid attention to rural El Salvador before the shooting began in the late 1970s. International attention was focused on the successful Nicaraguan rebellion against dictator Anastasio Somoza next door, and the Sandinista revolutionaries who took power in mid-1979, launching that country into a decade of hostilities with Washington, which funded a rural campaign of terror by counterrevolutionary guerrillas. In El Salvador, meanwhile, an ultraconservative coalition of landowners and military officers, alarmed by events in Nicaragua, relied on death squads and rural militias to repress a growing, Catholic-inspired movement for political and economic reforms. The relative international invisibility of El Salvador prior to 1980 provided a kind of carte blanche to the military government's excesses. When newly elected U.S. president Ronald Reagan "drew a line in the sand" and vowed to defend El Salvador's tiny upper class against revolution, that small country vaulted to center stage in the geopolitical arena. From 1979 to 1983 thousands of dissidents went underground to evade the state repression, feeding the ranks of the growing FMLN guerrilla army and their supporters.

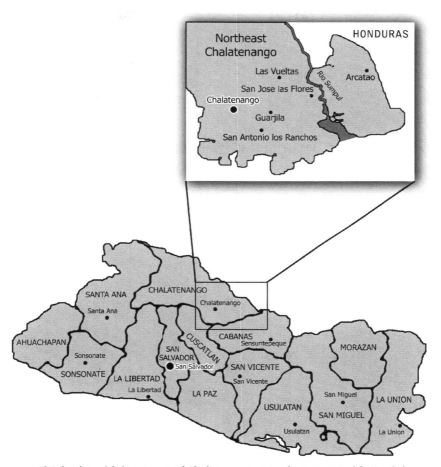

El Salvador with inset map of Chalatenango. Map by Roque Smith-Nonini.

The new U.S. military intervention spurred my initial involvement in 1982 when, as a young medical writer, I attended a meeting of doctors and nurses in a Washington, D.C., living room to discuss how to send medical aid to war refugees in Central America and publicize the destructive aspects of intervention for the public health. I was new to activism, but like many citizens I was moved by the bloodbath on the nightly news in the aftermath of Archbishop Oscar Romero's 1980 assassination and the rape and murder of four American church women in 1979. Reagan's portrayal of the conflict as a Cold War conflict driven by Marxist-Leninists led to confusing media coverage that ignored the role of poverty and longstanding class divisions in the region's turmoil. Many of my medical colleagues had been influenced by the 1978 Alma Ata declaration on primary health care, which asserted that development goals become irrelevant

if a population is unhealthy. Community-based health and other development
initiatives were central to the Catholic Church's Liberation Theology activism in
Central America, which condemned military repression against efforts to organize poor communities around the pursuit of reforms. By 1980, human rights critiques had gained traction in the media, but the notion that impoverished
peasants might claim economic rights to basic resources like food, medical care,
and a safe environment seemed like so much pie in the sky.

I made several reporting trips to the region, most on freelance assignments
for *American Medical News*, or with small delegations of U.S. doctors and nurses
volunteering with the National Central American Health Rights Network
(NCAHRN). We found that not only was it difficult to deliver medical aid to civilians caught in war zones, but increasingly the traditional "neutrality" of medical
work was threatened because the Salvadoran military and its affiliated death
squads viewed all civilian work with poor peasants as "subversive." It was not
until I moved to San Salvador in 1987 that I gained some understanding of what
Salvadorans euphemistically called *la situación*. So it makes some sense to start
with this experiential foray into chaos and the surprising (dialectical) "other"
side of a civil war—the human capacity to resist terror and to rebuild community. Like other foreign correspondents, my life in a middle-class neighborhood
of the capital was protected from the day-to-day vagaries of poverty and
violence experienced by most Salvadorans. It was on visits with colleagues to the
embattled countryside when the scales of privilege fell from our eyes, and we
were able, at times, to feel in our own bones the fear, moral outrage, and
courage of life in El Salvador's "conflicted zones," as the areas of leftist guerrilla
activity were known.

The extremes of terror and healing describe well the tenor of two excursions
I made to Chalatenango in 1989. This was the year that the ARENA party gained
the presidency, leading to a new military crackdown on dissident groups. During
the previous four years, the Salvadoran government, headed by the more centrist
president Napoleón Duarte, had been pressured by the Democrat-controlled
U.S. Congress to improve its dismal human rights record (ironically) so that
legislators could justify approving U.S. military aid for Reagan's war against the
insurgency. This scrutiny had created a political opening that was exploited by
Salvadoran dissident groups, which held numerous street protests and posted
ads in newspapers demanding peace talks, the release of political prisoners, and
social programs for the poor. Leaders of ARENA insisted that dissident labor,
human rights, and reformist groups were lackeys for the FMLN, which by now
was a full-fledged guerrilla army with an estimated ten thousand fighters.

Both excursions I recount here were illegal, involving long overland hikes.
By early 1989 the Salvadoran army had stopped issuing safe-conduct passes
(*salvoconductos*) for journalists to visit "conflicted" rural areas, and my experiences on both trips were tinged by an acrid overlay of fear that we would be fired

on by government soldiers. The first excursion, in February, was thrown together hastily. At a press conference, army officers had boasted that their elite (U.S.-trained) Atlacatl Battalion had killed eight FMLN "terrorists," and the army claimed to have "dismantled" a clandestine hospital in a place called El Coyolar, near the Honduran border. The army provided local media with photographs of confiscated medical supplies and the passport of a Mexican woman identified as Alejandra Bravo Betancourt, a doctor killed in the attack.

If the Atlacatl Battalion had intentionally destroyed a medical clinic, it was an egregious violation of international law, which states that health facilities and personnel should be protected in war. However, the Geneva Conventions were routinely violated by the Salvadoran military. At the time, I was preparing a report on such violations for *American Medical News*, and here was the army bragging about killing a doctor. None of my journalist colleagues planned to investigate because no one knew how to locate the site. Before dawn the next morning I set out with a photographer, whom I will call Terry, in a jeep headed north. We talked our way through an army roadblock, telling solders that we were covering an ARENA party election rally scheduled in the departmental capital later that morning. Instead, we turned west, passing through Dulce Nombre de María, and then north, winding around pine-covered mountains on a poorly maintained dirt road.

The road abruptly ended at the tiny village of Ocotal, only a few miles from the border. We had no idea where to go next. That afternoon we sat in on a "liberation theology"–style meeting led by a catechist where local youth planned a festival. Enthusiasm was muted as everyone compared rumors about the "massacre" at the FMLN mobile clinic and the alleged brutal murder of "Julia," a guerrilla doctor known to the villagers as someone they too had counted on from time to time when she was needed to treat sick or wounded civilians. The rumor was that a total of ten patients and health workers had been killed in a surprise ambush. Ocotal residents were angry but pleased that reporters had come from the capital to investigate.

We casually mentioned that we would need help finding the site. The catechist helped us set up canvas cots in the small church, where we spent an uncomfortable night being bitten by fleas. The next morning a young man knocked on the door and handed us a note directing us to hike to a hill outside of town. There we were greeted by "Manuel," a skinny ten-year-old in a ragged tee shirt and long pants who told us that he was an FMLN *correo* (messenger). Manuel took us in tow, and for the next three hours we struggled to keep up with him as he scampered across creeks and up steep hillsides like a goat with no apparent effort.

A half hour into our hike, woods gave way to a sunny meadow, where two streams of guerrilla fighters casually crossed the clearing in front of us on intersecting paths. They were young men and women dressed in jeans and fatigues and with backpacks and bright bandanas, each with the ubiquitous rifle slung on their back. They looked serious but friendly and nodded to us as they passed.

What we anticipated to be a short hike turned into hours of trudging up and down an endless succession of hills, each seemingly steeper than the one before. We took turns carrying Terry's camera gear. At midday we passed several abandoned villages, then skirted the side of a scorched hillside, and stopped at a lone adobe-walled house that Manuel declared our destination. Inside, campesino women worked around a fireplace, grinding corn and cooking red beans. FMLN combatants came and went on a rocky trail that emerged from a ravine behind the house.

Manuel ran off and came back a few minutes later with two robust, bearded guerrilla fighters, who introduced themselves as Miguel and Edgardo. The two sat down with us on a rock wall outside the house to answer our questions while polishing off two cans of sardines that we dug out of our packs as an offering. Miguel recounted that on the day of the attack he had watched in a helpless fury from a nearby ridge as Atlacatl commandos ignored existing trails and penetrated straight across a stand of dense scrub forest to reach the mobile open-air "hospital," which was hidden in a cave-like rock formation. "It was as if they had knowledge of the exact location of the clinic," he said (a fact that I confirmed years later from a former guerrilla who said the clinic's location had been revealed to the army by an informant).

Miguel was distraught that his *compañeros* had been unable to get a warning to the health workers, who had been temporarily left without an armed guard. The soldiers, undetected by the medical staff, had taken the time to set up an M60 machine gun looking down on the open-air medical encampment. Miguel and Edgardo confirmed the villagers' account of a ten-person death toll, which included the doctor, three nurses, and six patients, figures later verified by Tutela Legal, the human rights office of San Salvador's archdiocese, which sent a delegation to exhume the bodies. Two campesino men described how they had followed a blood-stained trail to locate the hacked up and naked bodies of "Julia" and a Salvadoran *sanitaria* (health aide), both of whom fled when the soldiers opened fire. One led Terry to their gravesite to take photographs.

Getting out of the conflicted zone proved more difficult than entering. After an exhausting five-hour hike, Manuel left us in the woods near Ocotal. The next morning as we turned onto the last stretch of gravel road leading to the Troncal Norte highway, we found our way blocked by two army jeeps with a bar lowered across the road. We spent the rest of the day detained in the fortified headquarters of the Army's Fourth Brigade headquarters while soldiers searched the jeep and belongings, asking us repeatedly where we had been and why.

The following June I found myself once again undertaking a day-long hike through a no-man's land of dense forest, rocky hillsides, and abandoned hamlets. Our goal this time was not to verify horrors but rather to witness the drama of former refugees determinedly carving a neutral zone by rebuilding bombed-out villages in disputed territory. Beginning in 1987 thousands of refugees, some of whom had spent years in refugee camps, returned in huge caravans to conflicted zones of El Salvador with the goal of resettling their abandoned villages. The new civilian presence in northeastern Chalatenango, a rearguard area for the FMLN (and our destination that June day), was a thorn in the side of the Salvadoran government. From 1983 to 1986 the army, guided by U.S. military advisors and armed with U.S-built aircraft, had bombed and strafed all traces of human presence in this zone. As intended, these "scorched earth" tactics had driven most peasants into exile or urban displaced person camps. The widely publicized return of civilians under the vigilance of human rights groups and United Nations observers greatly complicated the government's military strategy.

Our small contingent was made up of three journalists (a Salvadoran filmmaker, an Argentine reporter, and me), a local guide, a peasant woman, and her teenage son who rode a mule because he had lost a leg in a mine explosion. I remember that we circumvented a bomb crater and a burned patch of ground, the aftermath of an air raid, as we approached the settlement of Guarjila around 9 P.M. I was so exhausted I nearly sat down in the road.

Over the next two days, on visits to two resettlement villages, we were amazed to find that, despite makeshift housing and poor infrastructure, residents seemed to be socially thriving, with a strong sense of unity and determination to rebuild their lives. Evincing none of the wariness of strangers one often encountered in rural villages, the ex-refugees of Guarjila embraced us warmly, fed us dinner, and gave us space in the hut next to the community kitchen to spread our bedrolls on the ground. We stayed up late discussing politics with Antonio, a local guerrilla officer who stole into town after nightfall. The cook greeted him with a bowl of scrambled eggs and rice, and we joined him at the picnic table peppering him with questions about the war and frustrated peace negotiations. The night was pitch black, the only light coming from Antonio's cigarette and a small flashlight, which he turned off and on, carefully shielding the beam.

The next day I interviewed a man whose seven-year-old daughter had been shot in the side a few days earlier when a helicopter machine-gunned roofs of the village. Local health "promoters" operated out of a tiny shack with a handful of medicines, which were still treated as contraband at army roadblocks. Horses and mules were lent to us for the forty-minute journey to San José Las Flores, a more established village, where we learned that the local clinic had recently been forcibly occupied by soldiers, and several dental promoters had been captured and tortured by the army. Yet in the midst of these fearful accounts, we were being shown around by men and women with hopeful spirits, proudly ticking off their achievements—a new birthing room, a child care center, a cattle cooperative, and (marginally stocked) community stores. Here was truly a story of healing in the midst of terror. Both nights we attended outdoor dances—a surreal scene as young men, rifles clacking on their backs, swayed to poor recordings of American rock songs opposite civilian women in cheap polyester dresses; then the gendered norms were flipped as female guerrillas joined the dance in berets and tight khaki skirts.

We debated how to get back to the capital. I argued against hitching a ride since the few vehicles leaving the zone were routinely searched at government roadblocks. I feared the military would revoke my (army-issued) press credentials (given my previous arrest). We were lucky. Two jeeploads of European VIP's came to visit the resettlements, and they agreed to smuggle us out. At the roadblock we cowered in the rear when the soldiers asked to see IDs, but the driver waved foreign credentials and faced them down with splendid French arrogance. "In like bandits and out like diplomats," crowed my Argentine friend that night over beer.

Tension worsened in November 1989 when a guerrilla offensive brought the war to the capital. The military responded with raids on dissident groups and air attacks on urban barrios. Then an army squad murdered six Jesuit priests who were prominent social scientists at the University of Central America and advocates for economic reforms. The same week, I received telephoned death threats, as did another reporter.

In early 1990 I moved back to the United States. I did not return to Chalatenango until shortly after the U.N.-mediated ceasefire in 1992. Now a graduate student in anthropology, I was eager to discover what had become of the lay health workers who had so impressed me during that 1989 visit. It was a giddy feeling entering the former war zone in bright sunlight on a rickety little bus weighted down with sacks of corn, chickens, women, and children—light years removed from the tensions of the war. How strange to pass the site of the army roadblock under the old conacaste tree. No soldiers. No guns.

As we came within site of Guarjila's neat *bajareque* buildings, a campesino directed me to the new health clinic. The neat nine-room cinderblock clinic and adjacent small "hospital" easily qualified as the nicest buildings in town, with a bright interior lit by clear plastic panels in the roof. Women and children sat on benches inside, and three female promoters bustled about taking histories and peering at sore throats. Inside a woman physician from Boston was attempting to help but was hampered by her broken Spanish. I offered to translate. In the examining room a teenage boy lay on a table, his hand disfigured by a huge swollen abscess. Jennifer conferred with Lucia, the twenty-two-year-old health promoter, about the case and shook her head, suggesting that the boy be sent to a government hospital in Chalatenango, the departmental capital.

"No, I know how to take care of it," said Lucia. The physician stepped aside and watched as the promoter proceeded to give the boy an intramuscular injection of ketamine and waited until he fell asleep. Then she competently lanced the abscess with a scalpel and drained the pus into a pan. Throughout the procedure she kept a hand pressed to the boy's chest monitoring his heart rate. Afterward she started him on antibiotics.

Leaving the examining room afterward, Jennifer's eyes met mine with a look of amazement. She remarked, "Lucia even knew to give him Atropine and Valium to counteract psychological effects of the Ketamine. In the hospital where I work we would have called in a specialist!" While observing health practices in the weeks to come I learned that draining abscesses was a routine procedure for Lucia, who, as a former paramedic with the FMLN, had often assisted with complex surgeries in the field. The "popular" system was backed up by a small technical team of traveling physicians and nurses, but day-to-day health care in most villages, including routine diagnoses and prescribing, was the responsibility of competent lay promoters like Lucia, many of whom were only now, in the aftermath of the war, getting a chance to complete their primary education.

Healing the Body Politic

Introduction

Theorizing the Body and the State

Dialectics of Terror and Healing

In this book I recount a series of underreported struggles over health rights in El Salvador that date to the beginnings of the civil war in the 1980s. I examine the potential for a nondualistic theory of the body politic, or what Bryan Turner (1992) has called "a biopolitics of the somatic society." Used in this way, body politic refers to the implicit moral ecology and sense of social contract that gives meaning to representative governance and political legitimacy in nation-states. While much of my narrative focuses on a rural health movement that arose during the twelve-year civil war and its interactions with the post-cease-fire state, in a remarkable shift after 2000 the political agenda of health rights erupted onto the national stage in El Salvador, with massive street mobilizations to stop neoliberal reforms that have impacted national politics and resulted in one of the few cases in which the World Bank backed down from a privatization agenda. With the revival of health reform as an issue in American politics and the new emergence of the international People's Health Movement, health rights are becoming a centerpiece of global activism; this book aspires to inform those struggles.

My account traces a historical trajectory in which health and healing served as key sites of engagement during two decades of struggle over the nature of the Salvadoran body politic. I first visited El Salvador in 1985 as part of a small medical task force assessing damages sustained during a military invasion of the University of El Salvador's medical and allied health schools. I returned to document impacts on public health from the 1986 earthquake, and then moved to San Salvador in 1987 to report on the region for U.S. newspapers. My articles in *American Medical News* and the *Philadelphia Inquirer* on the military's attacks on rural clinics led to regular work as a stringer for the *New York Times* San Salvador bureau during 1989. After receiving death threats in a chaotic period of urban warfare in November of that year, I moved back to the United States and entered graduate school. I returned to El Salvador after the 1992 cease-fire to do ethno-graphic fieldwork on an NGO-supported community-based health system that had become established in the former war zone of Chalatenango. Between June 1992 and December 1995, I carried out eleven months of research on this "alternative" health system that evolved independently both of the country's poorly managed Ministry of Health and of large international development institutions. In 1995 my fieldwork expanded to cover controversies over multilateral development loans for health system reforms. In 2000 I began research on the 1999–2000 health strikes with research assistance from Susan Greenblatt, a health educator living in San Salvador. I continued research on the movement that culminated in the White Marches against privatization during visits to El Salvador in 2002 and 2007.

The first five chapters of this book tell a story of health work in a period of violent conflict. While thinking about health in the context of war, I have found the idioms of terror and healing helpful in two senses: as potent metaphors for the hopes and fears that buffet the human spirit under conditions of poverty and political repression, and as material anchors that ground the dialectics of struggle in existential realities of exhausted and wounded bodies—which are, after all, the substrates of poverty and war. In the process of seeing through the window of healing in an era of bloodletting, we gain insights into the symbolism built into cultural discourses about the body.

The urgency of life in wartime contrasts sharply with the trivial and vapid pursuits that increasingly dominate our lives in peacetime. A well-established trove of folk wisdom deals with life close to the edge. In his book *War Is a Force that Gives Us Meaning*, U.S. foreign war correspondent Chris Hedges asserts that despite the carnage and destruction of war, we remain addicted to it. "War is an enticing elixir. It gives us resolve, a cause. It allows us to be noble" (2002, 3). Because of its closeness to issues of life and death, Lewis Hyde observed, medical work is also "strangely vitalizing. Death in particular focuses life, and deepens it. In the face of death we can discriminate between the important and the trivial" (1983, 206).

Under these circumstances in which forms of violence and issues of vulnera-bility dominate consciousness and public discourse, bodies and communities at risk push aside other cultural forms, and power relations become focused around what Farmer (2004) has called the "materiality of the social." He distinguished this notion, from old debates about materialism (in which biology or economics is taken as a kind of bedrock that underlie beliefs and culture—Marx's base-versus-superstructure dichotomy), instead taking a position more similar to that of Jean and John Comaroff (1991) who assert that within anthropology there is a "growing agreement that the primary processes in production of the everyday world are inseparably material and meaningful" (8). Farmer points out that "adverse outcomes associated with structural violence—death, injury, illness, sub-jection, stigmatization, and even psychological terror—come to have their 'final common pathway' in the material" (308). Such impacts include damaged bodies and minds as well as experiences that shape the cultural worlds of the people that anthropologists study. I would add to his account the observation that these "adverse effects" on populations also shape wider political agendas, forms of production, human impacts on the ecology, and prospects for the next generation, and so must be thought of at multiple scales.

The importance of "praxis" or promotion of peasant engagement with political realities was, of course, central to the ideology of liberation theology that shaped Salvadoran resistance to military rule, including the politics of the Farabundo Martí Front for National Liberation (FMLN) guerrilla army. In many ways this ideological development, which influenced many countries in Latin America, did important work in reconciling aspects of Karl Marx's historical materialism with poststructuralist critical theory, as some researchers have noted (Lancaster 1988; and Escobar 1992.) The body has been a central actor—as subject and object, and as signifier—in the repression brought to bear on many liberation theology struggles and in the development of human rights movements and less studied movements, such as that of health rights.

But, as Turner noted, despite the fact that the body is "fundamental to any theory of action, too many modern analytical efforts either bracket out the body, or dismiss it as part of a set of environmental conditions" (1992, 245). Medical anthropologists have been among those to bring the body into focus in a material sense, including analyses of the processes whereby individuals or cultural groups exposed to violence somaticize trauma, developing symptoms that range from relatively common folk illnesses to rare syndromes and sometimes debilitating conditions that involve both physical and mental impairments (e.g., Scheper-Hughes 1992; Low 1994; and Green 1994). I met Salvadorans who attributed physical symptoms to either the routine violence of poverty—for example, *nervios*, with symptoms similar to what a biomedical doctor would call chronic anxiety; or to personal experience of war violence, for example, "*susto*" (psychological symptoms blamed on a traumatic fright). I also collected many testimonials from survivors who lost family members in violent attacks on civilian centers, and who used this form of human rights–centered narrative as a form of collective protest and witnessing directed at foreign visitors or NGO delegations (see also Stephen 1994; and Green 1998).

My focus in writing this book was not so much to collect accounts of traumatic experiences, an area that has been well studied, but rather to document new collective practices centered around health that sought to transform traditional relations of medical and political authority. For Salvadoran dissidents in Chalatenango, what I have dubbed "popular" health work involved conscious efforts to improve access to care and broaden community understanding and participation in health planning. The movement grew out of a more ecological and equitable logos than curative medicine; it promoted a set of practices that would interweave individual and social well-being in a context of radical democracy. Health advocates also sought to build systems that linked villages into a network that could guarantee some political, economic, and ecological sustainability. In this sense, I saw their project as asserting their rights to a kind of "moral ecology"—a social, economic, and political space that enables social development in the sense of a moral entitlement (Sen 1999) or with what Chalatecos referred to as dignity (*dignidad*).

Notions of illness and health are frequently invoked as metaphors for the body politic in nation-states (O'Neill 1985, 2004; and Turner 1996). Such metaphors serve as common idioms to establish moral criteria for inclusion or exclusion in normative social orders (e.g., Douglas 1984). The well-documented cultural power of the healer to cure, as well as to restore order and remove social ambiguity (Glick 1977; and Turner 1996), has been further enhanced in postcolonial settings by the status granted to Western biomedicine and the imperial hierarchies with which it is associated (Baer, Singer, and Susser 2003). This symbolic power, as with all power, cuts both ways, allowing health to be a revealing moral viewpoint on the material as well as the symbolic manifestations of violence while simultaneously making the healer's mantle itself contested, and subject to political appropriation and manipulation (Zola 1972).

But the invocation of disease or illness takes on new meaning in modern nation-states where biomedical institutions have become important brokers of power and knowledge. In these settings, biomedical ideas and practitioners have often helped construct and legitimize hierarchical social norms (Foucault 1975, 1980) while medicalizing social ills whose meanings might carry explosive implications if interpreted in another framework (e.g., exploitative labor relations or military pacification) (Frankenberg 1993; and Conrad and Schneider 1992). The philosophical orientation and analytic framework of *Healing the Body Politic* has been shaped by the burgeoning scholarship in progressive public health and critical medical anthropology that places medical institutions in a framework of power and seeks to analyze health under late capitalism (Singer and Baer 1995; Baer, Singer, and Susser 2003; and Waitzkin and Iriart 2001). But I also draw on critical interpretive medical anthropology that has sought to examine how healing and power are culturally constructed and shaped in tension between individual agency and structural forces (Scheper-Hughes 1992; Morgan 1993; Green 1998; and Quesada 1998).

My informants, in addition to health work, were also involved in ongoing struggles over labor relations, education, and land tenure that dated to the mid-1970s; it was state repression directed at this culture of dissent that led to the formation of armed struggle. As the violence of the late 1970s drew international attention, journalists, human rights monitors, and relief workers also became targets of terror. No argument is attempted here to privilege health work as a point of inquiry. Health services are not more essential to human life than a fair wage structure, for example. However, healing is somewhat unique in its apparent moral nature. Aware of this quality, health professionals and humanists have long advocated to keep medical services well separated from military operations. In practice, however, as the cases in the prologue make clear, this is seldom the case.

The War as Crucible

One does not ordinarily find models for rural development in war zones. But the massive repopulation of rebel-held areas in El Salvador that began in 1986 spurred numerous experiments in collective democracy, including new roles of civilians in participatory governance, collective stewardship of land and livestock, small manufacturing and craft cooperatives, collective struggles for disputed land, municipal childcare centers, popular education, and popular health (Binford 1996; Cagan and Cagan 1991; Clements 1984; Hammond 1998; Metzi 1988; and Wood 2003). Thanks in large part to support and training from the Salvadoran Catholic Church (which also supported health work in refugee and displaced person camps), the popular health network grew into the largest and most comprehensive community-based health system in the country. My use of the term "popular" is not meant to invoke traditional (indigenous) healing practices, although the Chalatenango health workers were more sympathetic to and conversant about traditional *campesino* beliefs than were Ministry of Health workers. Popular system lay workers did learn to grow, prepare, and prescribe about twenty herbal medicines that were considered biologically effective, and the system trained lay midwives.

The majority of medical and health practices, however, were similar to those promoted by the Hesperian Foundation for use in remote rural areas of poor countries—comprehensive primary health care (PHC) with trained village-based workers and a strong emphasis on prevention and public education. In fact, instructors used photocopies from the foundation's famous manuals "Where There Is No Doctor" (Werner 1977) and "Helping Health Workers Learn" (Werner and Bower 1982) in training courses. But the popular system departed from primary health care philosophy as a result of its roots in wartime curative medicine. The system included former FMLN physicians and many experienced *sanitarios*, or lay paramedics trained in the guerrilla army (like Lucia, the health worker described in the prologue). Given this capacity, and the absence of government services, a number of practices and procedures usually reserved for doctors were routinely carried out by the promoters, including minor surgeries and prescribing for common illnesses. (Chapters 6, 7, and 8 treat the popular system in more detail.)

Although popular clinics in the resettlements received supplies and educational assistance from the local Catholic diocese from 1987 until 1993, the technical team that coordinated services and training was a mix of secular and religious volunteers and health promoters and was not under control of the Church. The popular system did not even have a name for itself. From 1987 to 1993 seven popular clinics based in village centers and a wider network of remote health posts provided the only health coverage for around ten thousand resettled refugees in the mountains of northeast Chalatenango. After the war, once the Ministry of Health began its reentry to the zone in 1993, local people sometimes used the term "*salud popular*" to distinguish the system from the government-run services. So that is the term I chose for this account.

Shortly after the 1992 cease-fire, demand soared for more responsive health services in other rural areas of Chalatenango, and the popular system expanded training and helped start new clinics in areas that had remained under government control throughout the war. By 1995 more than three hundred popular health promoters served eighty communities throughout the department, and nongovernmental health promoters nationwide had formed their own union. Variations of "popular" health existed in other regions of El Salvador at the end of the war, especially in resettlement communities and in areas formerly controlled by the FMLN in departments of Morazán, Usulután, San Vicente, Cabañas, and Cuscatlán, but no other system compared with Chalatenango in terms of size, levels of organization, or sophistication of operations. Popular health took variable forms in different regions, but two things fundamentally distinguished it from government health services: its base in lay workers who lived in the communities they served and a commitment to a participatory model of primary health aimed at maximizing benefits and access to care for the majority.

Even before the war ended, the United Nations Children's Fund (UNICEF), which had negotiated an annual one-day cease-fire to vaccinate children from 1986 to 1991, recorded the success of Chalatenango's health promoters' in vaccination coverage, even in remote mountain hamlets. Several other indicators suggested health conditions in the repopulation villages had improved by the early 1990s. During the peace process the system was praised in public meetings and cited by representatives from the United Nations Development Program and the Pan American Health Organization (PAHO) (much to the embarrassment of the Salvadoran Ministry of Health) as a model for community-based rural health.

Economic Warfare

The reentry of the Ministry of Health to the former war zone in mid-1993 came after more than a year of controversial negotiations with advocates of the popular system who pushed for more responsive rural health care from the government. Limited by declining funding from NGOs, popular system negotiators finally settled for a compromise (which they later came to regret) with the conservative ministry, whose chief administrator disdained the popular model.

In some villages, ministry doctors prevailed and health promoters lost their positions. More organized villages insisted on a hybrid model in which government doctors were compelled to adopt many popular system "norms," but by 2000, most promoters had been marginalized by the ministry. A few were hired as health aides to run errands or clean ministry clinics; others in remote areas continued to work as volunteers with diminished institutional support.

The end of the Salvadoran war could be described as an end to routine state-sanctioned political repression, and in that respect the revolution was a success. The report of the UN Truth Commission (1992) that collected and evaluated evidence of human rights abuses from the war concluded that the vast majority of serious abuses were committed by the military or paramilitary agents acting on behalf of state authorities. Although the army remains intact and powerful, it is now far smaller and the peace accord ended large-scale state-sponsored repression. But the neoliberal peace offered few economic reforms that would improve life for the country's majority. Rural poverty has remained little changed from the late 1970s, and the peace accord, while authorizing limited land transfers to former combatants, left most social welfare issues to be worked out through national politics. Hence, from the perspective of a land-poor campesino in an economically marginalized place like Chalatenango, revolutionary gains at the national level were disappointing, and many felt that they had little choice but to continue political struggles for equitable development years after the peace accords.

That is why I have adopted a dialectical analysis (Ollman 1993) that emphasizes relational aspects of power as well as the ways that interactions between parties of a conflict shape a changing reality. Such a perspective places the war in a wider context and pays close attention to the roles of experience and process as well as historical contingency and contradiction. Given the unstable setting of this society in conflict and given the scope of my research questions about development and coercion, I opted against a traditional study of local culture and instead undertook a multisite ethnography. This book combines participatory-observation of the popular health system with oral history interviews, my personal accounts, other's accounts of journalistic and human rights investigations during the war, and historical research on the war and origins of poverty in El Salvador. Given the role of U.S. militarism and international players and institutions in health development and solidarity work, there is also a transnational analysis in most chapters.

As I analyzed my data on Chalatenango, three themes recurred in my informants' accounts: (a) an emphasis on the brute facts of economic scarcity that limited their life chances; (b) recurring effects from state-sponsored violence on their lives and political identity; and (c) evidence of a remarkably resilient sense of hope and collective agency—a development that many people consciously linked to the new forms of community that they had built in the former war zone.

Their collective projects of resistance and alternative development seemed always shaped as moral counterpoint to the harsh realities of poverty and war.

Many approaches to the study of social movements have been shaped by assumptions that collective action is rare, and that participation in mobilization runs counter to (presumably self-interested) human nature. Resource mobilization studies, most common in political science, tend to explain collective action as a function of the strategies of interest groups and have often focused most strongly on political leaders and issues of rational decision making and strategy (e.g., see Eckstein 2001) but tend to ignore the role of social knowledge and cultural agency that animates a movement. The poststructuralist focus, common in cultural studies and in many anthropological accounts since 1990, has tended to emphasize "identity" and the politics of difference over political economy (Laclau and Mouffe 1985; and Best and Kellner 1991). Deconstructionist approaches in this vein have emphasized the "hybridity" and "fluidity" of identities that members negotiate while participating in movements (e.g., see Escobar and Alvarez 1992), and scholars influenced by Michel Foucault have sought alternatives to idealistic (modernist) notions of culture as "shared meaning systems." By the mid to late 1990s, even in flagship anthropology journals, the slippery postmodern trope of "identity" was often applied in such a loose way that it became almost "coterminus with culture" and therefore limited in its explanatory power (Lewellen 2003). Underdevelopment in such analyses became reduced to a "linguistic construction," diminishing the relevance of historical or causal analysis or the roles of economic systems and institutions in the production of inequality (Best and Kellner 1991; Lewellen 2002). Certainly, I encountered anecdotes that support the poststructuralist claim that collective forms of resistance are tenuous and at odds with individual agency. If one relies on discourse primarily, conversations with organizers on the left, for example, are often fraught with doubts about various strategies, criticism of competing tendencies, and reports of disagreements over how to interpret any given political moment. But any long-term analysis of Salvadoran politics provides abundant evidence of repeated recourse to collective agency by advocates for social reform; the longer the timeline, the more this becomes apparent.

After spending close to four years of my life working in El Salvador as a journalist and anthropologist, half in wartime, and half during a time of peace, I became convinced that collective action there has not been a rare phenomenon. Tommie Sue Montgomery (1995) documents cycles of peasant uprisings against military-led governments dating back for most of the twentieth century, prior to the twelve-year civil war. *Healing the Body Politic* begins and ends with periods of mass mobilization before and after the war (in the 1970s and 2000s), which in both cases disrupted the national economy for many months and provoked militaristic responses from the threatened ruling oligarchy. I open the book by tracing the rising tide of activism dating to the late 1960s that was responding to top-down agricultural development programs that alienated tens of thousands of peasant smallholders from land. Similar enclosures of multiple public utilities that spurred inflated prices—this time resulting from neoliberal policies followed by World Bank pressures for privatized health services—prompted the White Marches of the early 2000s.

Another aspect of Salvadoran movements that only becomes clear in the long-term perspective is what Albert Hirschman (1983) called "the conservation and mutation of social energy" from one period of mobilization to another. For example, the thousands of Chalateco refugees who returned to their bombed out villages during the 1987–1992 resettlement movement were not new to political struggle. Many had spent one to two years living under protection of the FMLN guerrilla army prior to fleeing to refugee camps; others in more remote villages remained and collaborated with guerrillas throughout the war. Since the late 1970s these villages had been centers of liberation theology organizing. The radical priests' and nuns' emphasis on social organizing as a form of struggle for an equitable society was a philosophy adopted by the Fuerzas Pópular de Liberación (FPL), the FMLN faction that dominated in Chalatenango after 1980—in contrast to the Ejército Revolucionario del Pueblo (ERP) faction in the eastern department of Morazán, which favored a more military strategy and did not encourage civilian organizing until 1986 (Binford 1999). Prior to the exodus to refugee camps spurred by military sweeps in late 1983, the communities in rebel-controlled Chalatenango had set up civilian governing structures known as Popular Local Power (PPL) committees (Pearce 1986).

Upon reflection, the aspects of the popular health movement and the politics of the repopulated communities in El Salvador that seemed most salient were precisely the inescapable consistencies of their focus on a continuing "struggle" against a government with a history of threatening the peasantry, and their constant reference to being motivated by material issues of survival. Asked about their collective practices, campesino health workers and villagers insisted repeatedly that these evolved during their attempts to survive the military's "scorched earth" counterinsurgency campaign, which aimed to render the area uninhabitable (hence, inhospitable to guerrillas). They evinced deep distrust of the government. In conversations, and in my observation of popular health practices and strategies, the recurrent tensions around issues of structural inequity and references to government violence seemed to animate dissent, alternately forging solidarities around strategies and constraining possibilities for action.

Beyond Dualism: Dialectics of Social Materiality

In oral histories of the war, bodies and healing were frequently cast as iconic sites on a path of political conversion. Nancy Scheper-Hughes and Margaret Lock (1987) used the term "lived experience of the body-self" to refer to the experiential/personal body, which they distinguished from the social body (referring to its representational or socially constructed aspects), and from the body politic, which they saw as having to do with coercive operations of power on the body. While concepts of the lived and social bodies are more widely studied in anthropology, the body politic remains an underexamined concept.

Elaine Scarry's 1985 study, *The Body in Pain*, points up the profound individualization and social withdrawal that results from illness. Medical and other cultural anthropologists have used variations on the concept of embodiment to show how experiences of chronic stress, fear, or trauma may manifest through folk or cultural syndromes—for example, nervios, susto, or spirit possession. Individuals suffering from these syndromes exhibit a complex interplay of mental and physical symptoms, which have gained recognition in a cultural milieu, and may offer subjects an acceptable way to express anger or frustration over relations of power (Green 1994; Ong 1987; Jenkins 1991; Low 1994; and Nordstrom 1992, 1997). Similarly, "stress" (what might be considered a North American cultural syndrome) is often associated with other pathologies and is recognized as a "real" phenomena within medicine. But in many such cases, bodies seem to function as receptacles for, or reflexive objects of, political or economic coercion—in short, victims. Other than acting out in a local context, we see little mobilization that could enable reciprocity of action—there is an incomplete dialectic. We are left unable to imagine how or if social tensions become translated into creative action or political transformation.

Consequently, many cultural anthropologists, not to mention sociologists and political scientists, are likely to dismiss material effects of power on bodies as contributing to political praxis. At best, embodied violence becomes expressed through testimonials (Stephen 1994), although some would dismiss these as strategic devices (Stoll 1999); at worst, violence serves to inflict long-lasting psychic wounds that silence dissent (Bourgois 2002; and Desjarlais and Kleinman 1994). But there is likely a bias in this literature introduced by the fact that cultural work at the intersection of mind and body has most often been done by medical anthropologists whose entry point to the field is frequently through the clinic and is focused on patients and expressed suffering.

Are there other ways in which the material effects of political or economic coercion become channeled into social projects? My challenge in this project is to draw on ethnography and history to show the salience of bodies as both metaphors and mediators for material experiences in political practice—a first step, one might say, in theorizing a suit of clothes that gives shape to the ephemeral frame of the body politic.

Several theorists have broken new ground in this project and laid a framework for thinking. For example, William Dressler (2001) demonstrated in quantitative studies that "cultural consonance," or the sense that one's life is conforming to a positively regarded shared cultural model, is correlated with declines in blood pressure. This is in line with studies of placebo (Harrington

1997) and with predictions of Hahn and Kleinman's (1983) study of placebo and nocebo in which they predicted that cultural influences on physical health were likely to produce both negative and positive outcomes. In settings of political turmoil, Michael Taussig (1992) has illustrated the power of human rights testimonials, enacted through the activism of "mothers of the disappeared" groups in the aftermath of dirty wars in the Southern Cone and Central America, whose public rituals channeled "the tremendous moral and magical power of the unquiet dead into the public sphere" (48), challenging military rule. David Lan (1985) studied the role of native healers in helping to sanction political resistance in Zimbabwe, and more recently Carolyn Nordstrom (1998) studied ritual healing in Mozambique used to exorcise violent tendencies in the aftermath of a highly destructive civil war.

Pierre Bourdieu's work on practice theory and "structuralist constructivism" (1977, 1990) is perhaps the most extensive body of social theory that seeks to link these perspectives. Several other approaches to cultural theory deal with human practices and beliefs about material constraints and coercion, including the Marxist theory of alienation, Gramscian (and other neo-Marxist) theories of cultural hegemony, and concepts of moral economy and resistance (Wolf 1969; Scott 1985, 1990; and Roseberry 1994). Certainly anthropological studies of ritual healing are likewise exemplary models for exploring the material–social divide in ethnographic settings (e.g., Turner 1957).

But as Dressler (2001) has pointed out, contrasting the more macro-level structuralist perspectives of critical medical anthropology with constructivist scholars focused on negotiation of cultural difference at the level of the doctor–patient encounter, "there are obviously two different things going on in medical anthropology." Both he and Fletcher Linder (2004) allude to the so-called science and culture wars of the late 1990s as a moment when this divide became most apparent, producing a nonproductive or reactionary tit for tat between cultural researchers who defined the ethnographic field in a narrow, often emic-focused framework emphasizing "cultural difference," and those with a more critical orientation who sought to study inequalities in a wider context of power relations. The rise of Foucauldian analysis and the end of the Cold War generated debates in which theorists of resistance movements were accused of romanticizing struggle by creating ideal types (e.g., reified notions of community) or seeking premature closures through Marxist "master narratives." Conversely, critical theorists (of both the so-called interpretivist and structuralist schools) have criticized poststructuralists for essentializing culture and conflating evidence of class exploitation with forms of cultural difference (Starn 1991; Baer, Singer, and Susser 2003; and Lock 2001).

I take inspiration from Dressler's (2001) call for a "larger synthesis" that can better integrate these two distinct views of social life. There are many contributors to these academic divisions, from the alienation of living in a world of stark economic disparities to longstanding influences of anticommunist politics in the academy and the turf wars that afflict the academic disciplines. And certainly the dichotomy of structure and agency animates debate in many fields. In this project I undertake to write against the persistent influence of mind–body dualism in Western thought in shaping our habits of mind. This book seeks to highlight the material–social dialectics that lead humans to act in concert. It asks questions about the potential for a true community of science that contests predominant individualist and capitalist hegemonies on social well-being.

As social scientists we yearn to quickly wrest the material body back from medical science, so as to exercise our craft of meaning-making. We hastily stitch unruly flesh and blood back together with its symbolic counterparts in the effort to restore it to social relations. In doing so, I argue, we frequently marginalize the materiality of experience and subjugate it to the art of representation. Lacking the dualistic comparative of difference, we distrust the material body, for it is locked in the fastness of the person. We rarely consider that the very biological substrate we wish to dismiss has universal aspects, and that, since life experience integrates the personal with the social, those universal aspects also shape social and political representations. To emphasize that there are common aspects to suffering risks stating a fact that is patently obvious. And yet, short of the resort to poetic narrative, it remains highly unfashionable in social anthropology to link bodily experience to the wider political arena.

In approaching the experiences of Salvadorans, I found concepts of embodiment helpful in thinking about cultural life in a more dialectical way, which holds potential for better integrating social and material realms, and for bridging the gap between personal-scale interactions and those of larger national and global forces. It is in this context that I want to make a case for a more explicit anthropological focus on social "materiality." Placing the body at the center of the cultural field, Thomas Csordas argues, helps the researcher to "collapse the duality of body and mind" that confounds so much of Western thought (1994). Csordas is referring to a key concept in medical anthropology: the Western legacy of René Descartes's sixteenth-century philosophical division of mind and body. Descartes, applying an Aristotelian logic, brokered a kind of compromise between empirical investigations and monotheism that resonated with his beliefs and placated the Catholic Church (by setting aside the mind and soul as outside the realm of science) while facilitating objective study of the body (specifically, the dissection of cadavers). His strategic cleavage, known as Cartesian dualism, served to privilege mental processes and encouraged the reductionism that both plagues medicine (as a healing art) and underlies much of the analytical power in the medical sciences.

We have lived with the consequences ever since in the form of medicine's lack of holism and inattentiveness to the emotional, social, and ecological aspects of healing or to the agency of the patient. A key contribution of medical anthropology has been to demonstrate that Descartes's divide was a false one, since the mind–body is inextricably interpenetrated. Nevertheless, prevailing notions of objectivity, dualism, and reductionistic logic have become defining hegemonic tropes not only in science but also in economics, religion, and governance in the Christian, capitalist West, both in the ways that people (and institutions) understand the world and in how they act on it (Gordon 1988; and Kleinman 1995).

Of all disciplines, anthropology's focus on cultural experience and the ethnographic method makes it particularly well positioned to subvert Cartesian dualism. But anthropology, like all disciplines that hitch their wagons (however loosely) to the sciences, is intimately entangled in Western epistemology. (It is no coincidence that many medical anthropologists who work as faculty members of medical schools prefer not to do critical analyses of the powerful institutions or ways of knowing that surround them and sanction their scholarship.) But to be fair, no one educated in the industrialized West escapes the persistent forms of rationality that constitute our way of knowing.

In medical anthropology this debate has often played out through debates between researchers drawing on more biomedical or ecological theories on culture and health and those adopting more cultural interpretive perspectives, emphasizing that illness and healing are in part culturally constructed and malleable. Critical medical anthropologists (e.g., Baer, Singer, and Johnson 1986) have often adopted a more dialectical stance, mediating between or drawing insights from both the cultural and socialecological subfields while pointing out how both frequently fail to acknowledge the role of power relations, particularly under capitalism, in shaping illness and disease. In recent years there has been a rapprochement between these views, as medical ecologists and some cultural constructionists have incorporated more political analysis and critical theorists have expanded into studies of ecology. (As neoliberal economics expanded, for example, more cultural researchers have found political economy useful in understanding the relation between World Trade Organization (WTO) policies on intellectual property and access of AIDS patients to life-saving drugs in multiple countries [e.g., see Baer 1996].)

Csordas's (1994) proposal to collapse the false duality of body and mind is not a proposal to counter ideologies of biomedical or scientific hegemonies that privilege Western rationality with some alternate corporal or materialist focal point. Rather he sees the body as the place where language, experience, and practice meet. The body becomes "culture's subject" or its "existential ground." The key to integrating the material and social is to focus on the relationship between them (Strathern 1996). Embodiment thus gives us a way to express dialectical or "relational" thinking.

Bourdieu's emphasis on the role of experience (over mentalist models of cognition) in practice theory (1977) joins a distinguished cadre of Western philosophers and social theorists who have laid groundwork for thinking of the social and organic bodies as deeply integrated, including Jacques Lacan's assertion that the unconscious is itself cultural in that it derives from language-like representations (see Strathern 1996). Maurice Merleau-Ponty argued that perception is "intersubjective" in that it is selective and shaped by the (cultural) body as locus (Langer 1989). Francisco Varela coined the term "enaction" for this interface referring to the dependence of cognition on a person's cultural history as a "being in the world" (Varela, Thompson, and Rosch 1991). I would add to the list Jürgen Habermas's rejection of traditional rationality based in the "knowing subject" in favor of a socially interactive model for communication (1989) and Noam Chomsky's influential model of an evolved capacity for language (1968).

Emotions, which by nature thwart Cartesian divides since they are mediated and partially manifest through the body (as opposed to brain), are intrinsically bound up with these mechanisms. Emotional and other mental states influence the immune system, and emotionally laden memories tend to be stored more vividly, are prone to reoccurrence, and are often co-activated with areas of the brain associated with experienced events. Brain-imaging studies indicate that emotional centers of the brain become active when a person is ready to act on a moral belief (Gazzaniga 2005). While there seem to be many universal aspects to a "lexicon of emotions," ethnographies in non-Western cultures suggest that interpretation of emotional states is culturally malleable (Lutz 1988; and Scheper-Hughes 1992).

Psychological studies dating to World War II show that the emotions of hope and fear, which might seem quite distinct and opposed, are in fact functionally related. Soldiers returning from the war's frontlines tended to strongly associate their memories of greatest fear with strengthened trust in God or some similar notion of "providential" outcome (Allport, et al. 1948). Today researchers refer to open-ended, uncontrolled events that provoke existential anxieties (e.g., natural disasters, disease) as "telic event structures." Presented with such scenarios, humans (even very young children) tend to look for causal agents (natural or supernatural) to explain the event (Atran 2002), setting up a framework for moral reasoning. A multitude of ethnographic examples, many on non-Western social beliefs about causes of illness and rationales about healing, also demonstrate this tendency to appeal to supernatural agents for assistance with unexplained events or for dealing with the unknown or the future.

Interpretations of emotions and moral reasoning are always culturally and historically situated, but data from this growing body of work suggest that just as there are common patterns of emotional interaction, there are likely common patterns of moral reasoning about issues such as perceptions of equity, treatment of others, and decisions related to life and death. Emotional states play a role in this reasoning, as do issues such as whether events involve known individuals to whom one feels social ties versus strangers. Even when there is an

absence of evidence of causal agents, when humans confront powerful consequential events, we tend to invent explanatory scenarios that assign moral
responsibility.

And therein lies the potential for creative production, for empathy is also
strong. The highly social nature of healing in dozens of preindustrial societies is
evidence of this dynamic at work. The social welfare or order and integrity of the
group is, in fact, often invoked as a metaphor in healing ceremonies to stimu-
late recovery of the sick patient. Just as excitement or stress, prolonged exposure
to trauma, and fear adhere in consciousness, literally changing both our brain
chemistries and our motivations and feelings of self-worth, so also can hope and
solidarity function in a similar dialectic. Here is potential for moral–political
conversion and forms of collective action.

In Search of the Body Politic

The violence that erupted throughout Central America in the 1980s is emblem-
atic of conflicts that continue in many parts of the globalizing South—from
Chiapas to the Philippines. Importantly, an integrated understanding of globalization has only emerged as a historical explanatory framework (as opposed to a
purportedly scientific economic model) since the aftermath of the 1999 Seattle
protests and the Asian financial crisis. Debates over free trade have brought the
inequalities of the so-called Washington Consensus model of globalization to
the center of both scholarly and public debate, and in recent years we have seen
a groundswell of support for critical ethnographies of the industrialized West as
well as a renewed call for anthropology to reinvent itself as more "relevant" and
engaged with public policy. As we confront increasing evidence of the ecological and social impacts of global capitalism, it is clear that we also need to har-
ness our intellects to forces for social change. Material issues of access to
resources, quality of life, and the engagement of humans with the natural world
are at the center of these struggles.

Material issues related to the rapid expansion of global capitalism (which
causes creative destruction at the local level), accompanied by increasingly
apparent constraints on nonrenewable resources, have fostered a shift from a
conviction that "development" was possible (in the straightforward sense of
programs to improve quality of life) to a sense that it has been a failed undertaking, and, worse, has no epistemological basis. In fact, failures of social development are used to justify policies by the industrialized nations, especially the
United States, of withdrawal from those parts of the world where they have no
vital or strategic interests at stake. Meanwhile rhetoric about economic development has become distanced from any notion of rising tides lifting even a
minority of boats. Increasingly we have entered a period of ends justifying
means, of instrumentalist foreign policy, which lacks even the civilizing veneers

of "freedom and democracy" (much less economic security). Under the second Bush administration those terms became used in such a cavalier way as to render them without meaning.

Italian philosopher Giorgio Agamben (1998) captured the dissonance of this period of social exclusion in his widely quoted essay *Homo Sacer*. In these reflections on political sovereignty and the "sacred man," Agamben referenced a criminal punished by exile under Roman law, which effectively lifted the royal sanction that otherwise protected subjects under imperial justice. Such a person, Agamben noted, lost their political standing as a citizen of the realm, whose claims to rights were recognized by authorities. The exiled criminal was reduced from a politically endowed person integrated into social life to an unprotected peon who could be killed without sanction (a state he refers to using the Greek *bios*, or "bare life," to contrast with *zoe*, the life of a citizen; Redfield 2005). Agamben is alluding, in the neoliberal era, to the likes of refugees, squatters, political prisoners, or famine victims, whose lack of political identity or legally recognized status puts them at risk of exclusion from the protections of citizenship. This was the condition being resisted in El Salvadore when Chalatecos pursued mass repopulation of their bombed-out province and reasserted their status as protected civilians rather than peons or criminals.

Although Foucault took issue with Marxist materialism, he also argued for greater attention to the social materiality of bodies caught up in the structures of economic production. In *Discipline and Punish* he argued

> the body is also directly involved in a political field; power relations have an immediate hold upon it, they invest it, mark it, train it, torture it, force it to carry out tasks, to perform ceremonies, to emit signs. This political investment of the body is bound up, in accordance with complex reciprocal relations, with its economic use; it is largely as a force of production that the body is invested with relations of power and domination, but on the other hand, its constitution as labour power is possible only if it is caught up in a system of subjection (in which need is also a political instrument meticulously prepared, calculated and used); the body becomes a useful force only if it is both a productive body and a subjected body. (1979, 25–26)

Through his concept of biopower, Foucault theorized that industrialized states wield subtle levels of control over populations and reinforce their legitimacy through implicit social contracts authorizing centralized coordination of policies affecting population health, such as public health, and social and medical services. State-sanctioned professional management of "normalizing" knowledge about population health is critical to such power relations because it allows power to operate through subtle mechanisms of regulation both by consensus around a set of norms and by self-regulation (Foucault 2003; and

Hogle 2002). Yet such state hegemony has tended to be weak in a state such as El Salvador, which has historically invested so little in public health or social welfare. In his writings on the dirty war in Argentina, Guillermo O'Donnell (1986) described a "weak" state as one that is controlled by elites who resist redistribution of wealth. Leaders present to the public a vision of a national development project but continually fail to deliver on the promise of develop-ment. Confronted with dissent over this failure, leaders resort to force again and again as the major means of social control, presenting the government with an ongoing crisis of legitimacy.

International accords on civil and economic human rights, such as the Universal Declaration on Human Rights, evolved to address exactly the absence of political protections for human agency that occurs in military dictatorships and conflict zones. Despite critiques over the origins of human rights in Western indi-vidualism, these standards have gained acceptance among anthropologists and recent decades have seen steady growth in national governments' acceptance of civil and political rights (Messer 1993). Less work has been done on how such "rights" are perceived in affected populations, especially in settings of civil wars where the concepts have gained local currency and where local organizations have taken up the work originally begun by Human Rights Watch or Amnesty International. But to assume cultural dissonance over human rights a priori is as problematic as the imperial disregard of difference. As Lock (2001) observed, cit-ing Latour, "people everywhere are increasingly, for better or worse, partially modern" and thereby aware of the contradictions in Western constructions such as development, democracy, and human rights (488). Escobar's hybridity attends to this sophistication in the ability of even poorly educated people to accommo-date contradictory relationships and function strategically with a variety of both traditional and crosscutting forms of identity and alliances.

In Foucault's thinking, the industrialized state's reliance on biopower was based on the promise of autonomy and freedom that is tied up with the notion of social welfare and individual rights, and the state benefits from the ways that such empowerment becomes "fetishized," resulting in individuals becoming more subjugated to forms of authority (Hogle 2002). And so we must ask what this means for weak, semiauthoritarian states when biopower works its power in reverse, when the increasingly globalized promise of access to biomedicine and other increasingly normalized trappings of middle-class comfort so prevalent on television, in films, and in popular culture—fast food, a car, a job—become scarce at the same time that the state, facing neoliberal pressures, begins to back down on constitutional responsibility for services like water, electricity, and primary health care for the poor.

Hegemonic power is strongest in relationships that become normalized or taken for granted, and it fails most profoundly when populations are left bereft of services they formerly took for granted due to a breached social contract in a setting where disparities in wealth and power are widely acknowledged. In El Salvador, the breach in zones of war during the 1980s was far more profound because civilians perceived their own government as intent on their destruction. Combined with liberation theology's assertion that poverty was not God's will but a product of injustice, the suffering body shifted for Chalatecos from a symbol of normalized, generic poverty to an icon of political struggle.

John O'Neill (1985) sees reference to the "body politic" as a form of "radical anthropomorphism" that alludes to body imagery to reassert the human shape of lives threatened by impersonal social and political forces. It is posed as an alternative to the "logic of calculative rationality" for discussing the social order, which too often makes discussion of alternative conceptions of society seem utopian or irrational. In contrast, he argues, the body politic is a fundamental and "reasonable" concept that "provides grounds of ultimate appeal in times of deep institutional crisis, of hunger and alienation, when there is need to renew primary bonds of political authority and consensus" (68).

If we allow ourselves to pursue the implications of a material sociality, we cannot avoid the conclusion that experiential knowledge or "situated learning" embedded in our neural networks is also a social product. There is no background or neutral, physical environment where the drama is played out—the background is also social, and it changes. Hence the dialectic—which acknowledges the contingency of those choices. Seen in this way, what we speak of as individual agency is both constrained and enabled by social ties.

The resort to new forms of collective action as a matter of survival by Chalatecos under the profound circumstances of threat in which they found themselves does not seem so strange when we consider the dependency on social infrastructure built into modern life. In particular, modernity is constructed out of exchange of forms of capital that have, by entering capitalist markets, lost their ties to social relationships. Considering the individualizing nature of both modern and neoliberal economic development, and the role of coercion in enforcing the disenfranchisement of rural Salvadorans from social and material wealth, makes the turn to collective strategies for redress (or for material support) a logical move. My use of the term "moral ecology" in this study is intended to link the social and material fields in our thinking and situate human life in a wider context while restoring moral reasoning as a central logic of human relations. I read the Salvadoran demand for dignidad as a call for forms of development that contain a space for sociality and creativity.

Marx said man creates himself but not under "conditions of his choosing." While Marx sought to emphasize the material–political constraints of human choices, my point here is to emphasize also the profoundly social fabric in which exercises of productivity and coercion are carried out. I wish to animate our conception of the political field in a way that acknowledges the interpenetrated nature of material and social relations and provokes consciousness of the false dualism of Cartesian thinking that has so long infected our not-so-postmodern psyches.

The Plan of the Book

Part One, "Exclusion and the Politics of Bare Life," examines the politics of exclusion used to disenfranchise a large portion of the Salvadoran peasantry from claims to land or public goods, and peasant resistance to the repression in northern Chalatenango, a "zone of refuge" for dispossessed peasants. Chapter 1 uses a socioepidemiological analysis to explore the economic and political underpinning of peasant "ill-being" in El Salvador from 1978 to 1985. I draw the links between state violence and elite-backed policies favoring new export crops, which led to widespread dispossession of peasants. The chapter also explores the origins of racist sentiment in the official culture of violence as well as the role of geopolitical ideas about the "social body" in U.S. and Latin American national security doctrine. In Chapter 2 I examine the relationships among violence, poverty, and radicalization, drawing on oral histories, previously untranslated writings, and other accounts to examine how liberation theology practices of collective action, including health organizing, took root in rural Chalatenango. I argue that these practices were not only products of ideological influence (e.g., Christian Base Communities and the FMLN) but also essential in the communities' self-defense against the repression as rural areas became polarized and military "sweeps" targeted civilians. I address dialectical and pragmatic aspects of community, as opposed to the utopian notions often seen in "solidarity" accounts.

In Part Two, "War against Health," three chapters analyze the politics of health and medicine in the context of the civil war. Chapter 3 examines radical forms of productivity that emerged from the extreme conditions that existed in Salvadoran zones of war. It traces the seeds of the popular health system in northeast Chalatenango from 1978 to 1985 when the guerrilla movement, aided by urban supporters and international NGOs, developed its own system of wartime medicine while experimenting with new forms of pedagogy and organization.

Chapter 4 documents the impact on civilians from the most intense aerial bombardment ever carried out on civilian-occupied areas in the Western Hemisphere. I present data that I gathered to investigate violations of "medical neutrality" in the war from 1987 to 1989 with an analysis of state violence against humanitarian relief work in this setting of low-intensity conflict (LIC). I discuss the role of health rights and human rights as humanitarian narratives that shape hegemonic ideas about governance, and the potential for a "transnational" anthropology of state terror. Chapter 5, on psychological warfare, uses ethnographic accounts to examine biomedicine's powerful semiotics, with attention to the role of fantasies of order and magical cures in state political discourse. Medical and food aid were routinely used in an instrumental fashion to manipulate civilians by

the Salvadoran military and (after the cease-fire) by U.S. forces carrying out training exercises. I explore questions such as when these strategies achieve their goals,
when they fail, and how tactics of attacking civilians in rural areas square with the
LIC pacification campaign goals of "winning hearts and minds."

In Part Three, "Health against War," the focus shifts to ethnography of the popular health system that evolved after refugees and displaced peasants repopulated
northeast Chalatenango between 1986 and 1992. Chapter 6 analyzes practices of
"popular" health, comparing them with government-run rural health services,
devoting special attention to the key role of locally based lay promoters and to popular system innovations in training, medical prescribing, dental health, and use of
herbal remedies. Chapter 7 uses international health development criteria to
examine participatory aspects of the popular system and compare it with the community health program run by the Ministry of Health. I discuss debates over curative versus preventive approaches, and I offer a critique of the pessimism found in
much of the literature about the potential for participatory approaches to health.

In Part Four, "War by Other Means," three chapters examine political threats
to community health organizing during the neoliberal postwar period. Chapter 8
follows negotiations and confrontations between the popular system and the
Ministry of Health, lending insights on the ways that biomedicine functions to
reinforce state hegemony. Popular system advocates resisted the conservative
ministry's rigid, centralized, and medicalized model of rural health and fought
back in innovative ways, but gradually the popular promoters found themselves
marginalized by the ministry. Chapter 9 examines international lending in the
postwar period, with attention to neoliberal conditionality on health development. In this period the Ministry of Health offloaded many preventive services
onto NGOs without the funding or control they needed. I present a case study in
which pressure to lend from the World Bank, coupled with an ARENA health
minister's suspicion of NGOs led to funds being diverted from a well-designed
and managed community-based maternal and child health network to a poorly
designed and low-functioning rural program run by the Ministry of Health.
Chapter 10 brings the story full circle with the history of the health movement
that led, in 2002–2003, to the largest national street mobilizations since the
war. The health workers' strikes put the brakes on the president's (and World
Bank's) plan to privatize portions of the social security health system. The chapter draws on interviews with participants and leaders to examine how a technical issue such as health reform came to resonate with the general population,
and how two unions of radicalized health workers rose to national prominence,
reinvigorating a reformist political agenda.

These struggles in El Salvador over health rights of the poor majority offer
insights into the grave costs being paid by the most vulnerable citizens for
neoliberal policies, and to the explosive political potential of a biopolitics of
resistance that is able to cross over traditional political categories to create new

unities and present humane alternatives to the politics of profit. Throughout the Global South and in marginalized areas of the developed world, multinational lending and corporate-friendly trade agreements have sacrificed national patrimonies and enriched local elites at high cost to the bare life of those who no longer seem to matter in the global marketplace. In the aftermath of a civil war and two decades of ARENA's corrupt rule, the densely organized Salvadoran opposition is better positioned than many in the Global South to look beyond the glossy epidermis of modernism's sleek façade and offer a more wholesome broth for our common affliction. It is my hope that the struggles recounted here contribute to wider efforts to invent a more humane body politic.

PART ONE

Exclusion and the
Politics of Bare Life

1

Manufacturing Ill-being

An Epidemiology of Development and Terror

> They killed my husband and my daughter in 1980. She was with five other
> women—three cousins and two nieces. It was a massacre. . . . Someone went
> to the army as an *oreja* (informer). There were witnesses. The soldiers cap-
> tured them near the river and took them to my daughter's house. They took
> all the women's clothes and raped them. And they had little children with
> them! They hung them from a tree. One was pregnant and they cut the child
> out from inside her. Dogs were eating it when we found them.
>
> —Marta Ramos, former resident of Nueva Trinidad, Chalatenango

After the cease-fire when I began studying popular health in Guarjila, a resettled
village of northeast Chalatenango, I initially talked to patients I met at the clinic
and then asked permission to visit them at home for a follow-up interview. At the
end of one such visit in the open-air dining area of an elderly woman's *champa*,
I stood to put my notebook away when Marta Ramos, who had been describing her
granddaughter's persistent cold, suddenly grabbed my arm and sat me down again.
"*Escucha!* (Listen!)," she insisted, "I have to tell you this!" She erupted into the
bloodcurdling tale of the 1980 raid excerpted above. The story continued:

> They cut their heads off too, and threw them away. They burned my
> nieces alive with a pile of wood. They killed my husband the same day
> while he was working. If we hadn't run away we'd have been killed too.
> The *compas* [FMLN combatants] helped us escape. Then later we went to
> my daughter's house and found all the bodies. They burned everything in
> her house. All together they left twenty-one children orphaned. I was left
> with five children to take care of. It was so sad. We fled. We had to leave
> everything behind. We spent eight days walking and running, with noth-
> ing to eat or drink. We couldn't sleep. It was after that when we went to
> Honduras.

I had planned to separate research on the popular clinics from research on the war years. Stories like Marta's made me realize how tedious and irrelevant my questions about rashes and sore throats must have seemed to people who had lost family members under such horrific circumstances. It is easier for researchers—who, after all, live in enclaves removed from hunger and violence—to categorize their thinking than for people traumatized by mass murder.

The first years of the civil war in El Salvador are most accurately described as a period of state terror. Tutela Legal, the human rights office of San Salvador's Catholic Archdiocese, documented more than thirty thousand noncombatants murdered or "disappeared" from 1980 to 1985 in a context of indiscriminate military attacks on rural settlements, urban police violence against dissident organizations, and political killings by right-wing paramilitary groups or "death squads" allied with the military (see Porpora 1990; Montgomery 1995; and Bonner 1984). The violence produced a death toll not unlike (and possibly higher than) that of the infamous *matanza*, the 1932 army massacre of tens of thousands of Indian peasants after a small rebellion—an event (treated in more detail below) that is frequently cited as the prelude to fifty years of repressive military rule.

Reagan administration comments about the violence in the early 1980s tended to blame atrocities either on the chaos of battle or left-wing "terrorism." These explanations were contradicted by the UN Truth Commission report published after the war ended, which reviewed twenty-two thousand reported acts of violence, including political murders, disappearances, and cases of torture, most of which occurred during the first four years of the war. Of those giving testimonies to the commission, 85 percent accused state military or police forces, or allied paramilitary groups; only 5 percent accused the FMLN guerrillas of crimes (UN Truth Commission 1992).

The extent of the state violence far exceeded anything resembling a strategic military response to the guerrillas. Estimated at only a few hundred strong prior to 1980, the FMLN army grew steadily in part because of the repression; as options for public debate or protest were closed down by the police, many Salvadorans previously active in union or student groups took up arms and went underground as a last resort (Pearce 1986; and Wood 2003). In rural Chalatenango, many people who survived the scorched earth–type army sweeps of 1983–1985 told me it was safer for them to join the compas than to continue civilian life. By 1984 the FMLN had grown to an estimated nine thousand to twelve thousand fighters (Montgomery 1995), but at no time did rebels killed make up a significant portion of the death toll recorded by human rights organizations (see also Stanley 1996; and Wood 2003).

When the human toll is added to the equation, the era of progress in post-1960 El Salvador is converted from a success story to a holocaust. This chapter seeks to knit together the historical and transnational economies and power relations that created the public health emergency of contemporary El Salvador.

A number of medical anthropologists have explored the potential for a politically and socially conscious epidemiology that rises above the specialization and reductionism associated with biomedicine to address the wider social, economic, and political parameters of ill health (Hahn 1995; Heggenhougan 1995; Inhorn 1995; and Trostle 1986). Jaime Briehl sets out a rationale for such an undertaking, observing that "equity, justice, well-being, and health, issues at the heart of the practice of epidemiology, are the bases of a new more humane and democratic society" (1995, 911). Richard Levins argued that an integrated epidemiology should be interdisciplinary, reflexive, and quantitative but also "socialized" in ways that reflect class and other social inequities (1995).

In line with these ideals, I seek in this chapter to examine the social history of El Salvador, using an integrated sociopolitical epidemiology that assesses the role of militarism and modernization in poverty creation. A key question is how the country's stark divisions between the populace and a military state evolved, and how a sufficiently large number of people can be mobilized to take part in threatening or killing their fellow citizens. Almost by definition, genocide-like events occur only when a political system both promotes a set of beliefs stigmatizing a group of people and systematically initiates strategies of inhumane practices.

Most analyses of the war today agree that the conflagration that consumed El Salvador was about the distribution of land and access to resources. Several scholars considering Central America as a region have observed that war broke out specifically in those countries—Nicaragua, El Salvador, and Guatemala—that failed to institute social programs such as land reforms in response to popular pressure, instead resorting to military repression to contain unrest. In Honduras and Costa Rica, state-led reforms averted rebellions (Booth 1991; and Williams 1986). So to address genocide we must unpack the relationship between systemic violence (poverty) and state violence.

Unlike in Guatemala, where genocidal violence by the armed forces targeted the indigenous population in the Highlands, in El Salvador repression was more generalized throughout society and was indexed by class far more than ethnic identity. El Salvador's *mestizaje*, however, is of relatively recent origin and indexes a sharply stigmatized divide with all the fearful revulsion of racism. Such an elite remove and sense of entitlement in this setting with a tiny middle class contributed to the rise of militarism; conversely, the polarized social relations have contributed to an unusual level of class identity among the poor (Kincaid 1987; LaFeber 1993; Lungo Uclés 1996; and Montgomery 1995).

As William Stanley argues convincingly, violence became a currency of power in El Salvador, where, after 1932, the military was in effect granted a license to run a "protection racket" for the oligarchy (1996). The relations between the peasantry and the landowning class had many feudal aspects even as late as the 1950s, but the expansion of many large estates in that decade to grow cotton and sugar with modern methods began a rapid and consequential transformation of class relations. Landowners enjoyed a tight alliance with the government's five armed security forces, and the U.S.-promoted Cold War specter of "communism" provided a rationale for heightened repression to contain opposition to policies that impacted small holders. In a small agricultural state with a large population and limited arable land, modernization institutionalized what I call "ill-being" by greatly worsening chronic malnutrition, disease, and mortality for the vast majority of Salvadorans. However, for new export-focused agriculturalists, modernization was profitable, and close alliances with Central American strongmen indirectly served security interests of the United States, leading a succession of U.S. administrations to turn a blind eye to human rights atrocities.

Class, Fear, and *Ladinoización*: El Salvador's Apartheid

During 1993 I rented a room for two months from an elderly couple in the capital. Although they lived on the edge of Escalón, an upper-class neighborhood, the house was not particularly luxurious. It was surrounded, like its neighbors, by a high wall, topped by sharp glass from broken bottles. Don Pablo had once been active in the Christian Democratic Party (PDC), which supported social reforms, and he often argued over the afternoon meal with his son, a businessman who had joined the ruling ARENA party. The couple knew that I frequently traveled to a former FMLN stronghold for my research, but they asked few questions, which I appreciated, especially after meeting their son. One day Doña Elena took me aside and recounted a story of a Sunday afternoon excursion to the countryside that had been interrupted by car trouble. While waiting on the mechanic, she said, she had wandered over to chat with a peasant woman who lived in a champa by the edge of the highway. "You wouldn't believe how dirty her children were," Doña Elena said. "They had swollen bellies and ran around half naked, playing in the dirt. Their mother acted like that was normal. I asked her how they got along, and she said, 'Everything is fine.'"

"What do you make of that?" Doña Elena asked me.

"Maybe she was too proud to complain," I suggested weakly, realizing that she intended the story as an object lesson for her foreign houseguest.

"No," she said, "That woman really didn't see anything wrong with how they were living. They're different from us. They don't suffer as we do."

I had known that conservatives among the wealthy classes saw the peasants as lesser beings (e.g., see Rosenberg 1992), but it surprised me to hear this from the wife of a PDC supporter. Doña Elena, however, was giving voice to the extremity of class division in El Salvador, which is indexed by ethnicity and rooted in a historical legacy of state violence. John Sloan, writing about repression in Latin America, noted that the forms of nationalism that arose in much of the region are linked to "an inherited belief system that holds that most of the population—Indians, workers, urban squatters—do not have the capacity either to care for themselves or to influence public policy" (1984, 90). He argued that, unlike in Europe, in most of Latin America no strong traditions of liberalism existed to challenge military rule. Legal discrimination against indigenous people became less common after the wars of independence, and assertions of pride in mestizo identity were critical to the creation of nationalist identities. But even under liberal administrations that spoke of freedom and democracy, paternalism and social hierarchies persisted. Education, manners, and adoption of urban upper-class practices continued to mark status, often legitimizing discrimination that served to reinscribe ethnic difference (de la Cadena 2000). Gen. Guillermo Rodriguez Lara, the president of Ecuador, summed up the thinking of many regional leaders in 1972 with his claim, "There is no more Indian problem. We all become white when we accept the goals of national culture" (Stutzman 1980).

Hence, El Salvador is regarded as predominantly mestizo today, with only tiny pockets of people that lay claim to indigenous identity. But, importantly, the backing away from cultural markers did not occur gradually, as a result of mixed marriages and cultural assimilation, but in a relatively short period in the decade following the traumatic events of the 1932 matanza, when most peasants rapidly abandoned indigenous dress and culture in a move that many have interpreted as a response to the repression. Anthropologists have extensively studied indigenous identity in Guatemala and the Andes, with attention to the social and economic rationales of those who reject their traditions and adopt ladino or mestizo customs. But far less attention has been paid to "ladinoización" motivated by fear (But see Tilley 2005).

Tensions between the peasantry and El Salvador's small land-owning class can be traced to early colonial rule when native populations were forced to labor on export crops under the *encomienda* system, which allowed authorities to assign Indians and land to Spanish overlords. Indian labor had become scare (and hence highly valuable) due to the "great dying"—a combination of warfare, epidemics, starvation from disrupted trade routes, and the slave trade—that decimated the local indigenous population, reducing it from a high of five hundred thousand or more to seventy-seven thousand at its lowest point around 1570. The fortunes made through labor-intensive cacao production under this system in the sixteenth century helped consolidate the wealth of a small oligarchy and set the stage for reliance on monocrop production (Montgomery 1995). The cacao boom was followed by a depression in the early seventeenth century, during which elites expanded control over land, forming haciendas as a strategy to maintain cash flows. Indigenous communities received no compensation for land loss, but peasants were allowed to live on the edges of tilled fields as *colonos*, giving a share of each harvest to their *patrón* (Browning 1971).

The next big cash crop, indigo, helped haciendas remain profitable for 150 years. In the nineteenth century when European demand for indigo declined, many landowners turned to coffee. Inspired by the wealthy European states, liberal politicians adopted "developmentalist" policies aimed at privatizing land previously held by the Catholic Church and fostering entrepreneurial investments that would build a modern, secular economy (Edelman 1999). Remaining Indian land, much of it in fertile volcanic highlands, also came to be coveted by coffee growers, and in 1881 the state responded to the coffee lobby by abolishing the indigenous communal land system. The preamble to the decree reads: "The existence of lands under the ownership of *comunidades* impedes agricultural development, obstructs the circulation of wealth, and weakens family bonds and the independence of the individual. Their existence is contrary to the economic and social principles that the Republic has accepted."—Law for the Extinction of Communal Lands, Feb. 26, 1881 (Browning 1971, 205).

At the time, the native population made up 85 percent of the Salvadoran population, having only recently surpassed its preconquest size after growing steadily for four hundred years (Durham 1979; and Montgomery 1995). A predominant worry of elites had long been the threat of Indian rebellion (Paige 1994), and this scenario played out during the global economic depression of the early 1930s, when a rebellion led by El Salvador's small Communist party erupted in the Indian town of Izalco, in the heart of a rich coffee-growing region. The uprising culminated in the infamous 1932 matanza, in which marauding army and "civic guard" troops killed between seventeen thousand and thirty thousand campesinos (see Browning 1971; Anderson 1971; and McClintock 1985).

> Around Izalco a roundup of suspects began. As most of the rebels, except the leaders, were difficult to identify, arbitrary classifications were set up. All those who were found carrying machetes were guilty. All those of a strongly Indian cast of features, or who dressed in a scruffy campesino costume, were considered guilty. . . . All those who had not taken part in the uprising were invited to present themselves at the *comandancia* to receive clearance papers. When they arrived . . . those with the above-mentioned attributes were seized. Tied by the thumbs . . . groups of fifty were led to the back wall of the church of Asunción in Izalco, and . . . cut down by firing squads. (Anderson 1971)

Concerned about the peasant uprising, American navy officers in warships just off the Salvadoran coast offered military assistance to the government but were reassured by President Maximiliano Hernández Martínez that his troops had the situation in hand. (Given that Nicaragua, next door, was at that time occupied by the U.S. Marines, Martínez was no doubt eager to avoid giving the Americans an opportunity to station troops in his country.)

Shortly after the cataclysm, new laws were passed requiring adults over the age of eighteen to carry personal identity cards that would thereafter be required for most interactions with the state (persons of means could pay a patriotic donation and escape the requirement) (McClintock 1985). In the decade that followed, most campesinos stopped wearing traditional clothing (Anderson 1971) and gradually stopped registering new births as indigenous (Tilley 2005). Memories of the matanza became buried, whispered from generation to generation, a traumatic episode indelibly fixed in the Salvadoran psyche, its telling tempered by fear yet also serving to reaffirm solidarity. While teaching English in San Salvador in 1987, I was dressed down by a teacher for just describing the event to my students (see chapter 2). But Jeffrey Paige's (1994) study of elite beliefs about the matanza revealed very different collective memories among the oligarchy, for whom the event stands as a warning of what can happen when authorities let down their guard. The official story is one of anarchy and chaos in which mobs of communist Indians went on a rampage with no provocation and murdered thousands until they were brought under control by the heroic army.

> For the elite, the revolt combined their two worst nightmares, Indian rebellion and communist revolution. . . . In the aftermath of the insurrection racism and anti-communism merged into a single powerful ideology to justify repression and permanently block social change. . . . The ideological consequences of 1932 for the elite were paranoid anti-communism, dread of social reform, and the dehumanization of the left. . . . It also reinforced their belief that the poor were a separate species, ignorant, ferocious and credulous, easily "excited" by "communist" agitators. (Paige 1994, 24)

Indigenous identity survives in place names, words for foods, and household terms. By the 1980s only residents of a few towns actively claimed indigenous identity. The term "*indio*," when used, was almost an epithet meaning poor and uneducated. Yet the "othering" effect inherent to the rich–poor divide in El Salvador continues to carry the stigma and visceral aversion of racism. That the well-to-do in their walled compounds live existentially removed from the poor adds to a "political ethos" (Jenkins 1991) in which elites fear the peasantry. It is a common observation in political science that the level of repression a government employs speaks to the insecurity of its rulers (Sloan 1984).

The legacy of elite fear has bizarre manifestations. In her account of the lives of the six Jesuit scholars assassinated by the army in 1989, Teresa Whitfield told the story of a retreat held for upper-class students attending the Catholic high school in 1949 attended by a young Jesuit recently arrived from Spain who was shocked when the priest in charge asked the boys to "hand in their pistols." Within minutes they were standing guard over a pile of twenty-odd weapons. "And why did they have the pistols in the first place? Because they had a 'right' of self-defense against 'all those Indians'" (1995, 19–20). Ignacio Martín-Baró, a priest and University of Central America psychologist who was among those murdered, conducted opinion surveys among Salvadorans during the 1980s. His researchers asked upper-class children: "What would have to happen in order for there to be no more poor people?" Several answered "*Matarlos a todos* [Kill them all]" (Martín-Baró 1998, 68).

Toward an Epidemiology of Systemic Violence

This apartheid affected public life in a myriad of ways, including access to health services. Despite a clause in the constitution stating that all citizens have a right to health services, the majority, in fact, never have. Even today, more than a decade after the war, rural health is a shoddy affair in many areas. For decades El Salvador has ranked near the bottom in Latin America for public health indices, but Chalatenango holds a similarly low rank among the country's fourteen departments. More than half the department's population lacked any access to health in the 1971, and the department did not even have a hospital until 1973. In a 1985 session I attended at the Ministry of Health headquarters, an official estimated the physician-to-population ratio in Chalatenango at 1 doctor per 200,000 residents, and possibly less. For comparison, the physician-to-population ratio in San Salvador was 1:800 at the time.

Less than 15 percent of the labor force, most of them urban-based, enjoyed access to social security benefits for health services in the 1980s (and it was a recent achievement to extend services to this many), leaving the rest dependent on a health system that in rural areas consisted of a scattering of clinics that were shuttered most days for lack of staff or medical supplies. In visits to poor neighborhoods during the war mothers often asked me for help getting medicines for sick children. When I asked if they had gone to a public clinic, many scoffed at the suggestion. Typical complaints were that Ministry of Health clinics had no medicines or that the nurses there did not know enough to help.

In 1987 I rode along with a Salvadoran physician delivering medical relief supplies to a group of *desplazados* (displaced people) camped out in a church in militarized Suchitoto. Knowing that the doctor worked part time for the Ministry of Health, I asked him why peasants spoke so disparagingly of public clinics. He rolled his eyes and launched into a lecture on the problems of the health system, which ranged from shoddy training to shortages of medicines and low pay. Most doctors retained a relationship with the ministry for reasons of prestige and to maintain hospital privileges, he explained, but spent the bulk of their time practicing at private clinics and attended the public clinic for only a couple of hours a week, less frequently in rural areas.

The problem was that this left rural campesinos with few options in the event of a medical emergency. A 1987–1989 survey conducted by social scientists at the University of Central America (UCA) attempted to measure public use of health services nationwide. Asked what they did when they got sick, 73 percent of middle-class urbanites said they consulted a doctor, but only a third of respondents from rural areas or those living in urban barrios gave that response. Most

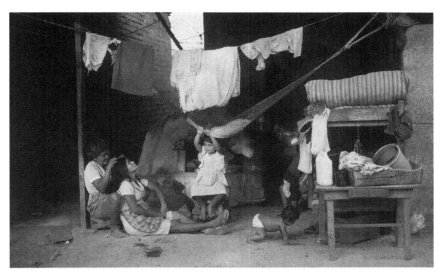

Displaced person camp in basement of church, San Salvador, 1985. Photograph by Sandy Smith-Nonini.

of them were more likely to look for medicines on their own or resort to household remedies. By the mid-1980s, around fifty Ministry of Health clinics had been closed down due to the war (Hanania de Varela 1990), and shortages of trained personnel and medicines plagued most remaining public clinics.

Marlene, a health outreach worker for the Chalatenango Diocese, helped me appreciate the hurdles that mothers with sick children had to negotiate. A mother of four in her late twenties, Marlene lived in a settlement nestled in a curve of the Troncal Norte, the highway running north from the capital. Throughout the war her village remained in government territory and was not particularly "conflicted." Marlene had separated from an emotionally abusive husband two years earlier and enrolled in church-sponsored health classes. Bright and articulate, she had risen rapidly in the Catholic diocese's health division, but Marlene still felt torn between her children's needs and her job. During an oral history interview, I asked her when in her life she first began paying attention to health issues.

> It was when I was dealing with my youngest child's illnesses. He had third degree malnutrition when he was three years old, and I thought he was going to die. He didn't get any good out of food. It just passed through him. His *pupu* was watery and it had whole chunks of meat in it. He lost so much weight, and wouldn't eat. Even if I just gave him water, he threw up. . . . It was like this for a year. I kept taking him to the ministry clinic in Aguilares—it was about a forty-five-minute bus ride. And I took him to the Chalatenango hospital, but the doctors just scolded me for not feeding

him properly. Finally one prescribed an antiparasite medicine called Virmix, and he started passing worms. Huge worms. And then he passed a kind of sack. I thought he'd passed part of his intestines and I was sure he was going to die. But when I touched the bag with a stick, it broke open and it was full of tiny worms. Ugh! It was so awful. After that he swelled up for a couple of days, but then he got better. So it worked. I don't know why it took them so long to prescribe that medicine.

The other problem was ear infections. Today, he's deaf in one ear because he had so many infections. None of the antibiotics or ear cleanings they gave him at the hospital worked. He had terrible earaches. He would complain, "Mami, my ear hurts. Please take me to the doctor." I took him to the Chalate hospital, to Aguilares. Half the time they didn't even give him a decent checkup. The doctors gave me antibiotics, but he always threw them up; they weren't doing him any good. Finally, I took him to Rosales Hospital in San Salvador. But I had the hardest time just getting an appointment. And they wouldn't give a follow-up appointment until two months later, even though the antibiotic didn't work. They said too many people were waiting to be seen. I remember one doctor asked how many infections he'd had and I told him, "Thirteen." He was shocked!

When I had to pay for antibiotics out of my pocket, sometimes I couldn't afford them. Luckily the diocese helped me. But the medicines weren't doing any good. One doctor told me the infection could spread to his other ear, so I was terrified he would end up totally deaf. I was pregnant at the time, and I was in bad shape . . . I only weighed 100 pounds myself. I was just desperate. At times I didn't know how I would survive with the children. You know, I first got interested in studying health when he was so sick. I noticed things like he never produced tears when he cried, and he had a dry mouth and kept it open all the time. It made me wonder. Now I know it was from the malnutrition and dehydration he had.

A family health survey of the U.S. Agency for International Development (USAID) found that diarrhea and intestinal disorders caused about half of all illnesses in children, and nearly a quarter of deaths for children under five in the 1980s. Preventable respiratory infections accounted for another 18 percent of illnesses. Poor rural sewage facilities and lack of potable water were the leading contributors to child morbidity (FESAL 1988).

Since international observers regarded Ministry of Health figures with suspicion, agencies like USAID and UNICEF often conducted their own surveys, extrapolating from a small sample to generate a national estimate. Depending on the source, one-year infant mortality rates ranged from 42 to 87 deaths per 1,000 live births in the 1980s, climbing higher as the war dragged on (see IDUCA 1992; and Fiedler, Gomez, and Bertrand 1993). As with all health statistics in El Salvador, there must be an urban figure and a rural one, and the latter was always the most egregious. Adult health was similarly precarious: Life expectancy of Salvadorans had long been among the lowest in Latin America, estimated at 56.5 years in the first half of the 1970s, but after the onset of repressive violence in the late 1970s, the estimate fell to an abysmal 50.7 years (IDHUCA 1992[1]). Perinatal mortality for women giving birth was an astounding 70.6 per 1,000 births in 1980 (Ugalde et al. 2000).

Statistics on rates and risk factors—this is the language in which epidemiology describes the human consequences of systemic violence. But this discourse so often fails to lift the analysis over the hump of causality, pointing us to remedies. Moreover, causality often remains trapped in the circular finger-pointing of unclean habits, cultures of poverty, and failures of education and medical compliance that blame the poor for being poor, all in the name of science. Measurement itself often becomes a higher priority than programs to address the problems. As Taussig lamented, "to measure meticulously malnutrition and poverty, when it is patently obvious to everyone that the state of deprivation is colossal, amounts to the most cruel fetish of scientific method" (1978).

I use the term "ill-being" in this study to subvert a way of talking and thinking about health that has become hegemonic in the West. The notion of "public health" usually evokes images of a set of benefits for populations accruing from the combination of economic growth-related prosperity and a welfare state that provides sanitary infrastructure, education, and basic health services. There is a hidden suggestion that progress, defined in terms of capitalist development and modern medical knowledge, brings with it these benefits, with the corollary that poor health is the natural condition of a place where capitalist development has not yet arrived. As Aviles (2001) noted, the epidemiological transition theory, which correlates disease patterns with levels of poverty and stages of economic development, has built-in assumptions that link health to the diffusion of Western values. This lends a sense of benevolence and authority to development institutions: surely if USAID is vaccinating children, then it must be pursuing similarly laudable goals when the same agency programs train and equip Latin American police forces.

While the roots of oppression in El Salvador date to the 1880s takeover of coffee land, less attention has been paid to the ways that twenty years of modern "development" economics contributed both to the institutionalization of state violence, and to the rapid dispossession of the peasantry from land. In the 1960s new lending for "Green Revolution" agricultural modernization helped transform El Salvador's economy, but the outcomes were a grotesque caricature of the promise as the shift to new export crops left hundreds of thousands of peasants effectively homeless or with too little land to support a family.

Cold War Development and the Creation of Poverty

The Central American states began experimenting with crop diversification in the 1950s as a way to mitigate overreliance on bananas and coffee. The 1930s depression had sensitized elites to how a dip in world prices for one or two crops could devastate a national economy. As land suitable for coffee came to be in short supply, landowning families began turning to sugar and cotton in an effort to maintain profit growth and diversify their interests. The advent of DDT to control malaria in wet tropical lowlands helped spur the spread of both crops.

Spooked by the Cuban Revolution and social uprisings in several Central American countries, the Kennedy administration invented the U.S. Alliance for Progress to foster noncommunist development in poor countries while promoting export of American technology and products. Through USAID, loans were made in the 1960s for road building, industrial infrastructure, and a variety of capital-intensive agricultural inputs such as fertilizers, chemicals for weed and pest control, and tractors. In El Salvador, cotton became the important new crop, and the formation of a powerful cotton cooperative by growers led to increased access to credit and finance through local banks (Bulmer-Thomas 1987; and Williams 1986).

As the Pacific lowlands came under cotton cultivation, these estates gradually took over half of the area's crop land, reducing the amount of land available for corn from 50 percent in the late 1940s to less than 30 percent by the late 1960s. The cotton yield doubled during the same period (Williams 1986). Many haciendas that had previously allowed colonos to grow subsistence crops on more marginal land now laid claim to this land for cotton. At first these changes created a new class of smaller growers as larger farms rented land for cotton to the better-off peasants, some of whom supplemented their earnings by picking cotton on large farms for part of the year. Once again, Salvadoran planters set records for productivity—formerly world renowned for high yields of coffee, now Salvadorans achieved similarly high yields in cotton.

But the boom and the new options for small farmers were short-lived. As occurred with Green Revolution technologies in other parts of the world, when chemicals killed off insects' natural enemies, new varieties of cotton pests emerged that were more resistant. Likewise, resistant mosquitoes produced a resurgence of malaria. And the high input crop literally began to wear out the light coastal soils, which were now more exposed to leaching and erosion during the rainy season. Peasants who had followed the advice of technocrats and adopted new fertilizers and chemicals for their corn and rice crops also saw declines in yields (Williams 1986).

Peasant land loss intensified as property owners, now heavily committed to capital-intensive strategies, began to require cash rents up front rather than allow peasants to pay with a portion of their harvest. In contrast to larger Central

American countries where new cotton lands were zones of in-migration for harvest jobs, in El Salvador, which lacked a land frontier, the cotton region became a zone of expulsion (Bulmer-Thomas 1987). The numbers of colonos in the area fell from fifty-five thousand in 1961 to only seventeen thousand in less than a decade (Pearce 1986). Many of the new landless joined the informal economy along roadsides or migrated to new shantytowns springing up on the outskirts of cities; others migrated to Honduras or Guatemala for harvest jobs or moved north and attempted to grow corn in the thin soils of pine forests and eroded hillsides. A minimum wage law in 1965 provided property owners with an added rationale for expulsions. Growers turned to mechanized harvesters to reduce labor costs, which contributed to a second cotton boom in the early 1970s. But this boom was shorter than the first one, and by the end of 1971 more than one hundred thousand harvest jobs in cotton had disappeared (Williams 1986).

Already, for more than a century Chalatenango had been a "peasant refuge zone" for small holders excluded from fertile coffee estates to the south, but the area's thin rocky soils and mountainous terrain was unable to support the new influx of people (Williams 1986). By 1975 the department had the highest unemployment in the country and the most out-migration to other areas. Land pressure intensified in 1969 when an estimated 130,000 Salvadorans who had migrated to Honduras were expelled, many settling in Chalatenango, during the "Soccer War" (so-named because the brief hostilities followed a heavily contested soccer match between teams from the two countries). The war arose in part because of a Honduran land reform plan. Conservative opponents to the reform, including powerful cattle ranchers, objected to allowing Salvadoran immigrants to benefit from the reform and demanded that the government expel them.

The Alliance for Progress development loans were supposed to hasten modernization and economic growth, which would create jobs and revenue, and spur national investment in the public sector, creating political stability. They included funds for El Salvador to set up mobile rural health units and antimalarial programs (Allwood Paredes 1960), and USAID assisted the Ministry of Health to build a network of rural health posts. It was during the 1960s that the Salvadoran government first required medical graduates to complete a social service year in rural areas. There were modest gains in public health as life expectancy crept from the mid-fifties into the sixties, and infant mortality dropped from 76.3 percent in 1960 to 66.7 percent by 1970, but most of these gains were lost after conditions for the majority worsened considerably in the 1970s.

Despite steady growth in exports and gross domestic product (GDP) during the Alliance for Progress years, El Salvador continued to lag behind other Central American states in social sector investments (Bulmer-Thomas 1987). Less that 5 percent of the population was eligible for social security health services, and in the mid-1960s El Salvador's per capita investment in health was only a little more than a third of that of Panama or Costa Rica. The modest gains in social spending disappeared entirely once inflation was taken into account (Allwood Paredes 1969). Despite rhetoric about the public good, the military officers who ruled the country continued to cater to the elite families that were the primary beneficiaries of the new programs.

The second most important export crop promoted by Alliance for Progress programs in El Salvador was cattle. While ranching was an old tradition, Williams (1986) recounts how the new export potential was gradually realized through development of new roads, refrigerated trucks, and modern beef farming techniques, as demand grew in the North for fast food. Modern beef production had been promoted since the mid-1960s by USAID, but it did not take off in El Salvador until after the Middle East oil embargo of 1973. As prices for fertilizer, chemical inputs, and interest rates soared, many cotton growers shifted to cattle, which had lower labor requirements. Also, in a poor market a rancher could hold onto animals for an extra year and wait for better prices to sell (DeWalt 1994).

Rising beef profits created incentives for ranchers to expand their pastures, and—unlike cotton, which had been developed on large estates—the cattle boom led landowners to encroach on land previously considered too marginal for export crops, which had traditionally been farmed by peasants. Furthermore, the low labor requirements for raising cows meant that, unlike cotton, the cattle estates offered few jobs to peasants as compensation for land loss. Between 1971 and 1980, the primary years of rising beef exports, landlessness rose steeply from 29 percent to nearly half of Salvadoran families (Bulmer-Thomas 1987; and Williams 1986).

Adding insult to injury, the 1973 oil shocks devastated peasant farmers, especially those who could no longer afford fertilizers and chemicals to improve yields on marginal lands. Since the mid-1960s, USAID had funded peasant cooperatives and a new national agricultural development bank, both of which had offered hope to small farmers, but after 1973 the pressure from organized peasants for cheaper credit and land reform gained ground rapidly. By the mid-1970s, peasants were engaged in land occupations throughout the cotton-growing region and in many marginal areas where cattle had taken over their cornfields.

The expulsion of Salvadoran squatters by Honduras in 1969 prompted a public debate over land reform that stirred up expectations among the peasantry. Unfortunately, the proposal was shot down by a powerful lobby of cattle and cotton farmers (Pearce 1986; and Williams 1986), and this reversal, followed by blatant fraud by the military in both the 1972 and 1976 elections, contributed to civil unrest. Several cases of military violence took place when soldiers fired on peasants conducting land occupations or on students demonstrating in support of peasant demands.

Export crop expansion had led to cutbacks in domestic production of food crops such as corn, beans, and rice. By 1975 El Salvador had become a net importer of food, but many peasant families could not afford to buy the food they had previously grown for themselves. The country now stood out in the region as having the worst situation for landlessness, and the lowest income per household (Bulmer-Thomas 1987).

It is worth emphasizing that the failures of social development did not come about as a result of failed capitalist economic policies. Rather, El Salvador's GDP rose steadily from the 1950s through 1980. The value of the country's exports more than tripled in value in this period. But this wealth congealed at the top and failed to trickle down. Policies that might have changed this situation failed to get off the ground. For example, a new law installing an income tax in the 1950s was undermined when the coffee and cotton sectors lobbied successfully to be exempted, resulting in a tax paid by less than 0.4 percent of the population and amounting to only 6.6 percent of national revenue (Bulmer-Thomas 1987, 122). By the end of the 1970s almost 39 percent of El Salvador's cultivated land was controlled by only 0.7 percent of the landowners while 87 percent of the landholders controlled plots of less than 5 hectares each, together comprising less than 20 percent of the nation's arable land (DeWalt 1994).

Despite the negative social impacts, agricultural modernization continued into the 1980s, repackaged as neoliberal free market policies. Conroy and colleagues (1996) traced the roles of the World Bank and USAID promoting another round of investment, this time in nontraditional agricultural export (NTAE) crops such as melons and broccoli. The pattern of export crops crowding out food crops became more exacerbated during the 1980s, which became labeled as the "lost decade" for development internationally after setbacks left most poor countries worse off in 1989 than they had been a decade earlier. Conroy and colleagues concluded:

> There is evidence that NTAEs have tended to undermine small farmers' economic position, drawing them into increased debt and sometimes leading to significant land concentration. At the same time the viability of traditional corn and bean cultivation has been undercut by trade policies, leaving the rural poor without the peasant safety net of basic grain production. . . . The developmental edifice built upon this cornerstone is beginning to show serious cracks. (1996, 2)

As public health workers know, malnutrition opens the immunological door to a host of infectious diseases and chronic problems, obscuring a precise etiology (Singer and Clair 2003). In the late 1970s Salvadoran workers who earned minimum wage on cotton estates were only able to cover about 85 percent of the *canasta básica* (basic basket of goods and services) to house and feed a campesino family (Arias-Peñate 1988, 270). Surveys found close to three-quarters of rural children malnourished during this period (Puffer and Serrano 1973). The relationship among land loss, nutrition, and health, however, was not recognized by the paradigms that shaped Alliance for Progress health programs. Discourses about health in the period of modernization included an overreliance on expert knowledge and curative care as well as paternalistic approaches in public health that emphasized hygiene and personal habits while neglecting the contribution of ecological or economic factors to disease incidence. A dominant discourse among international health specialists applied a simplistic functionalist logic that saw population growth as the major "cause" of poverty in El Salvador and other poor countries. The country is indeed more densely populated than its neighbors, with 5.5 million people during the 1980s in an area the size of Massachusetts. However, unlike Massachusetts (which had a comparable size population), El Salvador's relatively high fertility rates came to be cited as the main explanation for a multitude of social ills, ranging from the Soccer War of 1969 to erosion of land in rural areas and the civil war of the 1980s.[2]

The focus on population growth as the cause of Third World poverty dates to the 1960s, but the discourse reached its zenith with the Club of Rome's 1972 "Limits to Growth" study. USAID had already been criticized for distributing high-dose birth control pills in El Salvador and Puerto Rico before they had been adequately tested. Yet by 1979 around a fifth of USAID humanitarian assistance funds went for family planning, with an emphasis on promotion of sterilization and contraceptive use by poor women. In the design of the programs, little attention was paid to relationships between mortality and population growth, to socioeconomic and cultural influences on family size, or to how migration complicates demographic statistics (see Mazur 1994). As a result of such policies, national surveys in several Latin American countries show that by the end of the 1970s, between one-fifth and one-third of those women who used contraceptives chose sterilization. Around 40 percent opted for sterilization in El Salvador, the Dominican Republic, and Panama (Stycos 1984). Abuses related to these programs as well as rumors that the Yankees sought to exterminate minorities and the poor damaged USAID's reputation (and that of many NGOs) in El Salvador (CESA 1977). In later years this legacy undermined popular acceptance of well-designed health initiatives and more socially conscious family planning efforts.

Antipolitics, Militarism, and the "Organic State"

The other side of Alliance for Progress social development was a quieter, sinister legacy of military aid and training that converted what had been small, disorganized military organizations into centralized institutions with sophisticated forms of surveillance and networks of paranoid agents that labeled a wide range of civilian activities as "subversive." El Salvador's so-called protection racket state was preconditioned in ways that made its military receptive to Cold War ideology. Derek Sayer observed that social construction of nationalism in Latin America often worked through an engaged cynicism: "Individuals live the lie that is 'the state' and it lives through their performances" (1994, 374). To give an example, during the war in El Salvador foreigners seeking renewal of a visa were always at risk of an arbitrary denial. But most of us learned to seek aid from natives who had cultivated *cuello* (personal influence) with authority figures. In many cases "cuello" was simply knowing a friend or relative in a government office willing to "fix" things, usually for a price. It was taken for granted that politicians were corrupt to the point where a purportedly "democratic" politician (e.g., the Reagan administration's view of former president Napoleón Duarte) was subject a priori to suspicions that he was either a puppet for a stronger leader behind the scenes or a weak leader who would soon be overthrown. If a public official was not rich, then many would suspect that he (it was almost always a he) must be seeking power to get rich from the public till. A friend of mine from a poor barrio who was strongly critical of the ARENA party told me that he would vote for their candidate anyway because "Areneros are already rich, so they won't steal as much while they're in office." One dilemma of democratization in the postwar era is that so few believe electoral politics will change this modus operandi of "personalism."

This culture of mistrust crosses class lines. Both rich and poor learned to see pluralism or group autonomy as threatening stability and diversity as a possible prelude to anarchy. As a result, regardless of what set of political rules is adopted, at the first sign of discontent the guns are drawn, and those with the most to lose fall back on "coercion as the only workable means of social control" (Sloan 1984). Brian Loveman and Thomas Davies (1978) described Latin American militarism as a form of "antipolitics" because official histories of military *caudillos* have tended to cast blame on civilian politicians for all manner of social ills, including "backwardness," poverty, and corruption. Inside military academies, civilians were considered weak, venal, and self-interested. Only the honorable, self-sacrificing patriotic military could be relied on to maintain order and ensure economic progress.

Central American traditions of governing through such a hierarchical, corporate polity created a receptive setting in the 1930s for European theories of geopolitics—a fascist ideology that espoused an organic notion of the state. Germans had been prominent among Central American coffee entrepreneurs since the 1880s, and their influence in El Salvador led to closer relations with the Third Reich and a tripling of exports to Germany. President Martínez, who oversaw the 1932 matanza, was among the first foreign leaders to recognize Francisco Franco in Spain. Similar sympathies with Nazi Germany existed among Guatemala elites and the Somoza family of Nicaragua (Bulmer-Thomas 1987). After the United States entered the war against Germany, Central American leaders were pressed to support the Allies, but their continued attraction to fascist ideology even after the war contrasted with attitudes in the rest of the world, where such ideas became discredited. David Pion-Berlin describes geopolitical thought as "preoccupied first with the integration of underdeveloped and ignored regions with centers of power, and secondly with the establishment of tight political control over all subjects within the territorial confines of the state" (1991, 141).

These ideas also persisted in Southern Cone countries that became a haven for Nazis after World War II. Chile's Gen. Augusto Pinochet wrote a book in 1968 titled "*Geopolitica*," and his ideas influenced other regional military regimes, including Argentina, Brazil, El Salvador, Nicaragua, and Guatemala. In this organic analogy of the state, "states are thought of as brain centers of an organism and the public as cells who must cooperate if the 'body politic' is to survive. Rudolf Kjellen (1864–1922) took the organic metaphor furthest, claiming that states were conscious, rational entities with interests, prejudices and an instinct for self-preservation. As political life-forms situated in a hostile environment, they must prevail over rivals in order to survive" (Pion-Berlin 1991, 142).[3] This thinking strongly influenced the conduct of the dirty war in Argentina where security forces envisioned that they were saving the country from an alien infiltration of Zionist-Marxists (Suarez-Orozco 1992). U.S. National Security Doctrine (NSD) (also influenced by geopolitical ideas) became overlaid on Latin American geopolitics during the Alliance for Progress years. Under NSD, however, Latin American strategists shifted the focus of geopolitical theory "from the conquest of physical space to the conquest of political space" (Pion-Berlin 1991, 142). The most dramatic example of this shift is the U.S. promotion (and Latin American adoption) of counterinsurgency doctrine in response to Cuban internationalism. These strategies for combating guerrilla insurgencies and for infiltrating and undermining civilian organizations considered subversive, derived from civil warfare experiences of the British in Malaysia, the French in Algeria, and the United States in Vietnam.

In a study of the U.S. role promoting counterinsurgency in El Salvador, McClintock (1987) described a tight linkage between development and security, citing Secretary of Defense Robert McNamara, who regarded the Alliance for Progress as likely to succeed only if governments could "cope with subversion, prevent terrorism and deal with outbreaks of violence before they reach unmanageable proportions." A less zealous observer on the staff of the Senate Foreign Relations Committee described the programs as "stopgap measures to shore up existing governments, both democratic and dictatorial, provided they are reasonably friendly to the United States" (an assessment that seemed to rank modernist development policies little better than imperialist interventions of past decades; quoted in McClintock 1985, 14).

Beginning in 1962 the USAID, with CIA assistance, took charge of an aggressive program of police training in El Salvador and other Latin American countries, with a mandate that included "anticommunist" operations, surveillance, and interrogation. (McClintock 1987). Thousands of Latin American troops were brought to the United States for counterinsurgency instruction, and mobile training teams (MTTs) made up of Special Forces soldiers were sent to nineteen foreign countries, making use of a loophole in the law that allowed them to enter countries without notifying U.S. embassies abroad so ambassa-dors could plead ignorance of their activities. McClintock cites classified reports of MTTs in Central America training local troops in violent covert activities, including assassinations of civilians seen as supportive of communist activities (1987, 23). USAID also aided foreign militaries in setting up modern telecom-munications systems that allowed a centralized command to remain in close contact with rural units. The United States trained Central American militaries in the use of "civic action" programs designed as a component of psychological warfare in this period (32). These MTTs and civic action teams provided the blueprints for ORDEN, the large paramilitary spy network that emerged to pub-lic attention in 1968 when members attacked and killed striking teachers. Secretly overseen by military officers, ORDEN evolved into a nationwide net-work of spies and death squads by the late 1970s. Alarmed by public reaction to abuses linked to the programs in 1973, Congress banned police training abroad but left loopholes that allowed foreign soldiers to continue to travel to the United States for courses (McClintock 1987, 70–71).

National Security Doctrine ideas, combined with the geopolitical organic notion of the state, served to reinforce the paranoia of elites about the populace, which was often expressed in medical and epidemiological metaphors: Marxism—epitomized as Cuban adventurism during Che Guevara's ill-fated efforts to spark rebel *foci* in Bolivia—became an alien army, a social disease that must be elimi-nated by radical surgery in which the patient (society) must be confined and con-trolled during a long convalescence under the tutelage of military doctors (Sloan 1984). Argentine Minister of Foreign Affairs Adm. Cesar Guzetti likened his country's internal enemy to a contagion: "When the social body of the country has been contaminated by disease which eats away at its entrails, it forms antibodies. These antibodies (death squads) cannot be considered in the same way as the microbes. As the government controls and destroys the guerrillas, the actions of the antibodies will disappear. This is already happening. It is only a reaction of a sick body" (Simpson and Bennett 1985, 82).

Counterinsurgency doctrine, the operative arm of NSD, grew out of stereo-types about Marxist guerrillas that later proved to reflect poor intelligence. For example, military intelligence often took at face value rebels' exaggerated claims of popular support. This led in some cases to the willingness of officers in the Salvadoran military to consider, and even publicize, the need for extreme measures. A good example is the 1979 claim of one politically moderate colonel that "the armed forces are prepared to kill 200,000–300,000 if that's what it takes to stop a Communist take-over" (Bonner 1984).

A related belief of counterinsurgency doctrine was the conviction that civil-ians, being weak and "malleable" could be easily swayed by the disguised com-munist insurgents who had penetrated into the midst of the body politic. This idea can be traced to Col. Roger Trinquier, a leading French proponent of state terror in the Algerian war who argued that "humanitarian endeavors were wasted on a public that is infected by clandestine organisms that penetrate like a cancer into its midst" (1964, 49).

Other characteristics of counterinsurgency doctrine that colored military thinking in Central America are the beliefs that Leon Trotsky's prescriptions for a permanent war against capitalism must be met with a permanent counterrevolutionary effort. Hence, the battle is never won and, due to the anticipated nefarious tactics of the Marxist enemy, the boundary between war and peace, military and civilian become blurred. In addition, counterinsurgency doctrine held that foreign elements posed a constant threat of "penetrating" the state (the politics of *entrismo*) both through secret means and through the democratic processes. "Given the enduring nature of the threat, the state would have to be forever vigilant, and could do so only through an authoritarian political structure" (Pion-Berlin 1991, 148). Even anticommunist politicians who espoused democratic ideals posed a danger because they may have been duped by foreign supporters who have Marxist sympathies. Hence, patriotic vigilance also requires extraordinary means such as surveillance, smear campaigns against suspected Marxist sympathizers, and even assassination.

In the case of El Salvador, the historical legacy of militarism, combined with post-1960 U.S. anticommunist paranoia, helps explain how political terror became so institutionalized. The dominant military ideology both conformed to and helped perpetuate the polarization between the classes. Counterinsurgency policy generated further suspicion of reformist parties among conservatives. This was aided by widespread illiteracy among the peasant class (given an educational system every bit as hobbled as the health system) and the effective absence, prior to the 1970s, of a sizeable middle class in a position to challenge the oligarchy.

Toward a Political Epidemiology of Ill-being

U.S. foreign policy has long been shaped by the dominant social paradigms of each era—from Big Stick policies of the 1920s to modernization in the 1960s. Many anthropological critiques of development today emphasize the role of discourses and practices that engendered dependency on professional knowledge (Dubois 1991; and Escobar 1995). In this case, for example, such an analysis helps explain unforeseen outcomes from overdependence on technology in modernist development—for example, pesticide resistance and the oil shocks in the 1970s. Applied to development, discourse analysis is helpful for illustrating the ways that expert or hegemonic knowledge can come to substitute for power, and vice versa, so that either criticism of social projects does not arise or critics become easily marginalized. However, discourse analysis, with its frequent reliance on discursive evidence, does an inadequate job of explaining the (often rational and interested) material and coercive aspects of "top-down" forms of development (see Edelman 1999; and Aviles 2001). Years before translations of Foucault inspired American postmodernist analyses of development, William Durham used a social ecologist approach to demonstrate the shortcomings of the neo-Malthusian ideology behind modernist population control policies. In his study of the history of land scarcity in rural El Salvador, Durham (1979) found that "it was not so much the rapid growth of the population . . . as the simultaneous trend toward land concentration that created a scarcity of land for the majority," a trend that he traced from the turn of the century up until the decade following the 1969 expulsion of Salvadoran peasants from Honduras (48).

In Tenancingo, a rural community northeast of the capital, Durham found that the less land that families owned, the higher the likelihood that their children would die. Peasant families with 2.5 or more hectares had a 20 percent rate of child mortality whereas landless families in his sample experienced more than twice as many child deaths (48 percent). The relationship between land loss and child mortality was tightest for peasant families of recent generations, a finding that he attributed to the recent decline in their land holdings (families owned 1.10 hectares on average in the 1970s, compared with 1.43 hectares in the previous generation). Durham concluded that only the families with larger farms had experienced any discernible benefits from the limited advances in health and sanitation available to rural Salvadorans over the previous fifty years. He wrote: "The argument that more medicine and better sanitation are necessary to reduce the country's rural mortality rate, for example, ignores the fact that the people who most need these improvements are also the people who can least afford them. As long as land continues to grow scarce for El Salvador's small farmers, there is little hope that the mortality differentials documented here will disappear" (173). Durham's analysis tied hunger directly to the export crop policies of the 1970s:

> The scarcity of food and the scarcity of land in El Salvador are not the simple products of population growth. First, we find that food is scarce not because the land is incapable of producing enough for the resident population, but rather because large areas have been underutilized or dedicated to the production of export crops. Second, we find that land is scarce not because there is too little to go around, but rather because of a process of competitive exclusion by which the small farmers have been increasingly squeezed off the land—a process due as much to the dynamics of land concentration as to population pressure. Land-use patterns show that land is not scarce for large landholders. (1979, 54)

He also studied land use in Honduras, which has a far lower population density, and found rural peasants there to be actually poorer than their Salvadoran neighbors, due to poor soil and shifts in land tenure since the 1950s that had favored large cotton farms and cattle ranchers. As in El Salvador, he found little basis for assumptions that there was a simple relationship between population density and access to resources, and considerable evidence that export growth had negatively impacted peasants' life chances.[4]

A social epidemiology of ill-being is insufficient if it fails to unearth the historical and political relationships and chains of causality in which health statistics are often embedded. The accounts of development policy and counterinsurgency described here are intended to demonstrate how the material outcomes of social development, including rational capitalist interests in North and South, and more broadly U.S.-Central American relations, were often conscious and even explicit outcomes of a geopolitics driven by U.S. imperialist goals.

There was productivity in landowning classes expanding their estates to boost exports and in their reliance on repression to put down peasant uprisings and ensure a compliant population of surplus labor. An agricultural system based around seasonal labor during harvests runs most profitably when there is a "reserve army" of unemployed or underemployed people (Browning 1971). The willingness of this pool of migrant workers to work, when needed, at low wages is dependent in part on the workers not being able to meet their families' basic needs in other ways. This politics of exclusion allowed El Salvador to boast the highest yields in the world for coffee in the 1950s, and then to achieve similar world class yields in cotton only a decade later.

Few scholars of development would deny that most health workers involved in foreign aid programs are sincerely interested in relieving human suffering and helping to improve conditions of life for people in poor countries. And certainly the designers of most such programs are often well intentioned. But it becomes easier to appreciate the piecemeal nature of health development work, and the reasons it so often ends in failure, once the lens of our focus is widened to include the larger, more politicized scope of foreign aid. United States aid for health work in Latin America dates to the Rockefeller Foundation's initiatives to control tropical epidemics in lowlands and ports of countries that were important trade partners (Cueto 1994). In the late 1920s, U.S. military research on yellow fever, malaria, and other tropical diseases was specifically motivated by the impact they had on productivity of workers building the Panama Canal. A small program promoting the U.S. model of medical education to the region was expanded in the 1940s as part of Franklin Roosevelt's "Good Neighbor" policies aimed at countering German cultural influence. And U.S. funds for tropical disease programs rose again in the aftermath of the Cuban revolution. As discussed earlier, gains from Alliance for Progress health programs were limited in states such as El Salvador where elite-controlled governments failed to invest in social reforms. We can see how foreign health programs in nearly every case were grafted onto strategic political and economic policies, most of which were designed with the goal of strengthening U.S. regional hegemony through military alliances and trade relations that promoted the interests of Northern investors and farmers while deepening economic dependence in the South.

Given that health in such schemes becomes public relations as much as a goal in its own right, it should not surprise us when programs fail. The sad legacy of health development was documented in an epidemiological assessment of El Salvador that was carried out in a socially conscious way by progressive physicians and public health workers in 1998. Their report specifically cited malnutrition—noting that one in four children continues to be chronically malnourished, little changed over half a century of development programs (Colégio Médico 1999). Decade after decade, the gains of health work have been undermined by economic policies that remove poor farmers from the land.

The experience of El Salvador, while unusual in some ways (e.g., the degree of state coercion), is also common to much of the Global South. Anuradha Mittal (2001) reported similar patterns of shifts to export crops benefiting large landowners and national GDPs while dispossessing small farmers by the hundreds of millions in India, Thailand, Brazil, Mexico, Costa Rica, and Haiti. Carlos Vilas (1995) did a similar analysis for Central America as a region. Marc Edelman (1999) recounted how even in Costa Rica, the most prosperous country of the region, an economic downturn in the early 1980s combined with new free trade policies favoring loans for export crops undermined peasant livelihoods and prompted social protests. Nevertheless, he reported, the dismantling of state supports for subsistence farming continued through the mid-1990s.

The rationales for such free market development programs are justified in the North as a form of economic investment and do, in fact, result in capital flowing from South to North. USAID-promoted loans supporting export crops programs in Latin America to the U.S. Chamber of Commerce with promises that "for every dollar invested in Latin America three dollars come back to the United States in profits" (Lernoux 1982). A 1986 amendment to the Foreign Assistance Act forbade the use of aid to promote any commodity that would compete with a crop grown in the United States. Corn and other food crops fell into this category; as a result, credits fell for subsistence crops throughout the region (Conroy, Murray, and Rosset 1996, 23). By 1998, after thirty years of such "development," Latin American countries, rather than getting ahead, were falling further behind. That year the region's debt to northern banks came to $90 billion, and the imbalance of trade grew larger each year (IMF 1999).

Given this hypocrisy, it was a chilling epitaph to the Salvadoran civil war to hear Dick Cheney, on the occasion of the 2004 death of Ronald Reagan, describe U.S. intervention there as a free market success story. And it is distressing to see how free trade farm policies, the main logjam that once again stalled world trade talks in 2007, continue to worsen the inequities between poor countries and the North. When the majority of citizens are excluded from participation in a transnational economy and remain alienated from resources needed for basic social welfare, the concept of "public health" loses its salience as a meaningful concept.

2

Repression's Repercussions

Pragmatic Solidarity and the Body Politic

Todos nacimos medio muertos	All of us were born half dead
in 1932	in 1932
sobrivimos pero medio vivos . . .	we survived but half alive . . .
los asesinos presumen no solamente	the assassins presume to be
de estar totalmente	not only totally
vivos	alive
sino también de ser inmortales	but also to be immortal
Pero ellos también	But they too
están medio muertos	are half dead
y solo vivos a medias	and only half alive . . .
. . . Todos juntos	. . . All together
tenemos más muerte que aquellos	we have more death than they do.
Pero todos juntos	But all together
tenemos más vida que ellos.	we have more life than they do.

—Roque Dalton, "Todos" (1988, 124)

Encountering Chalatenango

My excursions to Chalatenango from the capital began with a two-hour ride on a crowded bus. The Troncal Norte wound around the foothills of the extinct Guazapa volcano, a rebel stronghold during the war. The bus stopped briefly in bustling Aguilares, where *pupusa* stands lined the road, and young women assaulted the bus hawking El Salvador's famous bean- or cheese-filled tortilla pies and *refrescos* (fruit drinks) in bright bulging plastic bags. Here was the birthplace of the Comunidades Eclesiales de Base (CEB) or Christian base communities. Jesuit priests, inspired by the new Catholic social theology, organized thirty-seven CEB Bible groups in this area beginning in 1972. CEB activists were among the earliest victims of death squad violence, as soldiers cracked down on the movement for labor and land rights (Cabarrús 1983).

Farther north the bus passed miles of sugar plantations in lowlands by the Cerrón Grande reservoir created by the dammed Lempa River. The reservoir bridge had been the site of a military roadblock during the war, where buses were stopped—men and boys were lined up outside, hands pressed against the metal sides while soldiers frisked them for weapons. Foreigners and urban-dwellers without army-issued safe-conduct passes (salvoconductos) were routinely turned back. Later the bus turned east off the *troncal*, stopping at the huge base of the army's Fourth Brigade headquarters before continuing to Chalatenango, a dusty market town and capital of the department of the same name. The town's small plaza was flanked by the local army base and a Catholic church. At daybreak hundreds of soldiers shouted cadence and squared off for calisthenics yards from the sanctuary steps. During the war, two camouflaged soldiers had guarded the plaza from a machine-gun nest in the church bell tower.

To the east the street climbed a steep hill, turning to dirt as it wound off among steep slopes lined with *milpas* (cornfields). Here, under a huge conacaste tree, the army had maintained a second roadblock, the more serious one that guarded entry to a "conflicted zone" (*zona conflictiva*), to use the lingo of the military, or a (FMLN) "controlled zone" (*zona controlada*) to local campesinos. In the 1980s no one passed this point except with army-issued salvoconductos, plus written permission on the day of travel from the Fourth Brigade commander (and sometimes the local commander as well)—a process that kept reporters, relief workers, and foreign delegations cooling their heels for hours in army bases waiting for approval.

To me, rural Chalatenango was both a beautiful and harsh place—even in areas unaffected by war, the natural wilderness of rolling hills, piney mountains, and fast-flowing streams was belied by the visible destitution of its people. In the north there are no cash crops except cattle, and farming is done on steep rocky *minifundia*—landholdings of medium-to-small farmers, many of whom rent plots to poorer peasant families. People who live in the hills above the town have smaller statures with bony frames. Salvadorans are famously friendly and outgoing. They will invite a stranger into their homes on a moment's notice and graciously serve up the last leg of chicken in the pot. They laugh easily, but their smiles betray gaps where rotten teeth were pulled. The road passed small wattle-and-daub houses with dirt floors, roofed with sheets of tin weighted down with old tires and rocks. Small children played listlessly in the dirt, their faces framed by the thin, straw-colored hair of malnutrition.

Leather-skinned men en route to their milpas walked the roadside carrying machetes and a few tortillas in a woven hemp bag. During the war no buses ran here. Both civilians and guerrilla fighters walked everywhere on rocky footpaths through hills dotted with hidden *caserios* (villages). The women at first seemed fragile to me, so thin and wearing cheap polyester dresses and plastic sandals, but they were dynamos. As I fell behind puffing on hikes up steep hillsides, they churned on with the endurance of long-distance runners, balancing giant baskets or water jugs on their heads. On a rest break during one such endless hike in 1989, an FMLN fighter consoled me with a pat on the shoulder, remarking, "In Chalatenango, there is no east or west, only uphill and downhill!"

Peasant Organizing and Repressive Violence

Robert Williams (1986) used the term "refuges" for marginalized areas, such as Chalatenango, that became destinations for peasants dispossessed by export crop expansions. By the mid-1970s the area had become a center for rural organizing, including CEBs, agricultural cooperatives, and peasant unions affiliated with the nascent guerrilla movement. But by 1978 the National Guard and death squads were carrying out a systematic campaign of repression, killing organizers with impunity. By 1980 many young men and boys were sleeping in the open and arming themselves with pistols to fight back, organized as the Fuerzas Pópular de Liberación (FPL), which became the largest faction of the FMLN. After the shooting war broke out in earnest in 1980, the army conducted a series of genocidal "scorched earth" campaigns over the next three years that made little distinction between insurgents and civilians.

In northeast Chalatenango the FPL responded in 1982 with a nine-month campaign to drive out the National Guard and secure the area. After that the army relied more heavily on air force support. The massive land operations gave way to paratrooper and Special Forces incursions, accompanied by aerial bombing or strafing of villages. By 1985 the armed forces had detonated three hundred pounds of TNT for every insurgent combatant. In such a densely populated country, this level of anticivilian violence took a terrible toll. By 1986 half a million Salvadorans were displaced within the country and approximately twenty thousand had fled to Honduran refugee camps. More than a million migrated abroad, most illegally, to the United States or other host countries.[1]

As it would anywhere, such devastation produced enormous despair and human suffering, disrupting campesino social life for more than a generation. Using Agamben's phrase from *Homo Sacer*, we might say that Chalatecos experienced a most brutal "entry of zoe into the polis" or the politicization of "bare life" (1998). The remarkable aspect of the violence here, and in other *bolsones* (pockets) around the country where the FMLN had a civilian base, was the unusual degree of popular unity and creative organizing that lent strength to the rebellion and challenged the army's anticivilian tactics, as well as official claims that residents of the zone were terrorists.

The most comprehensive account of organized civilian activity in northeast Chalatenango in this period was written by Jenny Pearce (1986), a British researcher. Pearce described how, after 1982, civilians in each village encouraged by the FPL elected *directivas*, or town councils, and governing representatives for three subregional zones, and they coordinated food production through both family milpas and collectives that depended on volunteered labor. Collective efforts were also undertaken in health, education, municipal security, and legal affairs.

Organizing persisted even after much of the population was forced out in the mid-1980s. Representatives of refugee and displaced person camps negotiated with the government and the United Nations High Committee on Refugees for the right of peasants to return in large groups to their homes in conflicted areas. Abandoned towns were first resettled by desplazados in 1986, and the first mass repatriation of refugees from Honduras took place in the fall of 1987. Thousands more would return, most in highly organized groups, in the last five years of the war (Edwards and Siebentritt 1991).

My first visit to the repatriated village of Guarjila took place only days after the first caravan of refugees arrived in October 1987. I made more visits there and to nearby San José Las Flores in the next two years as a foreign correspondent, then returned to both sites for ethnographic fieldwork in 1992. I collected oral histories of Chalatecos' experiences during the war, as well as accounts by health and other relief workers. I conducted interviews with forty-eight residents of the repopulations, including twenty local health promoters, most of whom traced their health activism to the late 1970s or early 1980s.

Historical documentation, combined with popular accounts, helped me reconstruct campesino experiences of social and political transformation. The tales progressed thematically in two ways: (a) from an emphasis on military violence to the hardships of life in the war zone (or a refugee camp), and (b) from an initial emphasis on the personal body as subject, to the community as subject. In fact, "community" (*la comunidad*) was probably the single word most commonly used by residents and health promoters to describe people and places in northeast Chalatenango. Reflecting the ideology of CEBs, community-building was a common goal of the FPL in the early 1980s (unlike, for example the Ejército Revolucionario del Pueblo [ERP] in Morazán, which put military aims ahead of civilian goals prior to 1988). There was also a practical aspect of claims to community for villages that were repatriated after 1986 since their status as civilian communities served as moral leverage with the military, which, by the late 1980s, was more hesitant to risk international censure by attacking the villages in the presence of foreign aid workers and international supporters who accompanied the refugees home and visited the area.

Of all disciplines, anthropology is the one most engaged in study of community dynamics. Relatively small egalitarian social groups predominated in indigenous cultures prior to the colonial era, whether living as foragers or horticulturalists (Boehm 1999). Yet the concept of community has often been romanticized and caught up in dualistic propaganda wars over communism versus capitalism, or in debates over the legitimacy of evolutionary ecology, political economy, or cultural paradigms. In much of the world, urbanization and the ubiquitous ideology of the market have disrupted public access to common resources and diminished communitarian values (Nonini 2007). During debates over postmodernism, theorists inspired by Foucault often squared off against neo-Marxists, insisting on identity-focused analyses that frequently cut across or diminished the significance of place-based or imagined notions of community. By the 1990s, it was a rare journal article in cultural anthropology that used the term "community" in an analytical sense. But awareness of the need to integrate the natural world and the economy into cultural paradigms has contributed to a growing convergence between scholars in evolutionary ecology and critical ethnographers. Increasingly works are appearing that seek to combine analysis of social systems with political economy and ecology in ways that are attentive to both local histories and pragmatic rationalities (see Bromley et al. 1992; Boehm 1999; Leatherman 2005; and Hornborg and Crumley 2007).

Several theorists have focused on the body as one way to integrate these dualisms. Mary Douglas (1984) observes that "the body is a model which can stand for any kind of bounded system" (115). Andrew Strathern (1996) notes that the ubiquity of folk models for treating the social with organic metaphors suggests there is merit to speaking of a "body politic." John O'Neill contrasts evocation of a political "body" with the "logic of calculative rationality" which, he asserts, "has dominated studies of the production and maintenance of social order." He sees the body politic as a fundamental concept, often evoked by societies undergoing upheavals because it "provides grounds of ultimate appeal in times of deep institutional crisis, of hunger and alienation, when there is need to renew primary bonds of political authority and consensus"(1985, 68).

For example, in El Salvador's civil war, as in the postintifada Palestinian struggle, martyrdom was both a tragic reality and a powerful central trope that crossed over the religious–secular divide in agendas for liberation. Archbishop Romero's famous statement, "If they kill me, I will rise again in the Salvadoran people," was prescient because his assassination indeed proved the final straw for many activists who gave up on politics as a route to change and went underground by the thousands in 1980–1981. The symbolic body's "reasonableness" is easily conveyed. The concept of solidarity, of standing together for common goals, is a variation on the same, and an alternative to the routine political avenues of party politics and nationalism that become corrupted by their association with repressive functions of the state.

Following Christie Kiefer (2000), I use the term body politic and community as "ideal types," keeping in mind on the one hand the hundreds of years of communal systems and ideologies that existed in the lives of a majority of rural Salvadorans well into the nineteenth century (alongside and posed in opposition to colonial expropriations) while on the other hand considering that a key definition of modern poverty, and characteristic of capitalism, is heightened individualism and an absence or decline in community.

When we consider the importance of place to conventional forms of community, it sets in stark relief the social costs of peasant dispossession from land and the pressing need to migrate for wage labor between 1960 and 1980, which constituted a massive assault on the social life of the Salvadoran rural body politic. In fact, these rifts forced rural citizens to invent alternative cultural survival strategies years before the shooting began. As Tommie Sue Montgomery (1995) has shown, despite five decades of military repression prior to the war, there were repeated cycles of peasant activism, which suggests it would be naïve to see conflict as a rare phenomenon. I argue that neither communal ideals nor the rational calculus of entrepreneurial pragmatics were novel concepts to Salvadoran campesinos. The question we may need to ask is why, in fact, those concepts are counterposed by many modern scholars.

A "Popular" Religious Pageant

Sometimes the story was told through dramatization. The most important holiday in each repopulated village was a festival to commemorate the anniversary of the community's return from exile. Guarjila's 1992 anniversary was celebrated with a procession of costumed clowns and big-headed "giants" walking on stilts to entertain the children, followed by a celebratory Catholic mass, soccer games, and a horse race. Each family enjoyed a holiday meal of chicken, courtesy of the communal chicken co-op.

The midmorning holiday mass was held in the *capilla* (chapel), which resembled an American picnic shelter with wooden benches under a roof, open sides, and a makeshift altar.[2] In lieu of formal Catholic ritual objects, the altar was decorated with flowers and colorful paper streamers. Rather than a homily, Padre Jon, the Jesuit priest, spoke a few words and then introduced a community theater group.

The play began with peasant women sitting in a circle slapping their hands together as if making tortillas. Suddenly the scene was interrupted by tape-recorded machine-gun fire. Men in black shirts with armbands that read "*soldado*" jumped onto the stage and pointed stick guns at the women. Some fell dead; others ran to the corners of the capilla and squatted down out of view. Then the soldiers themselves came under fire. From the sidelines emerged men and boys wearing jeans and with berets on their heads and red bandanas covering their noses and mouths. Two soldiers fell dead and the others ran away.

A woman began strumming a guitar, singing a ballad about martyred loved ones. Other women slowly rose from their hiding places, gathered their belongings and children, and began a slow procession down the center aisle and around the sides of the capilla. Some wore head scarves; others carried sacks of corn on their heads. They were reenacting a *"guinda"*—the local term for the secret mass flights of civilians from their villages to avoid the advancing army. Guerrilla fighters emerged to guard the procession, periodically firing at army soldiers.

The guitar player began a second song about sorrow and homesickness as the procession of women, moving slowly with bent heads finally stopped and huddled together under the watchful eyes of a line of new black-garbed soldados, suggesting their arrival at a Honduran refugee camp. The play was interrupted at this point by unruly children in the capilla who had climbed up on benches to see better. Their ruckus, combined with the clucks of an invading chicken, slowly built into a roar, obscuring voices in my recording of the play.

Cristo Rebelde

The repopulated communities were full of teenagers and children who had few memories of life before the twelve-year war, and little sense about urban settings or life in the capitalist economy. Carolina Velasquez, fifty-seven, of Guarjila, began her story with the indignities of migrant labor in coffee, but she traced the first talk of social change to the CEBs and FECCAS (Christian Federation of Salvadoran Peasants), a peasant union.

> Men and women used to go to work in the *cafetales*. It was a three-day walk. We would leave in October and stay there until January. But they robbed you. If you picked ten *quintales* they would only pay you for seven, if you picked seven they'd pay you for five. And we ate badly—huge tortillas with dirty beans. Many people got malaria and fever because we had to sleep in the open. And [there were] no toilets. They treated us worse than animals.
>
> The demands for change really began with the [Christian] base communities and with FECCAS, a few years before the war began. . . . [Nowadays] no one thinks about going to pick coffee again. It's not worth it under this bourgeois government. We need a change. We need a government that treats us right.

Elisabeth Wood found similar repeated references to CEBs predating other activism in her postwar interviews with Salvadoran campesinos in Usulután and Tenancingo, suggesting that the liberation theology organizing contributed to peasant willingness to engage in other political activism in the years that followed (2003, 119). The initial CEB organizing in Aguilares in 1972, and in Chalatenango and other rural areas after that, followed the spectacle of a stolen election by the military (to prevent a Christian Democrat victory) and coincided with the economic shock of the oil embargo and the loss of thousands of peasant jobs in the rapidly mechanizing cotton sector.

Liberation theology grew out of principles set out in the Second Vatican Council and adopted in 1968 at a conference of Latin American bishops held in Medellín, Colombia. The renovations, which openly stated the Church's "solidarity with the poor," followed longstanding debates among Catholics, primarily in Europe, over desires for a more worldly and socially conscious liturgy and policy. The new theology, articulated by scholars such as Brazilian Leonardo Boff and Peruvian Gustavo Gutiérrez, envisioned a more humble praxis in which priests, like Jesus, walked with the poor and interacted with them.

The movement drew inspiration from the Cuban revolution, and from disappointment with U.S. Alliance for Progress reforms, which had failed to raise living standards for poor families. Younger priests sought alternatives for alleviating poverty. Some had participated in Catholic Action, a project that helped set up self-help groups in rural areas during the 1960s. Establishing grassroots organizations such as CEBs in poor communities was also a way to address the growing shortage of priests in rural areas. Central to the new theology were dialectical or reflexive practices intended to build what Christian Smith (1991) termed an "insurgent consciousness" among the poor, or a wider understanding of the structures underlying poverty (seen as "structural sin") and a conviction about the need for fundamental political change. Religious workers were encouraged to live among peasants and establish forms of dialogue. Most CEBs began with literacy classes based around Bible stories, which were used as jumping-off points for eliciting participatory discussions of issues like hunger and land tenure (see Lancaster 1988; Lernoux 1982; and Whitfield 1995).

One of the more respected health promoters in the repopulated villages was Felipe, an articulate older organizer whose large family lived an hour's walk north of the main road. I asked him what people in his village had thought about being poor and about politics before the arrival of liberation theology:

> Well, there were two ways of looking at it. [Some believed] if you're poor, you're poor. You can't do anything about it. And some believed that poverty was because of God's will, that it must be because God wanted it that way. Likewise, whether children lived or died was up to God. If there was a bad epidemic, people would say it was something permitted by God. . . . The Church never denounced injustices in those days. Today, the Church is completely different in that it takes an interest in the conditions in the communities, and who is to blame for them. Now the people can't blame ignorance for being inactive.

As with previous outreach projects such as Catholic Action, the priests and nuns working with CEBs sought to identify and train lay leaders called catechists or "delegates of the word." Montgomery (1995) reported that fifteen thousand rural Salvadorans received training between 1970 and 1976 in regional centers for catechist training. Binford (2004) found that catechists from Morazán who attended these centers later joined the FMLN in significant numbers after the violence intensified. Felipe was one of those trained. He had been trying to attend school for years, initially thwarted by family needs and then by a National Guard crackdown on social activities suddenly classed as "subversive."

> I had eleven brothers and sisters. My father didn't want us to go to school. He saw school as a waste of time. I was the one [who was] most interested in school. My work was with cattle. I always had to eat on the run, in order to work and go to school. I was fourteen years old and I had only attended first grade some three weeks when the situation got ugly. The teacher couldn't come anymore because he was afraid. The National Guard was chasing him. Then guerrillas burned a bus near Arcatao.
>
> At that time we didn't really understand what was going on in the country. We knew that people had been passing through, interested in organizing the communities. My father didn't want anything to do with them at first. He understood about the repression we were suffering, but he was afraid of what would happen if they kept protesting against the government. It seemed like the repression was already on top of us. If someone got involved in anything, even given how little we understood of the situation, still they could kill you.

Two Mexican nuns helped set up a CEB in San José Las Flores, which later, along with Arcatao further to the east, gained reputations as centers of activism. Many of the priests and nuns who worked in CEBs were nonnative, according to Smith (1991), in part because local priests tended to see poverty as normal and were less motivated to seek social change. One effect of this, he noted, was that foreign workers, most from Spain or Italy, became exposed to extreme poverty for the first time, which was a radicalizing experience. After gaining acceptance from locals, their dual status as insiders and outsiders may have enhanced their cultural capital (social influence) from the perspective of peasants.

María Julia, an elderly resident from San José Las Flores, also traced the beginnings of the repression to the Christian base communities, but she insisted that it was the deteriorating economic situation and the fact that the campesinos were organizing themselves that most frightened the authorities.

> It was near the end of the 1970s that things got much worse—the prices of everything got so high we couldn't afford to live—food, medicine, insecticides, fertilizer—all of it was terribly expensive. Some of us went to meetings to discuss the Bible with three nuns in Las Piedras. We talked about the problems in our lives. It was the first time we had heard anyone from the church talk about liberation and organizing ourselves. We began to go to Chalatenango—to the very center of town—to demonstrate for lower prices. That's when the repression began. It wasn't a response to the church work as much as to the people's protests.

Miguél, a member of Guarjila's directiva, recalled that the violence in this period was directed specifically at civilian activists, and that it predated local guerrilla activity.

> It was the church that led us on the road. Chalate was one of the areas where the church was most active. Even where people never traveled outside their own *cantón*, there was substantial organizing. But even the "Celebration of the Word" by catechists was considered subversive. The officials said things like "communists had come to El Salvador," and that "they had to be annihilated." This was going on even in 1974. Ours was a strong movement. I remember going to marches in San Salvador. . . . [I was at] the one where they killed so many students. In that period the guerrillas hadn't yet organized themselves here.

An early center of the organizing was FECCAS, a peasant federation dating to the late 1960s that advocated peaceful methods for improving rural life. FECCAS, which had initially been affiliated with the Christian Democratic Party, was especially active in Aguilares. By 1975 the union had become closely allied with the FPL, which sought to build alliances with urban workers. A similar organization, the Union of Rural Workers (UTC), formed in Chalatenango in 1974. Other activism took place through the Fundación Promotora de Cooperativas (FUNPROCOOP), a Catholic foundation formed in 1967 that extended credit for seeds and fertilizers to more than seven thousand minifundistas. By the mid-1970s these loans were also assisting villages to build roads, schools, and clinics. Chalatecos made up a third of FUNPROCOOP beneficiaries, and the department housed a co-op training center for the program. By 1973, members of all these groups were feeling pressure to back down from their organizing (Pearce 1986).

A public outcry over the military-engineered fraud in the 1972 election led President Arturo Armando Molina to support a limited land reform, a move backed by reformists in the army. But the plan, made public in 1975, was denounced by the oligarchy, and large landowners succeeded in scuttling the proposal after a year of bitter national debate. Meanwhile, buoyed by talk of reform, thousands of landless peasants occupied idle land, a move that led to hostile encounters with army troops (McClintock 1985). Fernando, a health promoter and former CEB lay leader, described a 1978 land takeover near Arcatao, in the far north.

> The land takeovers grew out of the need of the people to cultivate the land for beans or corn. The landowners had taken a firm stand to not rent the land at low prices. That's when the people organized themselves. Around fifty–sixty people were at the first action, which was broken up by the Treasury Police. Four or five campesinos had pistols and a couple had *copetas* [short machetes]. With these few weapons they confronted police. There were only five soldiers, and they got scared and ran away.

They threw away their guns and the campesinos went and picked them up. And that was how the people got the first guns.

A seminal event nationwide was the July 1975 massacre of university students during a protest march in the capital. Eduardo Espinosa, secretary of international relations for the University of El Salvador in 2007 and previously a physician in the FPL, described to me how soldiers opened fire on the marchers as they crossed a bridge near the entrance to downtown. He had a broad view of the march from the fourth floor window of the hospital where he worked, which overlooked the intersection. Around thirty-seven protesters were killed. Wounded were taken away in National Guard vehicles and never reappeared. Firefighters used hoses to wash away the blood in the street (McClintock 1985). This unprecedented attack on families of the middle class spurred a massive response—fifty thousand joined a street demonstration on August 1. Several groups occupied the downtown cathedral for days and laid plans for a rural–urban coalition called the Bloque Popular Revolucionario (BPR), which soon became the dominant mass organization for mobilization. The BPR, which focused on rural areas, grew to about sixty thousand members by 1980 and became closely aligned with the FPL (Montgomery 1995; and Wood 2003).

In late 1976, tensions were high in the departments of Cuscatlán and Chalatenango after completion of a new hydroelectric dam on the Lempa River, which flooded low-lying land settled by hundreds of peasant families displaced by export crops. Government soldiers occupied Aguilares and northeast Chalatenango and began building National Guard posts in each municipality. The Guard worked closely with ORDEN, a rural network of militias and spies that was widely blamed for political assassinations. Rural membership in the secretive ORDEN had grown since its advent in 1968 because peasants valued the benefits the organization offered, including access to jobs, farm supplies, health benefits, and protection from police repression (Cabarrús 1983; McClintock 1985; and Wood 2003).

But ORDEN's growing reputation as a death squad led many peasants to drop out as the mass organizations gained popularity. One of the most notorious death squad killings was that of Fr. Rutílio Grande, in 1977. A popular priest who had organized CEBs in Aguilares, Grande was a friend of the newly appointed archbishop Oscar Romero; Grande's death was pivotal in Romero's conversion from a conservative with little interest in politics to a prophetic defender of the poor who denounced army violence in his popular Sunday homilies. Then Romero was assassinated in March 1980, during a period when the violence was escalating into civil war.

María Julia recalled the first local appearance of ORDEN after a series of demonstrations in the town of Chalatenango.

That was when the *militares* came here and began organizing ORDEN and deceiving [*engañando*] the people. They gave ID cards [*carnets*] and guns to members. That's why people joined. But they were nothing but civil patrols that went around threatening people, telling us not to go to mass, saying the church people were putting foreign ideas in our heads, crazy things like that. It was around then that they began harassing the church people and they killed Archbishop Romero. Also, two of the American nuns they killed had worked here in Chalate.

She was speaking of American churchwomen Maura Clarke and Ita Ford, who, along with Jean Donovan and Dorothy Kazel, were raped and murdered by Salvadoran soldiers as the women made their way home from the national airport on December 2, 1980. All four women had made trips to northern Chalatenango carrying food and medicine to displaced people and to people who had become stranded while fleeing the mounting violence. Donovan's diary in the eight months leading up to her murder was a chronology of repression against church workers and campesinos active in "*los bases*," as the Christian communities were called. Donovan "scrupulously recorded the names of the victims, the hour of the day, and the precise location of the rural repression" (Carrigan 1984, 149). One morning in 1980 workers arrived at the door of the parish house of the diocese to find an ominous sign: a drawing of a knife sticking in a head spurting blood and a message: "This is what will happen to anyone who comes to this house because the priests and nuns are communists" (Carrigan 1984, 231). That November a local army colonel told Ita Ford that the Catholic Church was "indirectly subversive because it is on the side of the weak" (Brett and Brett 1988, 297).

Most people I interviewed did not report seeing armed guerrillas in the Chalatenango mountains until around 1980. The murder of Archbishop Romero is cited by many former guerrillas as the point when they realized there was no longer space for open dissent and made the decision to go underground. The insurgent ranks swelled, and by the end of 1980 five guerrilla factions had unified to form the FMLN. Because El Salvador was heavily populated and had little impenetrable jungle or mountain terrain, there were few places for guerrillas to hide. In part for this reason, the rural organizing strategies of the FPL departed from the Cuban *foco* theory of revolution. Instead, wrote Montgomery (1995), they "lived among the people; they helped plow land and harvest crops; they provided medical care and other forms of assistance; they taught the peasants how to protect themselves" (115). Villages in northeast Chalatenango set up early-warning systems so one person keeping watch could alert the entire town of approaching troops, allowing the men time to escape. My informants described men and boys going up into the hills to sleep in these years because of fear that the National Guard or ORDEN would come in the night and take them away, a practice also witnessed by the American churchwomen who were killed (Carrigan 1984) and described by informants of Elizabeth Wood (2003).

In a relatively short time between 1973 and 1980, the same peasants whom Felipe had described as believing poverty and epidemics were the will of God made a remarkable transition—organizing themselves and demanding political reforms. The government blamed the Catholic Church for radicalizing peasants. When I asked Felipe why the people had changed their attitude, he gave a different answer.

> It was the repression that made the most difference. The National Guard feared they lacked peoples' support. People looked at them with fear in their eyes, and ran away when they arrived in a village to search for guerrillas. ORDEN was based in the cantónes. Some [members of ORDEN] complied with orders, and this was one reason lots of people fled—because they knew someone in ORDEN had a grudge against them. Others in ORDEN didn't follow their orders, and became involved in defense of the communities. During military operations, the Guard punished the communities to drive out those who were organized. And through these experiences the people became more inclined to organize themselves, and some became involved in the formal struggle in the mountains. Some fled, but others wanted to stay and do something to defend themselves. And this was a big decision.

Suffering and Transformation: *En Carne Própria*

During fieldwork in Guarjila and San José Las Flores, I often met residents for the first time when they came to the health clinic. I would ask permission to visit them at home for a more in-depth interview. I asked about health problems affecting other members of household. After discussing health issues, I usually asked, "How was your family affected by the war?" Here is a statistical summary of people's responses:

Eighteen out of the twenty-three residents (78 percent) reported losing children or other family members during the war, with an average of 2.5 family member deaths per interviewee. The total number of deaths reported in these families since the violence began was 58, and 95 percent (55 out of 58) of the reported deaths were due to violence.[3] I always asked if family members who had been killed or wounded were guerrillas or civilians; 84 percent (46 out of 55) of those reported killed from violence were described by family members as civilians while 9 (16 percent) were described as guerrilla combatants.[4] In addition, one woman reported that soldiers kidnapped her infant boy after a military operation in which they rounded up civilians for transport to a government-run displaced person camp.[5] She had not seen the child since. Three family members of interviewees were reported as wounded in the war. Eight of the twenty-three people interviewed (almost one-third) said their ability to work was impaired due to chronic problems that they blamed on effects of the war.

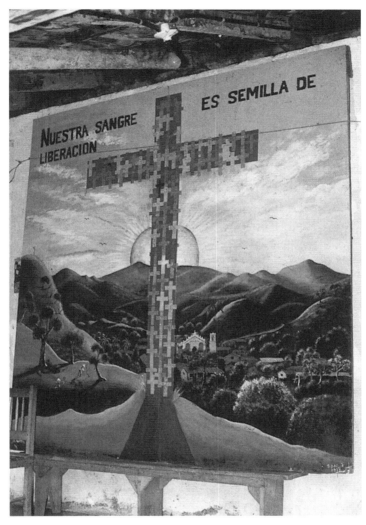

Cross on the wall of a church in San José Las Flores. Each gold cross represents a local family that lost someone in the war. The inscription reads "Our blood is the seed of freedom." Photograph by Sandy Smith-Nonini.

I often stopped to eat at a *cafetín* in Guarjila run by Tomasa Morán, thirty-five, a mother of four whose husband served on the town directiva. One day she told me how they came to spend seven years in refugee camps prior to the repatriation.

I lived in a *caserio* [hamlet]. The first massacres were in 1979. I lost a brother, a cousin, two aunts, and one child—all civilians. We fled in 1980 due to army operations. One day they killed my brother at our house. It was ten in the morning. Everyone ran away, those who didn't were killed. I fled with my parents and my one-year-old daughter Daysi, who didn't have any clothes on; she was freezing. We crossed the Sumpul [River] near Los Amates, and spent three days walking to Santa Anita, and then eight days more getting to San Salvador just to see if it was safe to go home. When we went back it was all burned. I wanted to cry. Our kitchen had been full of beans, corn, and rice. I couldn't even find any rags to use as diapers for the baby. We had nothing to eat, no milk for the baby, and my breast milk wasn't coming in. We walked for two nights to the border. ACNUR[6] gave us food in La Virtúd, Honduras, where there were about 2,000 in a camp. After that, I got really sick for about two months, with pain in my stomach [empache], vomiting, and a huge pain I couldn't stand; my whole body hurt. There was no doctor there. In 1982 we moved to Mesa Grande [refugee camp].

In more remote Arcatao, near the border, Felipe said that by 1980, the only remaining civilians in town were those who collaborated with authorities and lived near the National Guard posts, a description that jibes with a published report by Richard Alan White, a senior fellow at the Council on Hemispheric Affairs who visited Arcatao that year. White (1980) reported that only about twelve families out of four hundred households remained in town. He estimated two-thirds had left for refugee centers, and the rest had holed up in caves and high mountain villages. When White's party undertook a two-hour hike into surrounding mountains they found a small band of teenagers armed with pistols and roughly three hundred sick, undernourished children, women, and old people camped in a small village near the Honduran border. The Americans documented many serious illnesses among the refugees, including typhoid, yellow fever, dysentery, parasites, and gangrenous infections, yet the people told them that they feared excursions into towns on either side of the border to seek medicines because the Honduran army was cooperating with the Salvadoran military in its campaign against "subversives."

Felipe's family also fled that year, moving in with relatives near the southwest port of Acajutla. He was seventeen.

In the end we ended up with nothing. By then I was feeling more enthusiasm and supportive for the struggle. . . . I understood it as a Christian, but I couldn't really declare my feelings because most of my family would have opposed it. I had a small, very old radio, and I had always set aside time to listen to Radio Venceremos [the FMLN's clandestine broadcast].[7] I began to think about what we had been going through, and the great atrocities that had happened, and I gained a deeper consciousness. I began to think it was worthwhile to build a strong struggle to overthrow the capitalist system. I had a brother who was [with the FMLN] near the Honduran border. From around 1984 on I was determined to go to the countryside [to fight], but my mother opposed it.

Learning Pragmatic Solidarity: How Word Becomes Flesh

Many sympathetic accounts of revolutionary conflicts romanticize collective efforts whereas more critical accounts often seem influenced by idealized notions of democratic process, which assumes that the unity for collective action arises primarily from discursive processes such as ideological debates rather than through shared experience. In a discourse analysis of interviews with two women in a Chalatenango repopulation, Irina Silber (2004) described residents griping over fairness in distribution of aid from NGO projects, and she raised questions about idealized accounts of revolutionary struggles. When they spoke with foreign delegations during the 1980s, U.S. embassy spokespersons liked to deflect attention away from the government's human rights record, emphasizing instead FMLN factionalism and infighting. Although it is difficult to find comprehensive, unbiased accounts of life behind the lines in an insurgent struggle, there is much to be learned from historic accounts that capture "ethnographic-like" detail of daily processes, which carry insights into the role played by practical experience in transformations of social consciousness.

During the first two years of the war, the FPL made it a higher priority to protect civilians during guindas than to fight. But by 1983–1984 responsibility for these organized evacuations fell more on civilians, who had by then gained experience digging underground tatús to hide medicines and food, and preparing survival rations of flour and sugar for each person. Guarjila residents I interviewed and published accounts by witnesses depicted guindas as formative experiences in which survival depended on a high level of collective activity. The stakes were high, and participants talked about what had gone wrong and what had gone right for months afterward (Clements 1984; Metzi 1988; and Schaull 1990).

But the learning process was erratic. Wendy Schaull, a filmmaker, was trapped behind the lines in Chalatenango for ten months in 1984. In a book based on her diary entries, she wrote graphically of the fear and hardships of life under siege. She described how an unexpected army assault on the FPL rearguard in August caught civilian communities unprepared. After months of calm the civil defense planning was hasty and chaotic. During the guinda that followed, Schaull's account is full of despair as much from the lack of solidarity among campesinos as from hunger and exhaustion.

> It's the selfishness that's destroying me. Worse now than when I first entered the front because we are in a guinda. A number of people in this group packed rice, tortillas, potatoes, salt, candy, crackers, etc., when they

knew there was going to be a guinda. In the ensuing days they munched on their personal cache in front of anybody who was around. Some of us, in groups, had sugar. A few had absolutely nothing. . . . The unsharing in the midst of guinda has devastated me. (Schaull 1990, 81–82)

On the third day, as the danger receded, Shaull contributed to a small fund with a few others to buy bread in a nearby town. She assumed the bread would be shared, but when her friends returned with the food each one kept what he or she had paid for. She gave half of the bread she had bought away and suddenly "everybody was groveling for a handout." On the eighth day a civilian leader announced that from then on food would no longer be individual property but would be treated as collective. Interestingly, Schaull reported that after the guinda was over a fierce debate broke out about individualized versus collective food. A second army invasion took place several weeks later, forcing the population on another guinda, and this one proceeded in a more organized and communal fashion, with shared resources. Shaull noted that the success of the second guinda was talked about long afterward by campesinos.

Francisco Metzi, who spent three years in Chalatenango from 1982 to 1985 volunteering as a paramedic with the FMLN, gave a more idealistic account of the role of guindas in development of a communitarian ethic in the northeast region.

I'd wager, on one guinda or another, that we've all set aside something extra to eat secretly at night. But in the end, someone always finds you out, and you're left feeling ashamed, with your selfishness exposed.

The ideology that develops in a guinda forces you to share. It's the moment in guerrilla life when you're most conscious that survival is only possible by working collectively. Community is manifested in lots of ways: the organization of the retreat, the different columns assuming diverse responsibilities, commonly shared misery and hunger, and the very fact that some do the fighting so that others can get to safety. Nothing exists in and of itself, but rather, only as part of the whole. . . . Sharing becomes a strategy for survival. There is never enough for everyone. . . . One day you've got cigarettes, and others don't; the next it's your shoes that are falling apart, and somebody else knows how to repair them. You learn to give whatever the others need without keeping score, just as they aren't running a tab on you either. (1988, 140, 142–143, 145)

Notably, in both Schaull's and Metzi's accounts, collective practices are depicted as learned processes in response to dire circumstances. In both, there is mention of social sanction for not sharing but also a clear sense that the ethic was a rational strategy for ensuring group survival. Many in the West harbor notions about altruism as emotionally driven but irrational and contrary to human nature. Christie Kiefer (2000, 9), a community health researcher, points out that rules for cooperation, trust, and compassion are learned through informal education and social interaction. Studies of small-scale societies indicate that egalitarianism is maintained through ongoing vigilance and social sanction. Jacqueline Solway credits Alan Barnard and James Woodburn (1991) for coining the term "demand sharing" to describe the ways that participants in small societies are "morally bound" to share with colleagues (2006, 71). Raymond Firth (1929) also emphasized fear of social sanction as a primary motive for gift-giving in indigenous social groups.

As Lewis Hyde notes, this system of values is the reverse of the commodity exchange in that the gift moves toward the empty place rather than to turn a profit (1983, 23). Also, unlike a sale or trade, giving a gift tends to establish a relationship. When gifts circulate within a circle, they leave behind a series of interconnected relationships, resulting in a "decentralized cohesiveness" (xiv). Because gift exchange usually involves more than two people, it lacks the balancing of trade. Giving to a social circle becomes an act of "social faith" (16) because the circle structure effectively prohibits discussion of value; rather the gift seems to go "around a corner" (Hyde 1983). Participants, however, tend to feel a blind gratitude when gifts come back around the circle, providing for their own needs. For rural people, such moral economies are also moral ecologies. Latin American peasant models of exchange are based on a dialectical relationship with the land/Earth as well as based on social relations (Gudeman and Rivera 1990). Chalatecans, in spite of abandoning indigenous dress, still held the planting of the milpa with a quasi-sacred regard. (Even in the capitalist north, moral ecologies are deeply tied up with wider economic relations, as the environmental justice movement has demonstrated.)

I encountered this ethic on my first visit to Arcatao early in my fieldwork, when I took part in a group meal and afterward joined a line with the participants at the *pila* (outdoor wash basin) where each person, even the directiva president and guerrilla comandante, washed their own dishes, a practice that spoke to gender equity as well as collective sharing (see Schaull 1990). This was repeated at most gatherings of health workers, especially when organized by the diocese, although by 1995 the practice began to fade, as private cafetíns became reestablished in the villages once again.

These histories suggest that to understand origins of the ethic of solidarity in the repopulated villages, one must begin with the harsh lessons of the conflict and the process that campesinos went through of learning to trust their neighbors under fire. This, combined with a deep distrust of state authorities, helped to create conditions for much larger collective projects.

Self-Government: Los Poderes Populares de Liberación

Many who stayed in the mountains after 1980 told me that once the repression became intense they felt safer living near the guerrillas than trying to flee. After the FMLN's disappointing first military offensive in January 1981, FPL fighters retreated to rearguards in remote areas to regroup and train more experienced cadres. They gradually gained the advantage over the army, which at the time was staffed with poorly trained, unmotivated troops. Army soldiers preferred to fight only during daylight, and as a journalist I had heard many accounts in the late 1980s of army patrols in rural areas making efforts to avoid hostile confrontations with FMLN combatants while concentrating their operations on softer civilian or infrastructure targets.[8]

By late 1983 the FPL had gained control of twenty-eight out of thirty-three municipalities in Chalatenango, and nationwide the FMLN claimed control over a third of Salvadoran territory (Metzi 1988). Wood (2003) reported that Chalatenango guerrillas ranked second (after their comrades in Usulután) for the highest levels of government casualties in this period. The liberated zone provided the civilians and guerrillas with political space, and beginning in September 1983 the towns began electing new leadership known as Poderes Pópular de Liberación (PPLs) to replace former middle-class, or petit bourgeois, municipal authorities, most of whom had fled to urban centers. The PPLs were peasant-run structures based on principles of collective democracy, and these experiments in self-government were encouraged by the FPL. To some extent they also arose out of tensions between the demands of the guerrilla struggle and civilian needs. In a memoir, Metzi reported this account from an FPL organizer on the origins of the PPLs:

> We had to find forms of organization which corresponded to the aspirations of the people to participate in the war. There was a vacuum in that sense . . . with the new situation, when most of the young people had joined the guerrillas, and others had joined the militias and everyone was talking about combat and military struggle, the masses were more or less stuck in the middle: "Well, and us, what do we do here? What is our role? Our role isn't just to go on guindas." They had come out of the political struggle which had taken the form of economic demands for land, loans, markets for their produce; they had experience of an organization. But now they were in lands controlled by the people. From whom could they ask lands now or better salaries . . . ? We had to respond to this new situation. (1988, xv)

Municipalities like Arcatao and San José Las Flores, which had been resettled by civilians after the National Guard deserted their posts, held the first elections for these popular juntas.[9] Each such council had a president, a vice-president, and five *responsables* (representatives) who oversaw committees for production, trade, social affairs (including health and education), legal affairs, political education, and defense (Pearce 1986; and Metzi 1988). Jenny Pearce, a British political scientist who circumvented the army to gain entry to northeast Chalatenango in this period, reported that the FPL had subdivided the department into three subzones.

In subzone 1, where she conducted her research, there were seven PPLs in 1984 and a subregional government. Her extensive interviews with peasants showed that the civilian municipal governments were based on an ethic of participatory democracy and carried out debates about how to solve the problems of self-defense and daily survival in the context of what now was a full-fledged war. According to Pearce,

> The inhabitants of each locality were divided between three or four *bases*, or hamlets, which corresponded broadly to the old administrative units, cantónes. The highest power in each locality was the popular assembly, a general meeting of the whole population. Between popular assemblies power rested with the junta of the PPL. Candidates were proposed by each community and the junta was elected at assemblies of each base for six month terms. The bases would continue to meet in assemblies about every fifteen days to discuss problems with the junta. Every eight days there would be a meeting of the general secretaries of the mass organizations in the locality who were represented on the *consejo* [council] of the PPL and whose task was to mobilize the population behind the decisions of the PPL. (1986, 244)

Affairs at the subregional level were also managed by elected juntas, which facilitated coordination between PPLs. In 1984 Shaull witnessed a subregional election for civilian leaders in which twenty-eight local municipalities sent representatives to the town of Tamarindo to vote for candidates for each of the five positions on the junta. After the voting they held a two-day conference that began with the incumbent president, a woman named María, giving two detailed reports, one on the international scene, and one on national economics, politics, and social issues, each followed by question-and-answer sessions. After lunch incumbent junta members gave reports on successes and failures in their areas. On the second day Maria gave out mimeographed sheets outlining the new government's goals, with general and specific objectives. The participants divided into groups of twelve, and each group went off to discuss the plan.

> I went off with a group and listened for two hours. Again, all I can say is I was impressed. One *compa* who could read slowly read the first item for discussion. They went around the circle allowing each person to give his opinion (the group I was with were all male). Each of them had an opinion, actually several. Often times they would say almost the same thing as the other one, but they all wanted to speak. In the first half hour they had only gotten through three items and there were 30 yet to go through. Finally, a compa said, "Wait a minute, at this rate we'll never get through half. We have to organize ourselves better."
>
> "I've got an idea," said another compa. "We read each item, someone talks, if we agree with him, we don't need to talk unless we want to add

something." Everyone agreed. . . . They didn't get through the whole list but it was fascinating to watch them organize themselves more and more as time went by. (Schaull 1990, 24)

Schaull observed that campesinos took the process seriously and "got involved with gusto." She commented that prior to this, campesinos had probably rarely been asked what they thought about a government, much less had the chance to participate in one. For FMLN intellectuals and foreign visitors who wrote accounts of this period, the PPLs meant visions of a new revolutionary society. But for the Chalatecos, who had shared formative experiences in the CEBs and peasant unions, and in resisting the military repression, the PPLs no doubt appealed primarily as a practical response to the need to organize themselves for survival in the rugged terrain, under siege by their own government and cut off from the outside world. Kiefer noted that even in the absence of an secure established locale or ideal conditions for democracy, a "community of process" of the type described here can help establish forms of cooperation and the conditions of trust, out of which collective action for specific social goals can emerge (2000, 179).

Even before Schaull left Chalatenango in December 1984, the impact from two army invasions that fall had convinced many civilians to leave for Honduras. More left in 1985. But the experiences of self-government became reproduced in the huge Mesa Grande refugee camp in Honduras, where the refugees elected responsables in a similar fashion to the PPLs. When more than four thousand refugees defied government authorities to return from the Mesa Grande camp to El Salvador in October 1987 (approximately half settling in Chalatenango), one of the first things they did was organize work teams to clear brush for roads and temporary shelters and elect new representatives to a community council (Edwards and Siebentritt 1991).

Reconstituting the Body Politic

Many scholars of social movements have remarked on ways that liberation theology in Central America helped generate a "new historical subject" (e.g., see Gorostiaga and Marchetti 1988) on the part of the peasantry, previously regarded as an exploited class. Perhaps it is more accurate to say that the CEBs helped reconstitute a sense of community that had been lost, dating to the genocidal violence of the matanza in 1932 (Wood 2003) and the encroachments of coffee estates in the late 1800s. A key question is how new sets of beliefs and practices become invested with authority.

Marilyn Silverman and P. H. Gulliver (2006) have described hegemony as an ongoing political process with social and economic as well as discursive and cultural aspects. They note that peasant social transformations involve consideration of rationality as well as "common sense" (a set of taken-for-granted ideas, learned from social relations and daily experience). Or, as some might say, both Gramsci and Foucault have something to offer in understanding these processes.

Like the peasant intellectuals Steve Feierman studied in Tanzania (1990), the peasants of northeast Chalatenango were positioned in ways that allowed them to draw on multiple experiences and livelihoods. The migrant labor circuit initially exposed many of them to CEBs and to radical proletarianized peasants on the sugar cane plantations near Aguilares. Despite being extremely poor, their families still had a toehold on the land, making them similar to Wolf's "middle-peasant," (1969, 292) in that they were not wholly dependent on the cash economy; their principle identities and occupations were as subsistence farmers. This land base, however tenuous, combined with the recent experience of new land loss from Green Revolution crop expansion (see chapter 1) gave them a strong sense of place that they were willing to defend once their communities were threatened by army invasions. Their geographic isolation and the social space of the CEBs helped create conditions for "hidden transcripts" to emerge (Scott 1992). The common medium of oral testimonies about shared suffering likely aided traumatized individuals in developing a sense of belonging and identity that transcended the material limits of bodies, allowing for new forms of community (a metaphorical body), to emerge (Pandolfi 2007). This sense of shared suffering coupled with urgent common needs became a basis for planning political activities. By the mid-1970s, there were many overlapping networks—some having worked with CEBs, others with cooperatives or the large and rapidly radicalizing peasant unions (Wood 2003).

The surge of demands for land reform suggests that organized campesinos had developed an understanding and critique of modernist development schemes. However, the notion—increasingly common among some cultural theorists—that peasants categorically reject development per se seems overstated. What I heard consistently from my informants was a desire for external funds for infrastructure and programs to improve community life, but also a demand for democratic control over the forms that development would take. Marc Edelman who studied peasant protest in Costa Rica, concurs, arguing that terms like "development" are often appropriated by subaltern groups and given new meaning (1999, x).

Robert G. Williams argued that the negative effects on campesinos from agricultural modernization violated their sense of moral economy (see also Wolf 1969; and Scott 1976; 1985). While the paternalistic relationships between colonos and landowners had been highly exploitative prior to the 1960s, the classic patrón of that era was more responsive to peasant needs such as housing, food, or medical care for a worker's sick child. Relations were more personable, and day-to-day life for rural families was more predictable. In contrast, once investments in mechanized cotton or cattle diminished the need for labor and landowners began to claim land previously used for milpas, these relationships were severed in a relatively short time (Williams 1986, 67, 122). Indeed, some of the worst clashes occurred in lowland areas converted to cotton, and in areas where cattle ranchers encroached on marginal lands that had traditionally been available to peasants for subsistence cropping, which suggests that a violated sense of entitlement did play a role (Williams 1986; and Wood 2003).

Ironically, despite the revolutionary rhetoric, the values defended by the mass organizations actually functioned as a conservative bulwark defending traditional community values against the asocial (hence, amoral) anomie of the new intrusions of the modernized agricultural economy (Lancaster 1988). Similar to Wood's informants in Usulután (2003), the Chalatecos I interviewed stressed emotional and moral reasons for choosing to resist authority. The moral language echoed calls for justice in peasant movements elsewhere in Latin America, Africa, and Asia. Feierman notes: "When peasants organize political movements, or when they reflect on collective experience, they speak about how politics can be ordered to bring life rather than death, to bring prosperity rather than hunger, and to bring justice rather than inequity" (1990, 3).

Unlike Wood's informants, who lived in a region that was not fully controlled by either army, many Chalatecos who got caught up in the violence were assumed to be "subversive" by virtue of where they lived, and they had little opportunity to choose allegiances in a strategic fashion. While repression, economic hardships, and the CEBs, were all mentioned by people explaining their political motivation, Felipe argued, "It was repression that made the most difference." Chalateco oral histories support the conclusions of John Booth (1991) that in Central America it was not economic factors alone but also the repressive responses of governments to reform movements (which delegitimized the state) that resulting in the radicalization of the peasantry (see also Wood 2003; and Binford 2004).

A former FPL member insisted to me that moral outrage in the peasantry was also fed by a desire for revenge, an observation that jibed with investigations I did as a reporter on the war from 1987 to 1989. During a conversation about the army murder of the Mexican FMLN doctor described in the prologue, a European physician who had worked in northeast Chalatenango for many years confided to me: "When they murdered Julia, that was the first time I had the desire to kill." Wood's informants also spoke of revenge as a motive (2003, 116), especially in response to government forces killing family members (230). Revenge is common in human societies studied by anthropologists (Boehm 1999), and is further evidence that a body politics shapes collective social action and that "negative" reciprocities also contribute to solidarity. Sherry Ortner argued that social change occurs when rural people attempt to employ traditional social strategies to deal with novel phenomena and these efforts fail. "This change of context, this refractoriness of the real world to traditional expectations, calls into question both the strategies of practice and the nature of relationships which they presuppose" (1984, 399). Antonio Gramsci (1971) likewise saw contradictions between discursive and practical consciousness as providing possibilities for an assault on hegemonic power relations.

Stephen Leonard argued that the tradition of praxis distinguished liberation theology from other varieties of critical social theory such as feminism, traditional Marxism, and ethnicity-based intellectual movements, which, despite their rhetoric of liberation, remained more relevant to relatively privileged sectors in developed societies than to the poor or marginalized people they sought to represent (1990). Perhaps another reason that practice is so important with peasants has to do with the fact that exploitative relations have led them to distrust words. On initial visits to Chalatenango when I talked about my research goals, I hoped that people would tell me their history. But people often replied, "Stay with us a while, and you will see what our lives are like." The war, of course, heightened the need for trust. Outsiders could gain trust only by sharing the hardships and risks of peasant life.

When I asked Cristina, the health promoter in San José Las Flores, what community meant, she gestured around us at the village itself, at the health clinic, the school and the new houses, saying "Look at what we've built." Others responded by saying, "Look at what we've been through," citing shared rituals of guindas, the armed struggle, refugee camps, and repatriation. Popular health and other innovative practices were explained as part of the "struggle to survive."

In recounting his own process of *consientización*, Don Lito, a Chalateco peasant interviewed by writer María López Vigil, also insisted on integrating practice with beliefs:

> I say why separate the religious and the political . . . It always seemed to me to be the same thing. . . . In Chalatenango . . . [the people's] consciousness awoke with the Christian communities. It was . . . from there arose the commitment that they made. There are areas, yes, where it was pure politics. Big farms, haciendas, conflicts with patrons. But both the Christian community and the political fight depart from the same reality. It's not like the enemy [the government] now says: that the struggle was "invented," that it came from outside. No, it was born out of necessity. (1987, 76–77)

PART TWO

War against Health

3

Insurgent Health

How Liberation Theology and Guerrilla Medicine Planted the Seeds of "Popular" Health

> I believe the world is beautiful
> and that poetry, like bread, is for everyone.
> And that my veins don't end in me
> but in the unanimous blood
> of those who struggle for life,
> love, little things,
> landscape and bread,
> the poetry of everyone.
>
> —Roque Dalton, "Like You" (1983)

The power to heal is the existential antithesis to the power to kill, and healing has been a common site of religious and political transformation in many cultures (Glick 1977). In Marxist traditions, Friedrich Engels's 1845 study, *The Condition of the Working Class in England*, was the first scholarly effort to examine the health of the public as both materially related to capitalist expansion and a site for revolutionary struggle. For its part, Catholicism has traditionally regarded healing as representing the sacrament—"a sign of the healing Christ." Hence, health institutions have long been central to the Church's service to the community (Burghardt 1981). Contemporary Catholic teaching asserts that health care is a human right and an essential component of social welfare for the protection and promotion of human dignity (Quinn 1981).

Looking through the window of health in northeast Chalatenango provides insights to how new practices shaped collective identities. Popular health, as the system in conflicted areas came to be known after the war, arose in part out of necessity, and in part out of the openness to new ideologies created by the polarization and the influence initially of church workers and later of urban and "internationalist" health professionals who incorporated within FPL-controlled zones.

To reconstruct these fraught beginnings, I conducted oral history interviews with seventy-one residents of the Chalatenango war zone, including twenty-two lay health promoters (most former FPL sanitarios [paramedics]) and nineteen health professionals who worked in the war zone clandestinely (most of them former FPL internationalist doctors).[1] I also drew on memoirs of two internationalist volunteers, Dr. Charles Clements (1984) and Francisco Metzi (1988), and the diary of a U.S. pediatrician and nun (now deceased) who worked in Guarjila from 1987 to 1993.

The liberation theology movement led to a variety of local self-help and development initiatives, including health projects inspired by the World Health Organization (WHO) pledge to bring "Health to All," which emerged from the 1978 Alma Ata conference. The approach to health adopted by the social secretariat of the Salvadoran Archdiocese combined a focus on social causes of illness with Paolo Freire's (1982) hands-on, interactive pedagogy for adult education. Church workers in rural CEBs were frequently called on to help obtain medicines and provide emergency medical transport for sick or injured patients. In the polarized atmosphere of the late 1970s, demands for better health services were added to the Church's political agenda. Just as the CEBs laid groundwork for training lay catechists to address the shortage of rural priests, in health, lay volunteers were recruited to attend courses on basic sanitary practices and how to diagnose and treat common illnesses. In remote areas the same individual sometimes performed both catechist and health roles in the 1970s.

CEB Origins of Lay Health Organizing

Fernando, a soft-spoken, articulate man in his late forties, was one of the first health promoters trained by the church in the zone. In mid-1992 I caught a ride with him to San José Las Flores in the back of a pickup. It was dusk, and halfway between Guarjila and Las Flores a large flatbed truck in front of us lost part of its load of building materials in the road while ascending a hill after crossing a low-lying creek. There was no room to go around, so we talked for an hour and took turns holding a flashlight and helping the men reload the truck. Fernando reminisced about his health work prior to the war:

> There were some Ministry [of Health] clinics that had been built in rural areas. But the government doctors never talked to people about the causes of their illnesses. Some medicines they gave away free, but others had to be bought by patients. In [CEB] meetings we talked about the need for lower prices for *consultas* [doctor visits]. To see a doctor in those days cost two colones, but a man was only paid one or two colones for a day's work, so imagine, someone would have to work one or two days to pay for one clinic visit. So we encouraged people to stand together and demand lower prices.

I traveled from village to village to give talks about malaria, wounds, common illnesses. Sometimes I'd walk a half day to get to a cantón. We didn't talk in those days of latrines, or water purification. Some people responded well, especially the poorest people. Others were opposed. But hardly anyone we met supported the government. When we went to San Salvador to march our demands included lower prices for medicines and consultas. But every time we presented these proposals in a formal way to the Ministry of Health, they were rejected. Even as early as 1976 dead people had been appearing by the roadside.

Every day that passed the persecution got worse. It became harder to visit villages, due to fear, because we were threatened. There were no real guerrillas then, just the National Guard and their cantón patrols. . . . The guardia and patrols carried lists with names of people they saw as suspicious. They saw us as guerrillas, but we weren't guerrillas, just people who cared about the community. We believed that someday we were going to have a popular health system, and . . . the means to take care of our communities' problems. I did this kind of work from 1976 until 1980, when we were forced to leave.

After 1980 most government health clinics in the area were abandoned by their staffs, who feared traveling due to increasing clashes between army troops and new rebel groups. Then army roadblocks cut off the area entirely. In some parts of Chalatenango as the war disrupted daily life, the Church tried responding to health needs by contracting with international relief NGOs, but these efforts were difficult to sustain. Interestingly, the NGO doctors' motivation did not always align with liberation theology. Marla, a health promoter living near La Laguna, which remained under government control, recalled this shift.

Up until then the Church had worked with catechists, holding Bible classes, singing together. We were used to that. So it was strange, and a bit funny, when along came these two doctors sent by the Church who said they didn't know anything about the Bible. And one of them told us he didn't care to know! We didn't know what to think! But the army kept harassing the doctors, and people there were not organized. They were just afraid. Then the army captured the doctors . . . and after that they told us they couldn't keep coming because of the violence.

The FPL recruited some physicians and nurses after the University of El Salvador Medical School was invaded by the army and closed in 1980. Other internationalists were recruited through sympathetic foreign "solidarity" committees, mostly in Latin America and Europe. In addition to emergency medicine, the urban and internationalist physicians found themselves drafted as instructors for a series of irregular courses to train young campesinos as sanitarios for the guerrilla army, or as civilian health promoters.[2]

Several thousand campesinos either chose to remain or became trapped in northeast Chalatenango after the roads were blocked. The life of *las masas* (civilians living in guerrilla-held areas) was a transient existence. Cristina, one of the older health promoters in San José Las Flores, recalled that her family first fled their home in 1982. As about sixty civilians carrying food and small children set out on that guinda, Danilo, a community leader, learned that a local woman had gone into labor. It was common during a guinda for the combination of fear and exercise to bring on labor in pregnant women near term. Danilo frantically ran down the line of campesinos leaving town asking each one, "Have you seen Cristina? Have you seen Cristina?"

She laughed recounting the story of that hasty delivery in the midst of the frantic evacuation, noting that the boy, now ten years old, lived in the house next door to hers. Cristina's initial health training came from the Catholic Church and the National Red Cross prior to the war, but she attributed much of her expertise to practical experience and courses taught by FPL health workers during the war.

> There were no doctors with the compas [guerrillas] then [1980]. The civilians [who remained] reestablished our communities after the army left, but there were no medical supplies. We had to rely on the Frente [FMLN]. No one could even give injections. We had an epidemic of typhoid and two children died. Then I got it and I thought I would die! Finally we approached the compas and asked for training. I had been working with children, but I was drawn to health work. A foreign nurse working with them gave us a fifteen-day course. We had hardly finished the course when we had to hide in the hills because of another army invasion.

The next course, Cristina recalled, was taught to ten campesinos, eight women and two men, selected from their villages to be health promoters. The teacher, an FPL paramedic named Jorge, used David Werner's 1977 text *Donde No Hay Doctor* (*Where There Is No Doctor*) to prepare lessons. Topics included the basics of germ theory, recognizing and treating common diseases, doing injections, basic first aid such as using tourniquets and applying pressure on a wound, stabilizing a broken bone, using local anesthesia, and suturing wounds. Health committees were formed for each village to manage a small supply of analgesics, antibiotics, instruments for minor surgery, and bandages for small wounds. These were stored in a promoter's house or, during a guinda, hidden in an underground tatú (cave).

Internationalist Doctors and Clandestine Hospitals

The cultural gaps between educated professionals who joined the FMLN and the young campesino promoters were enormous, especially for foreigners, many of whom were learning Spanish while coping with immersion into the harsh conditions of rural poverty exacerbated by war. Large sections of accounts by Clements (1984) and Metzi (1988) are devoted to their problems of adjustment and establishing rapport and with young campesino women who staffed the clinics and attended their courses. During my fieldwork, from 1992 to 1995, it was apparent that the bond forged between the physicians and sanitarios (now called promoters) was tight. The physicians were always on the go—attending planning meetings, seeing patients, or delivering supplies. When one came into town, he or she acquired an instant coterie of promoters, community leaders, and the occasional ambulatory patient. To talk with ex-FMLN physicians I had to hitch rides while they made their rounds or follow them home at night. From their stories I came to appreciate that their rapport with community members derived from years of shared adversity and, for many, was hard won. Like several others, Octávia, a young Belgian physician, became involved during a stint volunteering in a Honduran refugee camp:[3] "I had been involved in the anti-imperialist movement since 1966. But I wasn't satisfied with the work [in Europe] because it was too theoretical. I wanted to find a way to contribute and to support the people I had met in the camp. My first break with my family had been to work in Honduras, and after doing that, the decision to work with the Frente was easier."

Octávia first entered northeast Chalatenango in January 1986 after a long overland hike from Apopa, north of the capital. She found Arcatao almost abandoned, with only one other internationalist physician in the area. In her early months she circulated among eight FPL bases, each holding about fifty guerrillas and civilians. "It took me a long time to gain people's trust. They didn't give me work to do at first. I went from base to base. Some thought I was too spontaneous—but no one who is not in an army is accustomed to following orders. Others thought I was too feminist, too anti-Soviet. . . . but little by little this changed."

Michaela, a middle-aged Danish physician who had volunteered with the FPL since 1983, befriended Octávia and encouraged her to develop a course in anesthesiology, one of her specialty areas. Through teaching the course, Octávia began to get to know the young women training in health whom the internationalists fondly referred to as *las bichas* (the girls). "We [physicians] were seen as intellectuals, and we became popular. We spent a lot of time with the bichas. We were never alone—they'd even go with you to the bathroom!"

One of the younger bichas was Carmen, a fresh-faced, energetic adolescent who had only completed fourth grade when the war broke out. Carmen hung out with her older sister, who took health classes, so she sat in on them as well. She was one of three to take Octávia's anesthesia course, which she recalled well when we spoke. The FPL relied on intramuscular injections of ketamine or epidurals for local medical procedures, Carmen recalled, although intravenous lines were used for major surgeries. "We had to do a rough calculus of a patient's weight and height, but we had no way to get exact measures. Luckily no one ever died of an overdose." Eventually Carmen ended up as an anesthesia specialist at the FPL's clandestine rural hospital and became practically inseparable from the two internationalist doctors.

Years later, after the cease-fire, Carmen was elected president of the promoters' union and went on to attend medical school. In 2007, when I last saw her, she was working in the San Salvador health office of Dr. Violeta Menjívar, an FMLN-affiliated mayor from Arcatao. "After studying medicine I realized how risky it was," Carmen remarked in that interview. "When a patient entered respiratory distress, for example, the doctor would have to stop [the treatment] and intubate because we [sanitarios] didn't know how to do it!" She recalled how new physicians arriving for the first time were "literally frightened" by the conditions they were expected to work in.

After the FPL drove the army out of the area in 1983, efforts were made to improve the clandestine hospitals. Several former colleagues chuckled over Michaela's zeal to round up volunteers to build a proper operating room. During our 1993 interview in Guarjila, her sunburned face and long white mane testified to Michaela's years in the countryside. She laughed, describing how the health team had raided bombed-out churches for wood and panes of glass to build a makeshift operating room in a champa that would have sufficient light. The team used limewater to whitewash the bajareque walls, and installed a plastic skylight in the tile roof. They rigged a system of bamboo tubes to carry potable water inside. A chest-high church altar became an operating table. A car battery and flashlights enabled night surgeries. Other champas held inpatient beds, called *tapexcos*, made of ropes or saplings lashed to a wooden frame. Michaela recounted daily routines that began with checking on wounded patients at 5 A.M., followed by breakfast, then surgical operations if necessary, followed by classes for the promoters in the afternoons. "Nowadays, I wonder how we did all that."

Broken bones were frequent due to mines and shrapnel from antipersonnel bombs with extender arms designed to make them explode before hitting the ground (see Clements 1984). Michaela, who had previously trained in trauma medicine, invented a method for healing broken bones using traction involving a nail through the bone at the foot and a large stone as a counterweight to elevate the leg. All guerrillas entering the FPL had their blood tested to learn their types in the event donations were needed for wounded companions (Espinoza 2007).

Carmen worked primarily at the hospital doing tasks such as making *suero* (rehydration fluid), washing bandages, bathing patients, and treating their injuries. The sanitarios sterilized gauze and instruments in a *baño amarillo* (yellow bath) by wrapping them in paper, then putting them in a powdered milk can placed inside a larger can filled with water. The can was then placed on a fire and brought to a boil.

"We lived in that hospital!" said Carmen, in a nostalgic moment during our interview in downtown San Salvador where she coordinated the mayor's municipal community health initiatives. "It was our house and our school. We all

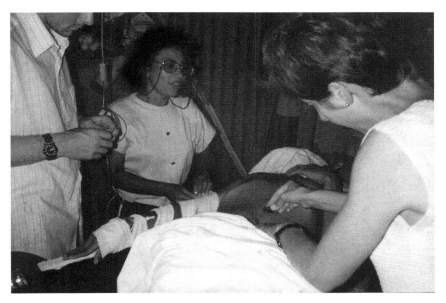

Surgical procedure in a clandestine FMLN clinic during the war. Photograph courtesy of El Museo de la Palabra y la Imagen.

shared the little we had. When someone finished a task, they would help others finish theirs. When patients got well and left, often they would come back to see us. It was a kind of school I'm not likely to see again."

Other sanitarios were assigned to more mobile units at graduated levels of health posts (*puestos*). The first post was held by one sanitario who accompanied troops into combat. Three or four sanitarios at the second post backed up those on the frontline. A third health post in a more protected position usually had a physician and a sanitario trained as an anesthetist with capability for emergency field surgery. The fourth post, at a more rearguard site, was a semimobile clinic with a staff and a cook where wounded patients could be cared for and more serious surgeries done. During less conflicted periods (e.g., much of 1983), the rearguard hospitals became more fixed, sometimes constituting a fifth puesto with greater infrastructure, like the one Michaela and Carmen described.

Margarita's health experience was mostly in forward posts. Originally from the town of San Isidro Labrador, she had just managed to complete seventh grade in school when war broke out and most young people in her area joined the resistance. After a three-day health course, the teenager filled a backpack with basic medical supplies and accompanied a fledgling FPL platoon during the 1980 offensive. She gained a reputation for being "*lista*" (capable). "I was stronger than most. They taught me techniques for rescuing a wounded person when we were under fire. I incorporated into our special forces unit and always accompanied them into combat. I was very lucky that nothing ever happened to me."

In 1985 an American nurse who had spent more than two years in El Salvador's war zones gave a detailed account of her work during an interview in New York City with me and Tom Frieden, editor of *LINKS*, the newsletter of the National Central America Health Rights Network (NCAHRN).[4]

> The part of Chalatenango where I first worked hadn't been invaded in two years. People planted, had stable villages. . . . There were families . . . schools, a whole system of hospitals. There was also a "step-down" place for [injured] people who could not go back to their homes. They made hammocks, mats for patients, fishing and farming supplies. We tried to keep people out of the hospital as much as possible. . . . Due to the war people needed to be in their homes and working . . . not in a dependent situation. The hospital was mostly for severe trauma and debilitating cases of malaria. We also used it for training, with the idea that many of the *brigadistas* (sanitarios) will go back to their communities after the war. We made our own IV solutions. We found an old man who had been sanctioned several times for making alcohol—[which was] not allowed in the [FMLN-controlled] zones—so we commissioned him to teach us to distill water. His implements looked just like glass lab equipment, except it was all made out of clay. (Frieden 1985)

During my fieldwork I got to know a gregarious ex-FMLN physician named Leo, who was widely known and popular in the repopulated villages. A Honduran by birth, Leo stood out among the campesinos because of his large stature and talkative nature. He remembered the period after the FPL gained control of the zone as a time when all the hospital supplies came overland from San Salvador, brought in "a little at a time, by foot, like the work of ants." The medical personnel depended on civilian networks to smuggle supplies, many of them from international solidarity organizations. The FPL-trained civilian militia aided communities by helping dig tatús into hillsides where medical supplies and wounded patients could be hidden during military operations (Keune 1995).

FMLN attempts to secure assistance from the International Committee of the Red Cross (ICRC) to evacuate wounded people from the war zones were usually thwarted by the Salvadoran military. On many occasions the agreed upon site for a rendezvous with the Red Cross was treated by the military as an opportunity to ambush combatants (see chapter 4). In the early 1980s the Salvadoran army had a reputation for not taking prisoners, and even after (post-1985) improvements in the human rights situation, evacuated patients often ended up under armed guard in hospitals, or in prison, even if they were civilians. So the FMLN, which had an official policy (and reputation for) abiding by the Geneva Conventions, relied mostly on civilian networks to secretly move wounded and disabled persons out of the zones. Some wounded combatants were sent to Nicaragua or Cuba to recover from serious injuries.

One of the few exceptions in terms of respect for medical neutrality was a policy of annual one-day cease-fires for immunization that the Salvadoran government and the FMLN agreed to beginning in 1985. The year before, the country's vaccination rate for children had fallen to 23 percent for polio, measles, and diphtheria, and pertussis. Measles was a special concern because it was a leading cause of child mortality, and an outbreak in 1981–1982 had resulted in 12,000 cases. UNICEF negotiated the accord, which had parallels in other Central American countries. In April 1989, only weeks after a new national outbreak of measles, I accompanied the UNICEF staff on a visit to Morazán, on the cease-fire day to observe guerrilla health workers vaccinating children. The cease-fire days were the only FMLN medical activity officially respected by the government, although soldiers attempted to exclude the media from covering the event. As we had passed through government roadblocks to enter the war zone that day, soldiers asked the driver of our jeep if any journalists were aboard. I shrank in my seat, but they took him at his word and waved us through. A photojournalist friend later told me that the army press office complained when a newspaper published her photographs of guerrilla health workers working alongside ministry nurses in Chalatenango.

Francisco Metzi, who volunteered as a paramedic in the zone, remarked on the fact that the rural population, accustomed to traveling long distances for medical care, came to regard the FPL's rearguard medical clinic as a community resource, referring to it as "our" hospital. He reported that on any given day there were one or more civilians in the hospital recovering from bouts of typhoid, malaria, or a cesarean birth. Although civilians living nearby were guaranteed access to medical attention, proximity to an FPL clinic also constituted a risk since hospitals were "prime enemy targets" (Metzi 1988, 35). Eventually FPL hospital teams were forced to become more clandestine and mobile. But maintaining secrecy proved difficult. "Hiding didn't work," said Michaela. "The people always knew where we were."

Metzi recounted an incident in which he and his team were resting in a supposedly secret hospital after finishing an abdominal surgery when a group of locals showed up with a woman in a *hamaca* (hammock on poles, or "guerrilla ambulance"). They explained, "We know we shouldn't come here, but the compa is really sick. So we decided to risk it. . . . The patient turned out to be a 32-year-old civilian with acute appendicitis. There was just one thing to do: put ourselves into high gear, wash and sterilize the instruments and prep her for the operation. It was 11 p.m. before we finished. If the people had waited, if they hadn't considered the underground hospital their own, the woman's appendix would have ruptured, probably killing her" (Metzi 1988, 36).

One of the worst incidents that Cristina described in San José Las Flores was a 1986 mortar attack that killed two civilians and wounded four others. She and Arlena, another promoter, ticked off the injuries: one head wound, an abdominal wound, one with a gashed leg, and another with multiple wounds in the stomach, forehead, arm, and leg. They put them in hamacas and sent them to the not so clandestine FPL mobile hospital. Cristina said most towns had a two-way radio on hand in case of emergencies. Civilian militia usually transported noncombatants to clandestine hospitals.

The need to train more civilian health workers burgeoned in 1983. Metzi reported that the civilian population in the war zone quadrupled from 1983 to 1984 as people who fled in 1980 learned that the National Guard and army had been driven out of the zone. Civilians slowly trickled back from refugee camps or hiding places (1988, 36). He noted that the influx of new people pointed up the striking differences in health between the ex-refugees and those who had stayed behind fleeing the army. Those who spent time in camps had managed to recover somewhat from their "life of chronic undernourishment" and usually had specific complaints such as infections (usually of the gastrointestinal, respiratory, or urinary tracts), parasitic infestations, or skin infections. In contrast, those who had hidden in the mountains came to the clinic looking pale and yellowish from anemia aggravated by chronic bouts of malaria. "Their hair had long since lost any semblance of shine, and they looked like walking skeletons. Their children were underdeveloped for their ages, their bellies swollen from worms." As the civilian population grew, he worked more and more in the outpatient clinic, where he said as many as twenty-five people often came for consults in a single afternoon (Metzi 1988, 36).

But civilians in areas removed from an FPL base, could not rely solely on guerrilla medical teams for health emergencies, and this became more of an issue when the FMLN adopted mobile tactics after 1985, frequently moving their hospitals and health posts. Fernando, the oral health promoter I met in 1992, was one of the coordinators in the mid-1980s who helped build a civilian health network in the area surrounding Arcatao and San José Las Flores. He traveled between cantóns, setting up *botiquíns* (first aid chests) in each one and encouraging campesinos who had a degree of literacy to train in health. Once health promoters were established in each village, he served as their liaison with FPL medical teams. Fernando was one of the few male health promoters I met who never "incorporated" as an FPL sanitario. "I've always worked with civilians. I've never been a combatant. There were huge health needs in the civilian population. The guerrillas had doctors. The FPL supported our civilian health work. But the problem was that [civilian] health promoters were never respected by the army."

He recalled an incident when planes bombed Patanera, a village that had a civilian presence but no guerrillas. Two women, a man, and a twelve-year-old were killed in the bombardment, and an eight-year-old girl was wounded.

The muscle tissue was left exposed on her arm, and when we took her back to the clinic we saw that we were going to have to amputate her arm, or she would die. It was difficult, but we couldn't just let her die. We had some general anesthesia, but we didn't have the right instruments. We only had a pair of tweezers and a blade. We didn't have a tool for cutting the bone, but we had a piece of a saw for cutting wood, and we cleaned it in boiling water for an hour, for fear of microbes, and we used that. We did have suture material—it wasn't silk, but we used it, first to suture the muscle, and then the skin. And it came out okay. She got well.

The issue of scarce medical supplies and whether combatants should have higher priority than civilians came up in community discussions in Guazapa, according to Clements, who reported the case of a rebel officer from a more militant faction than the local compas who argued that his troops deserved a fifth of the existing supply of medicines. He defended his case with revolutionary jargon, referring to his troops as "heroic." Then a local campesino replied, "That is an extremely important point of view. However, those heroic combatants to whom you refer have wives or husbands and children, mothers and fathers, whose well-being is on their minds. It is those campesinos who grow our food. Therefore we cannot say the priority for distribution of medicines is to the combatants." After more debate, the officer's proposal was voted down, in favor of sharing the medicines as they were needed (1984, 157).

When I asked Michaela to describe relations between guerrilla medical personnel and the FPL high command during the war, I expected to hear of a close relationship, given the strategic importance of medicine in a war. She surprised me, describing a relationship of constant tension. To illustrate she told of a period of intense fighting in 1984 when there were six FMLN hospitals in Chalatenango, all forced to be mobile by the government's new reliance on aerial strafing and bombing. At one point, Michaela recalled, the medical network was responsible for the safety of more than sixty patients in hamacas. "We were always struggling to resist orders [from the FPL high command] to move the hospital. We'd tell them that moving would ruin patients' healing bones. We'd beg them, 'Just fourteen days more!' Sometimes they told us to move anyway. But the jefes [commanders] were far away, so sometimes we just ignored their orders and delayed moving."

Once she allowed a patient with a bad head wound to stay outside the stifling hot tatú during a military invasion. "It was awful with everyone packed inside in the dark. You couldn't move or you'd smother, and you had to wait sometimes for many days. He said he'd rather die than stay inside. So I let him stay out. Later the [FPL command] wanted to sanction me. I laughed. I was the only surgeon they had there. What were they going to do?"

Another issue that strained relations between the medical teams and FMLN high command was the local perception that health and education were treated as low priorities by the Frente compared to strategic concerns like arms and food supplies. This, ironically, reflected these sectors' status in the country's federal budget, and Leo complained that health and education remained low in priority after the war compared to other areas in budgets of the Coordinadora de las Comunidades Repobladores de Chalatenango (CCR), the body that oversaw reconstruction in the Chalatenango resettled communities.

One Saturday in 1995 while returning by jeep from a health promoter meeting in a remote community, Leo and I had a long talk about the war years.[5] Since I knew Leo had close relations with the FPL, I asked him how the Frente's medical policies had fit with their military strategies. He seemed at a loss for my meaning, so I tried again. "How did the FPL make decisions about things like whether civilians should receive scarce medical resources? What was the structure for decision-making?"

Again, Leo looked at a loss. "Structures? I don't know what you mean. During the war we had the same kinds of meetings you've been observing. Our health policy [*política*] with respect to civilians was just understood—it was more a response to the need of the moment than to a set of rules." He was referring to the many popular health meetings I had sat in on. By then I had observed two civilian assemblies on health and more than a dozen planning meetings between promoters and ex-FMLN or church-based doctors and nurses where the collective ethic was to encourage wide participation in debates and decision making (see chapter 6).

I later learned that the PPLs in FMLN-controlled zone had helped instigate such dialogues, initially between civilians and the guerrilla army. The notion of participatory democracy between a guerrilla army and civilian supporters in an occupied zone during a war was certainly more of an ideal than a reality much of the time. Two or three ex-FMLN health workers I interviewed said frankly, "We all understood that winning the war took priority." Due to the strong influence of the FPL in civilian communities under their protection during the 1980s, it was unlikely that civilians who openly disagreed with FPL policies would rise to positions of power. Wendy Schaull's description, cited in chapter 2, of a talk about the international political situation given by a civilian woman who had just been reelected president of a subregional PPL suggests a sophisticated understanding that a rural campesino would only get from attending political education sessions organized by the FPL. But Schaull also discussed witnessing a forum at which villagers met with and offered criticisms to the FPL's top officers. Of the civilians she wrote, "these people had opinions and wanted to state them. They did it shyly at first but they were not intimidated when speaking to the *comandantes* even when they were being critical." One civilian said compas who were off duty and wanted to come into the village should report to local PPL representatives "so that we know it's a real *compa* and not an infiltrator." Another complained that compas spending the night in town should not shoot their guns to show off, adding "our children are already traumatized by the bombings—we don't like to hear guns going off for nothing." The comandantes agreed in each case and promised to talk with the troops (Schaull 1990, 24–25).

I asked informants in Chalatenango if they remembered debates over whether civilians should have equal access to scarce medicines. Several said this had never been an important issue. "It was the other way around," according to Leo, who joked about the "control" civilians exercised over the hospital in the form of "Comandante Maiz and Comandante Frijoles"—a reference to the critical role that corn and beans grown by civilians played in the war effort. On my prompting, he acknowledged that the FPL medical system's relations with the civilians were "a kind of exchange, since we loaned them our expertise," but he said, "it wasn't formally established, it was more like a union." Others said debates over use of medicines had, in fact, taken place when supplies were tight but had always been resolved in favor of the FPL serving civilian needs. The best use of doctors' time was a related question. Octávia remembered a European internationalist physician who had argued strongly against a post-1985 policy of the Frente calling on medical teams to do more outreach to civilians. "I always wanted to do more work with the communities, but Felix would ask, 'How *can* we . . . !' He wanted to focus on winning the war so that the health promoters could go to school and become professionals. But in the end, he supported me."

Just as the FPL physicians treated sick or injured civilians, promoters based in villages sometimes cared for wounded combatants. Several sanitarios and civilian lay workers, including Cristina and Carmen, assisted physicians in surgeries. At a time when no physician was available, Carmen once performed emergency surgery alone on a teenaged guerrilla whose hand was nearly destroyed by a bullet. While it would have been far easier for her to amputate his hand, she painstakingly reconstructed the two fingers that remained attached, which allowed the young man to retain use of his hand years later.

Clements, a Quaker and pacifist, found that despite his intentions to serve civilians, it became difficult in practice to separate civilian from guerrilla needs because the two were so intertwined. Without the FMLN combatants, he wrote, civilians would have had no protection and intelligence during guindas to escape the army sweeps; without civilian-run agricultural and fishing cooperatives, no one would have had enough to eat. He concluded that civilian networks for sending messages, transporting wounded, and smuggling medical supplies were just as essential as the compas with their guns (1984).

Likewise, Metzi's experiences in Chalatenango turned out to be a far cry from his initial "romantic . . . paternalistic vision" of single-handedly saving lives in revolutionary struggle. He wrote, "I never dreamed of meeting experienced doctors like Bernardo, who performed complicated operations assisted by teams of five or more. Nor did I ever imagine that the majority of my patients would be civilians. It never entered my mind that training others would become my most important job of all" (1988, 195).

In interviews with civilians, I heard stories of friends or family members whose lives were saved by the physicians and sanitarios, who several commented had "made great personal sacrifices." Mobility was the key to survival during an army invasion of the zone, but residents knew that when other compas moved out, doctors took personal risks by staying behind to care for immobile patients. Indeed, my informants could tick off a long list of former health colleagues, including internationalists, who did not survive the war. My questions about whether civilians were treated any differently from combatants seemed to shock Cristina. She replied in consternation, "How could they let the civilians die? The Frente doctors were always there for us. If there was no civilian population, where would they recruit more combatants? How could they eat without the civilian population? We were all the same family." Later, when I learned that Cristina's companero had been a combatant, I appreciated the literal sense in which she meant this.

When I reflected back on Michaela's comment about the distance between the high command and the mobile hospitals and the many examples I heard of local level decision making in Chalatenango, I realized why Leo was puzzled by my questions about FPL policy. Accustomed to more conventional notions of military hierarchy, I underestimated the degree to which guerrilla warfare relies on ongoing flexibility and innovation at the grassroots. This situation, which placed humanitarian-minded professionals in a setting where they lived and worked with relatively uneducated peasants—all under great pressure to solve problems of survival—created a highly unusual set of conditions for health development.

In Search of a Popular Pedagogy for Health

Probably the most effective teachers of health promoters in the war zones were other campesinos who shared their cultural background. But the shortage of lay workers with more than a few years formal education meant that courses were often taught by internationalists and Salvadoran professionals from urban settings. Clements (1984) and Metzi (1988) give detailed accounts of their frustrations in initial interactions with the young women (and a few men) they trained as sanitarios. Beyond problems of language and cultural style, basic concepts like germ theory were challenging to explain. In her anesthesia course, Octávia said that she had to start by teaching mathematics so the sanitarios could calculate dosages. They were slow to learn division, so she developed a system for them to simplify equations and rely on multiplication instead.

Unaccustomed to abstract learning based on didactic methods, the young women's eyes would glaze over during physicians' explanations. Carmen laughed, recalling that the worst were courses with Leo, who insisted on introducing promoters to Marxism, which she found deadly boring, at the same time as he taught them public health. (He was the exception among the FMLN physicians I met, most of whom rarely used ideological language.) Given her close relations with the popular system promoters, I was surprised when I first asked Michaela about her relations with the sanitarios after she arrived in El Salvador. With a loud laugh, she lit up the first in a chain of cigarettes, and said, "They hated me! Sometimes the promoters were so mad at me. I was very demanding. Eventually they got used to me. I was fascinated with them. They were like sponges in water. They got the hang of things rapidly without understanding the theory. We had a woman in the pharmacy who couldn't read or write and yet she knew all the medicines. She tasted them and studied the boxes. She never mixed up the aspirin with the penicillin. I don't know how she did it!"

What worked best for public health instruction, the physicians found, was teaching by example—a technique that was extended to how promoters engaged in community education. The physician and other community leaders had to dig and use latrines themselves to effectively promote use of latrines. Before one seminar, Metzi reported finding and reading a copy of Paolo Freire's *Pedagogy of the Oppressed*, which advocated an interactive approach to teaching illiterate adults (1988). This excited him in theory but left him frustrated about how to put notions such as "problematizing reality" into practice. In classes he still fought to keep the promoters attention. Rather than engaging with the material, they treated him with deference during lectures, and broke up in shy giggles when he asked them questions. Then he made a breakthrough:

> In the middle of class one day, it suddenly occurred to me that I was looking at the problem completely backwards. It wasn't these young women who should sit back and absorb what I taught, but rather, I should learn from them. After all, these women were the local experts who had suffered all their lives from the very diseases we were studying . . . I began to see the human body and health care the way these peasants understood them; this proved to be the key to making my work more useful." (43)

After that he began to learn the local lingo for parts of the body and for culture-bound illnesses or beliefs such as *ojo* (evil eye), "hot and cold" dietary rules (humoral medicine), and perceptions that it was dangerous to get wet too soon after work, before the body cooled. He began to take local explanations into account in treatments. Prior to a guinda, communities often slaughtered animals for food (otherwise the animals would be killed by the army), so Metzi and the promoters took advantage of the slaughters to practice dissections. When they lacked the peasant vernacular for an internal human organ, they substituted the local term for anatomical parts of animals—for example "air gut" for large intestine and "water gut" for small intestine (53). Michaela told of a similar technique she tried with sanitarios who assisted her in surgery: "I didn't know what surgical instruments were called in Spanish, and neither did they. So we invented names for them so the promoters and I could work together during surgery. One day this Italian doctor joined us during surgery and it was a real surprise for him. He didn't know what we were talking about!"

Metzi also used local realities as metaphors for medical explanations. He recounted a lesson he developed on overuse of antibiotics. An enduring problem in El Salvador is peasants' tendency to see pills and injections as magical cures, a problem that is exacerbated by lax state regulation. So patients self-medicate, buying prescription drugs from street-corner pharmacists. Metzi looked around for materials at hand and placed piles of red and green peppers, pieces of tiles, and pebbles on a table. He told the sanitarios:

> "Picture the center of the table as the inside of the intestine. The green chili peppers are the healthy bacteria, and the red ones represent bad germs that cause infection. The pieces of tile are parasites and the pebbles, viruses." I told them to imagine that the intestine was a battlefield in the [FMLN] controlled zones. The green chili peppers represented the compas. The red chili peppers would be the enemy invading with tanks—the parasitic tiles. The viruses, or pebbles in this case, were special armored cars, against which we had no weapons. To illustrate a healthy intestine . . . we scattered green chili peppers, or good bacteria, the *compas* of the intestinal flora, with just a few tiles and red chilis as "infiltrators," which were kept under control by the strength of the flora. "When there's an invasion—an infection, that is—the intestine fills up with red chilis, or bad bacteria. If we start to mortar-fire with tetracycline, what happens? Who dies?" I tossed a tetracycline capsule on the table. The compas stared at me in awe.
>
> Rosa spoke up: "The chili peppers. Both red and green."
>
> "Right," replied Metzi, "Both are vulnerable to the shrapnel. What happens to the armored vehicles and tanks?"
>
> "Nothing." Fernando was catching on. (Metzi 1988, 54–55)

In addition to courses taught in the warzones, the FPL sent sanitarios to a clandestine location called the Escuela (School) on the outskirts of the capital. Both Hector, the urban-based Salvadoran physician who directed the Escuela, and his students wore masks with cutouts for eyes during class to protect their identities. On occasion Hector, a former professor of medicine at the University of El Salvador, also traveled to Chalatenango or San Vicente to give medical courses. He described the development of a "popular pedagogy" as the equivalent of "learning another language." In addition to using *Donde No Hay Doctor*, Hector developed his own teaching materials with hands-on activities and Salvadoran slang. Civilian promoters who attended an Escuela course were expected to give similar talks when they returned to their villages.

Esmeralda, a regional health coordinator in Arcatao during the early 1980s, recalled that when there were shortages of medicines, health teams focused on environmental sanitation. "We gave talks on standing water, latrines, hygiene, and child care." She said the promoters also sought out the old people to learn what they knew about "*medicinas del monte*," or natural medicines. They began routinely using bark of the quina tree (which contained quinine) for malaria, *chichipence* or sábila (aloe vera) for skin infections, *ruda* (rue) for fevers, and teas of *yerba buena* (mint) for cough.

Health Work Is "Women's Work"

In the war zone most lay health workers were women despite the fact that instructors of courses insisted that anyone who showed interest could train in health. The FMLN had a higher proportion of women combatants than other Latin American guerrilla armies, and the FMLN encouraged women to adopt nontraditional roles. But traditional notions of "machismo" were still very much intact. In reflecting on the high numbers of women in health, my informants noted that most men had already "incorporated" into the FMLN as combatants, leaving primarily women as candidates for health training. Antonia, a Spanish nurse, said, "I think it was machismo. Men considered health women's work. In the hospitals the sanitarias were expected to do everything, wash clothes, cook, and take care of people. Those were traditionally women's tasks."

In contrast, Leo saw the glass as half full, claiming that women were more inclined to have the patience and aptitude to attend courses. Health work helped move women into new social roles, and liberated many from patriarchal oversight. Yet during my fieldwork observing health classes, it was clear that many young women beginning training, especially those from outside the war zone, were shy and lacking in self-confidence. An instructor would give a lesson and ask if everyone understood, and new promoters would dutifully nod their heads "yes" but then grow mute when asked to repeat what they had learned. But more experienced female promoters were often as outspoken as the men, and many became dynamic leaders.

Leo, who was married to a health promoter, insisted to me that the women's demeanor was misunderstood by foreigners. "The shyness of the promoters has to do with the way women are educated. They are accustomed to listening for a long time before they say something. They would rather be absolutely sure of themselves than be wrong. It's not timidity so much as a sense of reserve. I see it as a virtue. Gringos often take the promoters' shyness to be ignorance because promoters will say, 'I don't know much.' But in fact, they know a lot. They just don't talk about it."

During the war one outcome of the gendering of health was that female sanitarias who frequently spent months traveling with a platoon of mostly male combatants sometimes became pregnant, despite FPL policies promoting the use of birth control pills or IUDs by female combatants. In the last months of a pregnancy, the Frente would help a woman combatant either settle in a civilian community or leave the war zone to deliver the baby. Margarita, who worked for years as a sanitaria close to the front lines, left the zone in this manner. She described a three-month ordeal in 1987 involving hikes to five different clandestine locations, with fifteen-day stays in each place, before eventually making it to the Mesa Grande refugee camp in Honduras just ten days before giving birth.

Exile and Repopulation

By 1985 continued military operations had driven most remaining civilians in northeast Chalatenango into internal or external exile. While enclaves of civilians still remained, repeated army invasions (now conducted from helicopter airlifts) disrupted campesinos' attempts to return to their towns. San José Las Flores's entire population fled during an army invasion in January 1986. After a long guinda, the villagers took refuge many miles to the west in the church of Dulce Nombre de María only to again be surrounded by soldiers who sought to arrest the men. Catholic officials from the capital intervened with the army and negotiated the group's move to Calle Real, a displaced person camp near the capital. At that time an estimated one in ten Salvadorans lived either in exile, many in refugee camps in other countries or as "displaced persons" in internal exile (Edwards and Siebentritt 1991).

Many sanitarios lived in the Mesa Grande camp in Honduras for two or more years after fleeing Chalatenango. The PPL governing structures and the health organizing continued in this new setting. Each promoter was assigned to a *cuadra* (block) of families in the camp, whom the promoter assisted with hygiene, sanitation, and medical care. The collective organizational forms they brought from the war zone led to a clash with doctors from the French-based relief agency Médecins sans Frontières (MSF) who worked in the camps. Several promoters and Octávia (who volunteered in the Colomoncagua refugee camp in 1982) complained that MSF doctors were "arrogant" and inclined to give orders. Promoters also became frustrated at the MSF doctors' narrow focus on acute problems and their reluctance to offer training classes. At one point in Colomoncagua, refugees banded together and barred the French doctors from the camp, precipitating a round of negotiations to resolve the problems.[6] Octávia saw ideological differences as part of the problem because MSF held to a view of medical neutrality that precluded taking sides in a conflict. The refugee camps were difficult places to be apolitical. Many refugees felt threatened by the Honduran army, which periodically entered the camps to arrest people. And the FMLN treated the camp as a rearguard, where pregnant or wounded combatants could convalesce, and where they could recruit new fighters. Margarita said sanitarios in the camp periodically left to assist with FPL operations in El Salvador.

In 1986 the organized sectors of refugees, backed by international solidarity groups, began a campaign for permission to repopulate areas abandoned due to military operations. There was precedent; a year earlier, in 1985, after unusual negotiations between the government and the FMLN, a group of peasants had successfully repopulated the town of Tenancingo (in Cuscatlán Province) despite army opposition. In 1985, under pressure to show the U.S. Congress that the country was becoming democratic, President Duarte relaxed draconian laws against dissident activities. Among the new "popular" organizations that sprang up in the capital was CRIPDES (Christian Committee for the Displaced of El Salvador), which advocated for interests of displaced peasants. Six months later, after many negotiations between CRIPDES, the Catholic Church, and relief organizations, a group of one hundred Chalatecos left the Calle Real camp near San Salvador in a caravan of buses to repopulate San José Las Flores. Accompanied by the press, international volunteers, and Church workers, they succeeded without army intervention. In just a few weeks the town's population grew to four hundred as others emerged from hiding in the countryside. After this the Church and solidarity groups began sending aid and providing foreign "accompaniment" to the *repoblados*. Among the projects was a series of health classes for local promoters, carried out by the ICRC, which sent emergency vehicles and supplies for the health post.

This success inspired refugees in Honduran camps to lobby the United Nations High Commission on Refugees (UNHCR) for support of a larger repopulation effort in 1987 involving four thousand refugees, half destined for Chalatenango. The Salvadoran army opposed the refugee return, and President Duarte, who was elected as a moderate but held little power over the military, only gave permission at the last minute, after it was clear that the refugees' vow to return by October had become a major media event (Edward and Siebentritt 1991). I was among the reporters who flocked to the border for the crossing.

On the Honduran side a line of buses stretched for two miles, stopped dead in the hot sun. Every adult refugee was interrogated at the border, a frightening ordeal since many had lost their *cédulas* (personal identification cards), in the course of fleeing the army. Once they stopped, the old metal buses became stifling ovens, so hundreds of men, women, and children milled around, many squatting in the shade of the buses as the hours passed. Overhead racks and the floors of buses overflowed with bundles of belongings, cackling chickens, and sacks of corn and beans. In a bus parked off to one side, a relief worker and refugee health promoters assisted a peasant woman giving birth in the midst of the tumult. Although international volunteers had accompanied the refugees from Mesa Grande and planned to stay with them, they were refused entry at the border, adding to the refugees' anxiety. After crossing the border, there were more waits at army bases inside El Salvador. The road to Guarjila turned out to be impassable, and the ex-refugees had to walk the final miles behind men with machetes chopping the undergrowth. To add insult to injury, when the civilians arrived, they found the former village site surrounded by soldiers.

Years of poor nutrition, overcrowding, and unsanitary refugee camp life, combined with the five-day ordeal of the return trip, spawned a myriad of health problems among repatriates, including diarrhea, tuberculosis, impetigo, and parasitical diseases. Many mothers carrying small children complained that their breast milk had "stopped falling" due to the heat and the stress of sitting all day and then sleeping in the same cramped seats at night. A dirt-floored storage shed was outfitted for double-duty as a health clinic. When I visited two weeks later, the young health promoters had little on their shelves besides aspirin, some antiseptics, and bandages; they worried aloud what they would do if one of the men constructing houses was injured or someone was bitten by a snake.

Groups of refugees continued to return to Chalatenango in the years to come. The refugees asked the Catholic Church for food aid during the first year until crops were productive, and for help to train health promoters and rebuild and supply health clinics at the repopulation sites.

Health, Solidarity, and the Political Body

Health was not the highest political priority for either the FPL or the community PPLs during the war years. Winning the war and feeding the population took precedent (and indeed, protection offered by the rebel army and the harvest were fundamental to the population's health). In most settings, "health" is thought of as a normal state—the absence of disease. It is not health but injury or disease that calls the body to personal (and public) attention (Gadow 1980). In the Chalatenango war zone, death and disease displaced the normal in the 1980s and set up a high degree of visibility and social regard for popular health activities. Health workers became leaders addressing basic needs—such as potable water, latrines, and waste disposal—that the war turned into emergencies. The violence in the aftermath of liberation theology organizing led to wider awareness of the causes of rural poverty and government responsibility. Health teams went door to door on vaccination campaigns and traveled to remote hamlets to help villagers organize themselves for self-help.

I first encountered "scientific" confirmation of the effectiveness of health networks in guerrilla-held territory during my reporting on the annual vaccination day cease-fire. I was shocked to learn from UNICEF officials that their surveys showed the best vaccination coverage in El Salvador (at 85 percent) in the areas that were FMLN occupied. I had assumed that the devastated landscapes and abandoned towns in these areas and the danger of air raids would have precluded positive health indicators. The UNICEF project officer attributed the feat to the high motivation of health workers in rebel areas and their extensive grassroots networks among the peasantry. He blamed the ministry's low rates of coverage (for example, only 57 percent coverage in the capital) on its personnel lacking a capacity to organize at the neighborhood level. It seemed that in rural El Salvador, Foucault's (1980, 171) "technology of populations" had been turned bottom up.

The visibility of healing is of course tied to its relation to existential issues of life and death. Elaine Scarry (1985) argues that war, through the act of injuring, converts the body into a political artifact with a symbolic agency. Bodies so altered by violence evoke the memories of other altered bodies, keeping the past in the present, and continuing to name the author or authors of violence. Healing fits the criteria that Victor Turner (1974) laid out for a "root metaphor" or a conceptual archetype that establishes a linkage between the known and the unknown, and lays out a pattern of relationships and action that can serve as a template in a process of social change.

The genocidal tactics of the Salvadoran military aimed at the *masas* constituted not only attacks on personal bodies but on the corporate body of the rural peasantry. This common threat, ironically, served as a unifying force as residents of communities that had previously been divided by personalistic and patron–client tensions reconstituted themselves and fostered collaboration for survival (see also Binford 1999, Wood 2003). Anderson argued that communities should be distinguished, "not by their falsity/genuineness, but by the style in which they are imagined" (1983, 15). Collective acts with visible humanitarian effects, such as the networks that built and supplied the clandestine hospitals (which saved lives) came to epitomize the social struggle and give hope to those who took part.

A key purpose of terror and "low-intensity conflict" is to generate fear, chaos, and anomie, effectively destroying the social solidarity and trust that underpins community life (Nordstrom 1992). Through these tactics, a military regime seeks to control civil society. The assumption behind theories of counterinsurgency warfare is that all civilians are controlled by either one side or the other. Hence, groups that remain outside of official control are suspect, from the view of the state, and political warfare is intended to heighten civilians' dependency on authorities for protection and subsistence. Central to this strategy is the negation that civilians have rights to self-determination (Sinclair 1995). Thus, even humanitarian aid to displaced people becomes a military concern. In addition to surviving physically, Chalatecos who went into in exile after 1985 realized that to regain their homes, they needed to confront the image being presented to the world in which there were no dissenting peasants, only terrorists (who deserved the violence directed at them).

People involved in social movements are simultaneously engaged in formation of new cultural identities that "are not given, but constructed . . . [a process that] involves negotiation and conflict" (Escobar and Alvarez 1992, 11). These processes involve not only issues of meaning but also material risks and sacrifices.

As Orin Starn has noted, scholars "should be able to explore the politics of rural identity without losing sight of the often quite elemental matters of scarcity and survival that drive people to act" (1992, 93).

Health organizing and other community-building practices—which date to the 1970s CEB grassroots development efforts—represented both survival strategies and forums in which the peasants experimented with reimagining themselves. A mural on the walls of the San José Las Flores church testified to this in its call for "a new heaven and a new earth." The massive repopulation was one manifestation of this long process. International attention that followed the caravans of buses back to their villages in 1987 made it far more difficult for the army to claim that there were no civilians in northeast Chalatenango. The rebuilding of communities reasserted an alternative social order led by people reputed to be dupes of terrorists, lacking their own agency. It is ironic that the experience of government repression helped create conditions for such agency—recalling Taussig's assertion that traumatic historic events such as military conquest can become objectified as magically empowered imagery, capable of both causing misfortune, and also of relieving it" (1986, 367).

Lyon and Barbalet argue that the body in society can be thought of as "institution-making." They see emotion as a means "whereby human bodies achieve a social ontology through which institutions are created" (1994, 56). Studies of neurological states of people under stress also suggest that hormones such as acetylcholine affect beliefs. A study of Israelis forced to seek refuge repeatedly from SCUD missiles during the first Gulf War found that those who felt most helpless were most likely to engage in "magical thinking," such as prayer or superstition.[7] Material realities of war were ever-present in Chalateco accounts. "We did these things out of necessity," residents told me again and again.

Healing, whether physiological or social, is a reassertion of hope, order, control, and self-sufficiency, and a repudiation of fear and dependency (Dow 1986; Lyon 1990; and McGuire 1994).[8] It is in that sense that popular health should be seen as a ritual of healing for the political body. The new roles and structures of radical health work helped create both new identities and a hopeful alternative social order. The new "popular" rituals were the semiotic bone structure of what Lyon and Barbalet (1994) call the "corporate body." And the examples they cite— "the body of the church" (which exists as congregation and a community), and the "body of armed men" which make up an army—are particularly appropriate for the case of peasant rebellion in Chalatenango. These authors argue further that " 'body' in these cases is more than a mere metaphor. . . . The Christian congregation and the army corps are made up of human bodies of particular types of disposition, brought together as a unity at particular times through cognitive and affective orientations. Indeed, the role of feeling and emotion in the creation of a corporate or collective body is through engaging aspects of the individual body in a particular and direct manner" (1994, 55).

Although I did not realize it at the time, this is what was being demonstrated before me in the drama I witnessed in 1992 at the popular mass celebrating the fifth anniversary of Guarjila's repopulation. After a hiatus due to the children's chatter (where I interrupted this story in chapter 2) the audience quieted down and the play resumed with a scene at the Honduran-Salvadoran border where women refugees argued with the black-garbed soldiers. "We are tired of being in jail! We want to go home!" The soldiers denied the women permission to pass and threatened to kill them if they persisted. A chorus of actors cheered the women and booed the soldiers.

In the next scene the women paraded down the center aisle of the outdoor chapel singing a folk song about being reunited with their families (a reference to relatives who had stayed in Chalatenango to fight with the FMLN). A campesino man then stood up and offered a statement of support for other Salvadorans who were still struggling to return to their "places of origin." He held out a tortilla, which in the liberation theology mass stood for the host in communion, and concluded the dramatic enactment with these words:

> Our people have struggled to give our children a new life. And we're going to keep struggling for justice, lives of dignity and peace. All our children today over the ages of eight or nine years old can read and write. These are the achievements we celebrate today. Today we can say, "We are the FMLN!" All our achievements have literally grown out of the blood of our fallen family members. Just as the bread of the Eucharist is the blood of Christ, the blood of these martyrs has literally come back to us in these tortillas which represent the accomplishments of the community.

4

Low-Intensity Conflict and the War against Health

We looked for peace, but no good came, for a time of healing, but behold, terror. . . . the wound of the daughter of my people is my heart wounded, I mourn and dismay has taken hold on me. Is there no balm in Gilead? Is there no physician there?

—Jeremiah 8:15, 21-22

The prologue of this book recounts my 1989 investigation of a Salvadoran army ambush of an FMLN mobile clinic. Witnesses and forensic evidence concurred that a U.S.-trained Special Forces unit quietly mounted a 60-mm gun on a ridge above the camp and methodically machine-gunned ten patients and health workers while soldiers chased down Mexican doctor Alejandra Bravo Betancourt and a lay nurse who fled the scene, raping, torturing, and killing both of them (Smith 1989a). While one of the more egregious cases, this was only one among scores of documented violations of international law protecting medical neutrality in the war.

Protection of "health rights" during conflicts is a subcategory of the broader human rights guarantees that, after World War II, the majority of nations codified through the Geneva Conventions. I investigated reported violations of "medical neutrality" between 1985 and 1989 in two Central American wars. My first visit to El Salvador, in 1985, was with a small task force of U.S. medical workers to document the army's invasion and four-year occupation of the national university's medical and dental schools.[1] I also took part in three mobile task forces investigating attacks on health clinics in rural Nicaragua by the U.S.-allied "contras" who sought to overthrow the Sandinista government (see Smith 1987, 1988). I moved to El Salvador to work as a freelance foreign correspondent in 1987, and over the next two years I wrote a series of articles on violations of medical neutrality in the Salvadoran war (Smith 1989a, 1989b, 1989c, 1990).

Gathering evidence on events in El Salvador's countryside was difficult not primarily because of the hostilities themselves but because of army restrictions on travel to conflicted areas. For example, a photographer colleague and I were arrested by the army for entering the Chalatenango war zone to investigate the case

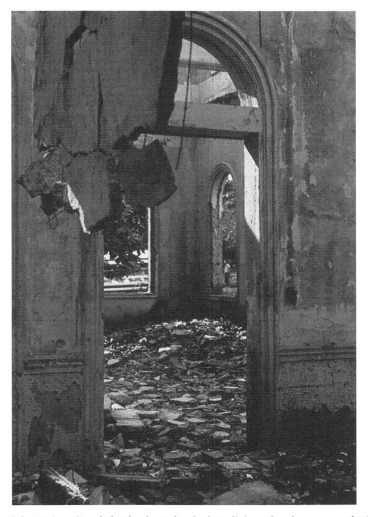

Ruins of the University of El Salvador School of Medicine after four years of military occupation, 1985. Photograph by Sandy Smith-Nonini.

described above. But rules for reporting for the mainstream media further complicated what qualified as "news." Reports from civilian survivors of targeted paramilitary and army violence arrived in the capital regularly during the war. Thousands of cases were carefully documented by local and foreign human rights organizations, but only a few such cases in any given year became news stories—and these usually involved either multiple witnesses to a massacre or foreigners who became victims. As a foreign correspondent it was difficult to cite Salvadorans as witnesses to crimes because they were rightly fearful of having their names published, and because editors of U.S. newspapers frown on anonymous sources. My editors often did not consider such reports credible because they contradicted official sources about El Salvador's reality (see also Pedelty 1995).

In a survey of *New York Times* coverage of the Salvadoran elections in 1984, Edward Herman (1984) found that 80 percent of sources cited by reporters came from U.S. and Salvadoran government officials, and only 0.8 percent came from peasants. The organized opposition was only quoted briefly, calling the elections a "farce" but was never allowed to elaborate on why.[2] After my report on the ambush of the FMLN clinic, I was recruited as a stringer for the *New York Times*, but I was frankly told by my boss that when I investigated a human rights case in which witnesses blamed the government, I needed to track down twice the number of witnesses compared to stories about crimes blamed on the opposition. When I asked why, I was told, "Because the U.S. State Department calls our Foreign Desk to complain about stories like that."

So much for the media. Can social science do any better? Sadly, as this book goes to press a new issue of *Medical Anthropology Quarterly* carries an article by Marcia Inhorn, the outgoing president of the Society for Medical Anthropology, lamenting the poor record of medical anthropologists at documenting impacts of war on health (2008). Using the Iraq War as an example, she gives a list of reasons why—ranging from realistic fear to ethics review boards, sources of funding, and issues of access. I would add to her list that medical anthropology is still getting over some theoretical hurdles. We remain caught on the horns of a dilemma—we have not yet reconciled the degree to which our restricted, local-centric concepts of culture lead us to repress body counts, as well as the macropolitical/economic machinery within which war-making takes place.

Humanism and Foucault's "Moral Orthopedics"

When I began graduate study in anthropology, I was surprised to discover that many in the field questioned whether there was a cultural basis for human rights. This derived in part from the discipline's respect for human diversity and its tradition of "cultural relativism"—which, as a hedge against scientific racism, privileges specificities (over commonalities) in analyses of social life. Anthropologists had long documented the destructive effects of colonial regimes and Christian missionaries on native cultures and common property regimes. Indeed, international law and human rights did not gain wide acceptance until after World War II, and the concept has been shaped by Western individualism and capitalist ideals. The Geneva Conventions privileged rights to personal security from kidnappings, imprisonment, torture, and harassment of political dissidents over the broader interpretations of civil/political rights, economic rights, or cultural rights favored by socialist regimes (Donnelly 1989).

Postmodernist skepticism about Western humanism was a factor in many scholars' embrace of Michel Foucault's theories, which linked modern notions of liberty to the individuation resulting from "disciplinary" institutions such as schools, prisons, and clinics during formation of European states. Foucault detailed a historical process as states replaced monarchs whereby the populace acceded to a process of "self-subjection" (under guidance of new social sciences), giving up to the state certain freedoms (personal sovereignty). This process of citizen-making, under the guise of new, scientific authorities such as doctors and psychologists, enabled insertion of state power "more deeply into the social body" (1979, 82). Foucault's "instrument-effects" referred to the unintended (but not necessarily disinterested) outcomes that resulted from disciplinary regimes lending legitimacy to the state. Such regimes benefited from this more efficient (and less politically risky) approach to maintaining order compared with reliance on coercion. Foucault's historical accounts depict how processes of individuation (dressed up as humanism) resulted in "normalization" and a pathologizing of difference, effectively producing docile conformist bodies. The influence of professionals in this production of "moral" self-surveilling citizens becomes invisible as politics takes a backseat to the public good of disinterested science (Hook 1997).

Although Foucault alluded to the liberating aspects of citizenship that serve as the trade-off for loss of personal sovereignty, he devoted most of his writings to a micropolitics of the person at the mercy of institutions—in short, depicting people as unwittingly turning themselves into "objects." Notwithstanding Foucault's many contributions to social theory, in the "new world order" triumphalism of the 1990s his analysis of modern states was frequently lifted out of its setting and used to support a political cynicism about collective forms of social change in any setting. In this chapter, I draw on human rights discourses and practices to contest the claim that humanist politics inevitably succumbs to repressive power. I draw on Foucault's concept of instrument-effects, a term that he uses to keep subjecthood and causal relations open-ended or ambiguous, to emphasize the multiple articulations of power. Hook describes the shift in subjecthood for the conditioned (civilized) body as creating a sense of "diffusely managed souls" through a process that Foucault referred to as "moral orthopedics." Docile bodies and moral souls seem to be Foucault's way of sidestepping both the suggestion of a Marxist or Weberian political community and the trap of mind–body dualism (for he was very attentive to the material aspects of bodies in power relations, and frequently alluded to a social body, albeit a passive one) (1997). But as Marcelo Suarez-Orozco (1992) noted, Foucault fails to account for torture in the post-colonial world. Nor does his analysis offer insight into why physicians and psychologists, the same professionals held up as social regulators in European states, became preferred targets of military violence in Latin American dirty wars.

Most scholars of contemporary El Salvador acknowledge that the combined experiences of liberation theology, repression, and revolutionary struggle created new forms of subjecthood in portions of the peasant population. I argued in chapter 2 that these processes strengthened forms of collective morality, but no doubt the emphasis on participation and assertiveness in base communities and the FMLN also rewarded forms of individual initiative. However, the question I ask here is, given that "diffusely managed" moral souls are instruments as well as effects (subjects as well as objects), what happens when subjecthood emerges in a challenge to a (still militarized) state that has to a degree modernized economically but eschewed social reforms, and, as I show in the following, a state that is cannibalizing its nation. I argue that emergence of the modern "regime" of human rights constitutes a transnational form of moral orthopedics that can be turned back on the repressive state.

Anthropologists themselves have exercised power in this way. Elaine Messer documented a progression of anthropological thought on human rights from early skepticism and concerns about cultural relativism to a more recent acceptance at least of minimal standards of human rights (1993). Many scholars have acted as human rights advocates in organizations such as the Guatemala Scholars Network and Cultural Survival. Many also helped develop ethnographically informed arguments for expanding human rights to include cultural or indigenous rights, economic rights, and the right to help plan and benefit from development. Anthropologists working in unstable political regimes have increasingly called for scholars to do a better job of what Taussig (1992) called, "writing against terror." (See also Binford 1996; Farmer 2003; and Starn 1991.)

Institutionalized violence has a long history in Latin America, even constituting a regional literary trope. But the hegemonic relationship that remains underexamined in the United States is the role played by the U.S. government in shaping regimes of state terror. The more than forty instances of U.S. military interventions in Latin America in the twentieth century noted by *New York Times* reporter Larry Rohter (1994) must now be amended to include the U.S. role in the ongoing human rights debacle in the "drug war" in Colombia (Kirk 2004), the 2002 coup against Hugo Chávez's elected government in Venezuela (Golinger 2008), and the 2004 coup against Haiti's president Jean-Bertrand Aristide (Democracy Now 2004). Sociologist Douglas Porpora went so far as to argue that the Reagan and Bush administrations' Central American policies warranted classification as a "Holocaust-like event" despite the fact that the death toll was an order of magnitude removed from the Nazi genocide, arguing that the Jewish vow "never again" loses meaning if citizens of democratic countries do not recognize and resist inhumane policies (1990). By financing and helping orchestrate the Salvadoran government's war against the FMLN, to the tune of over $7 billion in economic and military aid over more than a decade, he argued, the United States assisted in the systematic murder of men, women, and children who were noncombatants—journalists, priests, nuns, teachers, labor organizers, students, political figures, and others. "Roughly one percent of El Salvador's population was so destroyed" (1990, 7). Estimates of total political murders at the time of the cease-fire ranged from forty thousand to fifty thousand (Murray and Barry 1995), with seven thousand "disappeared" (probably dead) and a total death toll around eighty thousand (Montgomery 1995). Porpora made similar arguments about U.S. backing of the contra war against Nicaragua (at a cost of thirty thousand lives), itself following a civil war with a similar death toll against the U.S.-allied dictator Anastasio Somoza. Washington also supported (to a lesser extent) the Guatemalan military's genocidal war against the Mayan population (one hundred thousand civilians killed since 1960). What the Holocaust and U.S. Central American policy during the 1980s had in common, according to Porpora, was that in both cases powerful governments pursued policies that resulted "in ongoing, systematic murder and in both cases, the populations served by those governments (e.g., Germany and the United States) allowed it" (9).

Civilian casualties and suffering from wars have risen steadily in recent decades, and the skewed casualty lists say a great deal about hegemony in the world. Marcia Inhorn cites the recent restudy of the now famous *Lancet* article assertions on civilian mortality in Iraq, which resulted in a *raised* body count to 655,000 (Johns Hopkins Bloomberg School of Public Health 2007). When compared with numbers of U.S. military deaths in Iraq, at 4,183, the Iraqi toll is clearly a fraction of the Iraqi dead (Inhorn 2008). The skewed figures recall the current body counts in the Israeli invasion of Gaza, with 5 Israeli dead versus 500 Palestinian dead and 2,500 wounded, 20 percent of whom are estimated to be civilians, according to UN relief workers (Nissenbaum and Bangali 2009). The UN High Commission on Refugees (UNHCR) estimated that refugees and people displaced by violence worldwide totaled more than 50 million (Agier and Bouchet-Saulnier 2004).

Much like the skewed death tolls in El Salvador, the current wars represent what Giorgio Agamben has dubbed the increasingly prominent "state of exception" to the civilized state. He compared the modern refugee to *Homo sacer*, or the "sacred man" of Roman law—referring to a person formally exiled and excluded from civil rights, who could be killed by anyone without risk of sanction. Refugee status, according to Agamben (1998, 2000), results in one's biological life (zoe) becoming separated from one's political life (bios), or citizenship, with all the protections that once entailed. Yet, he argues, from the state's standpoint, a refugee crisis constitutes a standing affront to the "fiction" of nationhood; hence, those displaced by internal conflict are often viewed as threats to the state despite their civilian status.

This chapter seeks to "write against terror" by making an argument that human rights, including health rights, should be seen as "humanitarian narratives" that are essential components in the common project of imagining an international body politic—a project in the global age that we are already bound up in and cannot reject (Laqueur 1989).

Humanitarian Law and Medical Neutrality

The Salvadoran human rights record lends support to the thesis that military strategies that the United States funded and promoted in El Salvador during the 1980s violated Geneva Conventions protections for civilians and humanitarian services, and contributed to genocidal policies in the rural countryside. Three types of abuses are treated here: (a) aerial bombing and other attacks against civilian infrastructure and populations in rural areas, (b) targeted military attacks on FMLN mobile hospitals, and (c) military harassment impeding health-related and other humanitarian relief activities in rural villages repopulated by organized refugees.

The data in this chapter is somewhat unique in that it was gathered primarily through interviews with (and about) personnel working in medical and health-related services. I see respect for health work as a kind of "litmus test" for respect for human rights in general. (But it is important to point out that human rights abuses were directed at many kinds of civilian work, including union organizing, religious work, and popular education in the Salvadoran countryside.) The Geneva Conventions of 1949 and Protocol II (pertaining to civil conflicts) specify that medical units and transports shall be respected and protected at all times and shall not be the object of attack. The conventions and protocol specifically prohibit anticivilian policies such as destruction of crops or interfering with relief aid for civilians. Nearly all governments publicly claim to respect medical relief work. Both El Salvador and the United States are signatories to the conventions. The reality of civil wars, however, is that medical neutrality is poorly monitored and only weakly enforced. Since the 1970s, the International Committee of the Red Cross (ICRC) has tended to emphasize protection of political prisoners over medical neutrality per se in civil conflicts. The committee's personnel make periodic trips into conflicted areas and document medical neutrality violations observed, but one of the ICRC's understandings with governments of host countries is that such violations are kept confidential. As "guests" in the country, ICRC personnel claim that they are in no position to do more than mediate privately between warring parties about violations. (The French humanitarian organization, Médecins sans Frontières [MSF], which worked in Salvadoran refugee camps, favored a similar stance of official neutrality but has tended to be more vocal in protesting abuses than the ICRC [Redfield 2005].) While the ICRC enjoys great moral authority—few governments wish to become international pariahs by kicking out the Red Cross—in fact disputes rarely rise to this level. The ICRC chose not to defend medical neutrality on the premise that more lives are saved by maintaining an ICRC presence in countries at war, even in the face of repeated violations of the conventions (Armstrong 1985; and Blondel 1987).

Besides the ICRC, no international body exists to monitor these abuses. As a result, violations of medical neutrality receive relatively little attention internationally—they fall between the cracks of human rights and relief work. However, a variety of NGOs document these violations, and a considerable body of evidence suggests that violations of medical neutrality are common in civil wars (Cliff and Noormahomed 1988; Geiger 1993; Kiefer 1992; Lundgren and Lang 1989; Sabo and Kibirige 1989; and Weissman 2004). During the 1980s I volunteered with the National Central America Health Right Network, which documented such abuses (NCAHRN 1986; Physicians for Human Rights 1990; Smith 1987, 1988, 1989a, 1989b, 1989c, 1990; and Third Public Health Commission to El Salvador 1985).

Data on health rights abuses from both the Salvadoran and Nicaraguan civil wars showed that the vast majority of violations were carried out in the context of counterrevolutionary warfare using low-intensity conflict (LIC) strategies promulgated in the United States. Two clear categories of attacks emerged: (a) those by police and army units against NGO-sponsored civilian health efforts, and (b) those by the army and air force against rural clandestine health activities of the antigovernment rebels. Most targets were community-based projects serving marginalized populations. A tendency for community-based health workers to fall under fire in situations of civil strife has been noted by other scholars (Heggenhougan 1984; Green 1989; and Stark 1985). Jean Herve-Bradol (2004) went so far as to claim that humanitarian action during a conflict inevitably clashes with the established order and is therefore seen as subversive.

The finding that health activities, particularly when community-based, are not respected as neutral in counterrevolutionary warfare is consistent with the premise built into LIC strategy that no social activity is politically neutral. It is also a testament to the inherently political nature of community health work as a public activity. If, as I argue in this book, the project of healing both represents the political body symbolically and is formative in the sense that healing plays an important role in "community-making," then it follows that in a political struggle the control over, and definition of, health services become issues of contestation.

Anticivilian Warfare and the United States

The invasion of Iraq was famously justified by President George W. Bush on the grounds (later proved false) that Saddam Hussein had weapons of mass destruction and that, given Hussein's previous use of chemical weapons, banned under the Geneva Conventions, he could not be trusted. Few pundits weighing in on Bush's Iraq plans recalled the U.S. Air Force's wholesale destruction of the fleeing

Iraqi army during the final days of Desert Storm, a massive and blatant violation of laws of war. As I write this, news stories in the *New York Times* testify to heightened tensions in both Iraq and Afghanistan over alleged continued U.S. disregard for civilian casualties, which long ago passed the death toll of the 9/11 attacks on the World Trade Center and the Pentagon, and the plane crash in Shanksville, Pennsylvania. The U.S. "war on terror" since 2001 hurt the country's moral standing globally, but most scholars lay blame at the door of the Bush administration rather than seeing U.S. policies of covert and overt aid to repressive governments in a longer term perspective.

In El Salvador, human rights organizations in 1982–1983 noted a repeating pattern of increases in civilian killings immediately following approvals of military aid by the U.S. Congress (Doyle and Duklis 1990). After 1982, several U.S. and foreign medical workers based in the Salvadoran countryside reported that the Salvadoran Air Force used U.S.-supplied planes that indiscriminately bombed areas where rebels were active. Stanley (1996) reported that the bombardment became much more intense by late 1984 after the Reagan administration, alarmed by right-wing threats against the U.S. ambassador and concerned to boost election prospects for its favored presidential candidate, Napoleón Duarte, finally began to lean on Salvadoran army officers to clean up human rights abuses. The quid pro quo with the armed forces, according to Stanley, was a boost in U.S. military aid and training.[3]

Ramon Flores, a former Salvadoran medical student who worked in a displaced-person camp near the Guazapa volcano, witnessed the air war.

> People died because they did not receive care in time. Frequently after a bombing more than fifty badly wounded people would come, mostly children. More were stuck in the countryside, alive, but unable to walk. It was necessary to go out and find them. We had to care for these people with virtually no equipment and no trained personnel. I became sensitized to a reality I had not lived before. There would be stories in the paper about a great triumph of the army in such and such a zone. I began to see it was not as the newspapers said: Fifty terrorists killed. [Often] there were no guerrillas, only women, children and other civilians. If this was a triumph, then one had to ask what was being accomplished. (Frieden 1985)

One of the most credible reports came from Dr. Charles Clements, the U.S. physician introduced in chapter 3 who spent a year taking care of primarily civilian patients on the FMLN-occupied Guazapa volcano, twenty kilometers north of the capital. Clements reported that in early 1983 air raids had become "almost daily" events. In his 1984 book *Witness to War*, and in interviews I did with him that year in Washington, he gave detailed accounts of assisting whole villages to flee army operations by hastily improvising mixtures of diazepam, orange juice, and sugar to tranquilize infants so they would not cry and draw the fire of nearby troops. In prior army "sweep" operations there, he said, government troops had systematically killed any civilians they encountered, including children, old people, and livestock, even shooting holes in pots and dishes in an effort to make civilian life near the guerrillas impossible.

A former air force pilot who served in Vietnam, Clements investigated the aftermath of a firebomb attack in the Guazapa war zone and treated a woman with a third-degree thigh burn from a sizzling, sticky material that coagulated muscle and fat—much like napalm. In 1985 I photographed burn scars on the shoulder of a former Guazapa resident who described being hit by a napalm bomb. Dr. John Constable, a senior burn specialist from Massachusetts General Hospital, traveled to El Salvador in 1984 and examined patients whose wounds he described as "classically consistent" with napalm injuries (Biddle 1984). In a 1983 interview with a legislative fact-finding mission, Col. Rafael Bustillo, commander of the Salvadoran Air Force, reported that the military had in the past used Israeli napalm in rural areas. He credited U.S. advisors with "weaning the military away from napalming our own people" but underscored the importance of incendiaries to the war effort by commenting that "if we had not used [napalm] I would not be sitting here" (Biddle 1984).[4]

Clements (1984) also reported treating civilians with severe burns from U.S.-made white phosphorus rockets. Ignited by contact with air, white phosphorus embeds deeply in tissue where it can smolder for days, causing an extremely painful wound that often leads to death. Little could be done for victims except to attempt to put out the fire by continuously packing the wound with mud. In 1984 one of Clements's former patients, a thirty-eight-year-old peasant woman, described her daughter's death from this weapon known locally as "white fire" (*fuego blanco*): "That little plane kept flying overhead, searching. . . . that afternoon they massacred a lot of the people. That was when my daughter was wounded. I've never seen anything like the burning from the pieces that fell from the bomb. She got white blisters and then they turned red and then purple, and her leg got really hard and this awful smell of rot came out of it. There was nothing we could do" (Smith 1985).[5]

Confronted with allegations of supplying anticivilian weapons, U.S. military spokesmen insisted that white phosphorus rockets were only used only to "mark targets." But Clements contended that any evidence of civilian presence, including health clinics and schools, had become targets in Guazapa, which was designated a "free fire zone" by the Salvadoran army (1984).

Don North, a filmmaker and former ABC reporter in the Vietnam War, visited Clements in the war zone and produced a 1984 film titled *Guazapa* that documented an air force attack on a guinda of fleeing civilians. In our interview Clements called the routine attacks against civilians in FMLN-occupied rural areas "one of the grossest violations of the Geneva Conventions since Pol Pot's brutalities in Kampuchea." Janis Zadel, an American nurse who spent three years in FMLN-controlled areas, gave this account of the air raids:

> We had to leave the first hospital I worked at because of the bombing. The hospital was totally destroyed. A *brigadista* [paramedic] and her boyfriend were killed and a doctor was very seriously wounded. . . . Another bombing raid destroyed a clinic where I was working. Everyone was evacuated safely, but we lost a fair amount of medicine. Strafing from helicopters was even more scary. Pilots don't fly low and strafe unless they know their targets are all civilians, since a good shot with a high-powered rifle can kill the gunner. We were strafed frequently. (Frieden 1985)

In 1984 at medical aid meetings I attended in the United States, we began to hear requests for burn medicines from health workers in the Salvadoran countryside. Medical Aid for El Salvador, based in Los Angeles, launched a campaign to send Silvadene, an expensive antibiotic salve that was almost unavailable in Central America, for severe burns.

This kind of anticivilian warfare, called a "scorched earth" campaign by U.S. military advisers in Vietnam and El Salvador, was talked about openly at times by Salvadoran officers. In 1985 Col. Sigfrido Ochoa, commander of the army's Fourth Brigade in Chalatenango, held a press conference and announced that "To help cut civilian contact with the rebels, the program in Chalatenango prohibits civilian movement or residence in twelve free-fire zones. Air strikes and artillery bombardments now are being carried out indiscriminately in these areas" (*Dallas Morning News*, January 21, 1985; see also Montgomery 1995, 152). In an analysis after the war, U.S. military strategists confirmed the army's use of scorched-earth tactics in FMLN-occupied areas after 1985 but asserted that no civilians were present (Bracamonte and Spencer 1995). (In fact, routine bombing from 1983 to 1985 was precisely the reason so many civilians fled the rural areas.) A diplomatic cable sent from the U.S. Embassy in San Salvador to Washington noted that civilians killed by bombs were "something less than innocent bystanders" since they lived in rebel-controlled areas.[6] The bombing tactics were denounced in Americas Watch's 1985 report "Free Fire" as a flagrant violation of the laws of war.

In one eight-month period from 1983 to 1984 the Red Cross reported a surge of one hundred thousand persons fleeing the countryside (Montgomery 1995). In 1986, after increasing public criticism, the strategy was modified to reduce indiscriminate bombing and focus attacks more on areas where the population was closely identified with the insurgents. Such tactical bombing "to soften up the masas" prior to an army operation, was common in Operation Phoenix, a new LIC strategy showcased to reporters in 1986 as evidence of the Salvadoran army's newfound respect for human rights. Under this program, the army forcibly removed (instead of killing) civilians in guerrilla-occupied areas and transferred them to government-run camps (Montgomery 1995).

Although the bulk of abuses of international law were carried out by government troops, the FMLN also endangered civilians in rural areas in 1986 when guerrillas began planting homemade land mines in response to new army strategies. At the time, a new influx of U.S. transport helicopters allowed the army to drop platoons behind FMLN lines. Although the FMLN claimed that civilians knew the location of minefields, human rights data gathered by three progovernment agencies showed between 116 and 172 civilians injured by mines in the first six months of 1986. Americas Watch, which carried out one of the studies, concluded that FMLN mines caused more casualties than army mines due to poor warning systems (1986).

Premeditated Attacks on Medical Workers and Patients

In the late 1980s I collected dozens of reports of clandestine mobile clinics being targeted by army attacks. The army tacitly acknowledged that guerrilla-run clinics were targets when on several occasions its own press office claimed responsibility for attacking and "dismantling" FMLN mobile hospitals (for example, destruction of the El Coyolar medical unit described in the prologue). Other evidence that medical work was targeted came from multiple reports of intercepted radio communication between government pilots and headquarters. During an army invasion of the FPL rearguard in August 1984, Metzi (1988) reported, "One of the *compa* radio operators intercepted an ominous enemy transmission from the pilot of the circling plane: 'I've located the hospital. Send in the bombers'" (130). Schaull (1990) reported actually listening to such live radio exchanges on the FPL receiver. She reported that soldiers requested "an A-37 to bomb Tamarindo, and specifically, the hospital." The attack left the hospital in ruins, but there were no casualties because it was successfully evacuated.

Only two months after the El Coyolar incident, the armed forces press office again issued a report claiming credit for a surprise attack on an FMLN hospital, this one in a remote area of the department of San Vicente. Photographs provided to reporters by the army showed two dead bodies laid out side by side, dressed in camouflage gear with rifles laid alongside them.[7] The two were labeled foreign mercenary doctors and later identified as Dr. Gustavo Ignacio Isla Caceres, an Argentine medical doctor, and Madeleine Lagadec, a French nurse. On Radio Venceremos the FMLN said that patients at the hospital had been evacuated before the invasion but that the two foreign health workers, along with three Salvadoran paramedics and four teachers, had been captured alive before being murdered by paratroopers. This was confirmed in a 2007 interview I conducted with a former FMLN paramedic who said she helped evacuate patients during the attack. The U.S. Embassy called a press conference, which I attended, at which photos of armed guerrillas that the Salvadoran military claimed they found at the site were displayed. U.S. ambassador William Walker disputed FMLN claims of the site being a "hospital," claiming there was no building or structure at the site (the paramedic described a house in which Lagadec and a wounded patient were hiding when paratroopers arrived). After an autopsy was performed on Lagadec's body in France, the nurse's family made public a forensic report that supported their claim that she had been summarily executed at close range with six bullets after capture, and that she had been dressed in other clothes after the murder because the camouflage fatigues she was wearing in news photos had no bullet holes (suggesting that the military photos of the two in uniforms with rifles by their side had been staged). They cited similar evidence from Argentina that the doctor was also murdered at close range.

In a report on medical neutrality for *American Medical News* that I wrote that spring, I listed four other reports of army attacks on FMLN clinics in the previous year, which I had been unable to fully investigate, and several cases in which the army interfered with NGO relief aid to populations affected by the war (Smith 1989a). In one case a Spanish medical doctor was wounded in a war zone and European diplomats assisted to secretly evacuate him from the country to protect him from military reprisal or arrest, according to diplomatic sources.

In a recent memoir, former FPL physician Eduardo Espinoza (2007) related a wartime incident in San Vicente when he and four colleagues carried out an emergency cesarean section in a clandestine hospital while under mortar attack. Each successive round landed closer to the hospital, and finally, just after the surgical team fled the building carrying the patient, a round destroyed the hospital. Espinoza wrote that because proper targeting with a mortar involves an assistant using binoculars to correct coordinates after each firing, the medical team concluded that the hospital had been the objective of the bombardment.

With few exceptions, the FMLN respected government health facilities. Exceptions included a case I investigated in 1989, an FMLN mortar attack on a San Salvador military installation in which a projectile missed its military target, badly damaging a Ministry of Health clinic. One civilian was killed and ten health workers were wounded. Also, during a firefight in Zacatecoluca the same year, both government and guerrilla troops entered a hospital building endangering patients and workers.

Repeated requests by the ICRC to evacuate severely wounded guerrillas were turned down by the Salvadoran government. During the early 1980s the army did not take any guerrilla prisoners and was reputed to kill wounded rebel fighters. Under human rights pressure, this began to change by mid decade. A few small evacuations of wounded took place after 1987 following negotiations between the FMLN and newly elected president Napoleón Duarte. The right-wing ARENA government that succeeded Duarte in 1989 discontinued the policy, prompting a group of one hundred wounded and disabled guerrillas to occupy a downtown cathedral for three months to protest the blocked evacuations.

In a concentrated year-long documentation effort following the November 1989 guerrilla offensive, the Seattle-based International Commission on Medical Neutrality documented assassinations of four health workers (blamed on the government) and two sick persons (blamed on the FMLN); disappearances of seventeen wounded persons, five medical and allied health students, and one lay health worker (eighteen of which were blamed on the government, with four cases unclear); and arrests or detentions of one hundred sick or wounded persons, twenty-eight lay health workers, six medical students, five paramedics, and twenty-five salaried health workers (all by government forces) (ICMN 1991).

Health Rights in the Repopulated Villages (1987–1992)

After the 1987 return of refugees and displaced people to northeast Chalatenango, soldiers at roadblocks confiscated health education materials, which they classed as "subversive materials." For this reason health promoters began traveling to the city for training. Two cases of abuse that I investigated were linked to urban training of Chalatenango dental promoters. In July 1989 the army raided a house in San Salvador, arresting a Brazilian oral physician and nurse team and a Salvadoran promoter in training. The foreigners were deported, but before leaving they reported to the press that they had been held blindfolded with no food or water during three days of interrogation. The physician said he had been kept awake all night by screams from the next room where his student, a dental health promoter, was being beaten. "It seemed like a school of torture. They were experimenting with different methods. The officer in charge kept saying things like 'Good. That's it!' and 'You're getting better.' to the younger soldiers who were beating Victor," reported the physician, who had previously worked for Medicos del Mundo. In an interview with me, the nurse denied army charges that the two belonged to a "terrorist cell" and said that they were affiliated with the Catholic Archdiocese, which I confirmed. She said that during their ordeal a Treasury Police soldier told her, "You work with poor people and that makes you suspicious" (Smith 1989c).

Two months later, in September, the National Guard raided a San Salvador health clinic, capturing twelve oral health promoters (most from Chalatenango) and eight patients. After pressure from the Church and human rights groups, they were released a week later. They reported being held for forty-eight hours blindfolded and without food, with their hands cuffed and raised over their heads. They said they were forced to do extended calisthenics, hit with clubs, and punched on the heads by soldiers wearing brass knuckle–like metal rings on their fingers.[8]

In January 1989 the Chalatenango Diocese began training health promoters to document health and human rights violations in the repopulated communities. In 1995 I analyzed the diocese's reports for the final three years of the war. There were

reports of seventy-one popular health workers detained by the army for long periods, usually at roadblocks, despite the fact that most carried cards identifying them
as health workers. Eleven health workers were threatened, twenty were arrested
(including a vaccination team carrying a letter from the Ministry of Health), and
eighteen wounded civilians were detained or arrested, including two U.S. reporters
wounded by mortar fire. Six health clinics in repopulated villages were attacked by
army fire, as was an International Red Cross ambulance. Five clinics were searched
by soldiers, who often stole or destroyed medicines.

In this period there were repeated incursions of Salvadoran army troops into
the repopulated villages and forty-six reports of army soldiers opening fire in or
near the new civilian settlements. Ninety-two repatriated refugees were wounded
or killed by warfare in a two-year period, with army soldiers blamed in 70 percent
(or sixty-six) of the cases, the FMLN blamed in three cases, and the origin of fire
unknown in twenty-three cases. In addition to banning entry of medical and
school supplies, the army also blocked food deliveries from January through
August 1988, forcing several resettlements to adopt food rationing (Sollis 1992).
During a July 1989 visit to Guarjila, Mariana, a local health promoter told me

> Right now we have a very serious shortage of medicines. The clinic is prac-
> tically empty. Some of us bought a few items in Chalatenango [the town],
> but right now we're even out of aspirin, which is very much in demand to
> lower fevers of children. It has been three months since the army road-
> block let anything pass. We don't even have injections to stop hemorrhag-
> ing in women giving birth. Dr. Ana [a Catholic pediatrician] visits when she
> can get through. But lately no doctors have been allowed to arrive.

> Although the Church obtained permission from the military high
> command to bring in medical supplies, shipments were often turned
> back at roadblocks. In July 1989, the Army captured a truckload of medi-
> cines on its way to Chalatenango and arrested two Church employees,
> who were interrogated for four days. In August 1991 foreign nurses and
> physicians working for the Diocese were turned back at a roadblock and
> shown a copy of a blacklist supplied by the Armed Forces High Command
> that included their names, plus those of three popular health system
> workers and five foreign development workers in the repopulations.[9]

Humanitarian Narratives and the Body Politic

Anthropologies of the body provide a theoretical toolbox for probing the nature of
the credibility and legitimacy accorded human rights documentation. Two aspects
stand out: (a) the universality of the body, and hence the compelling nature of
claims based on suffering (Scarry 1985), and (b) the appeal to medicolegal civil
authority that can be traced both to the eighteenth-century revolution of empiri-
cism in European medicine (Jewson 1976) and to the subsequent incorporation of

medical expertise into legal proceedings and juridical authority (Foucault 1975, 1979, 1980).

While cultural differences exist as to permissible forms of violence, a moral economy of violence against persons appears to be ubiquitous in human cultures, as does the quest for revenge (Boehm 1999). After interviewing scores of witnesses to such crimes, I became convinced there was validity in the claim that stories of human rights abuses resonate across cultural, class, and national boundaries. The power in such stories derives from the universal existential contingency of consciousness embedded in a human body that can be injured. Such testimonies are "humanitarian narratives," a term that Thomas Laqueur coined to describe the compelling nature of medical case reports. In his study of the advent of medical case narratives in the eighteenth century, Laqueur pointed to their reliance on empirical detail as a sign of truth, and their basis in "the personal body, not only as the locus of pain but also as the common bond between those who suffer and those who would (should) help, and as the object of a scientific discourse through which the causal links between an evil, a victim, and a benefactor are forged" (1989, 177).

In expanding his observation to human rights testimonies, I would argue that in addition to enhancing credibility, there is an individualizing or personalizing effect of such reports owing to their reliance on testimonials of victims and witnesses. Like the "humanitarian narratives" of medical cases, a human rights story particularizes suffering, thereby promoting a personal relationship between the reader/listener and the victims; also the narrative specifies a particular cause–effect matrix that points to a means for relief. When this story is interspersed with legalistic presentations of evidence for the alleged abuse, the accounts gain their full power in public relations.

In a civil war, the impossibility of investigating many reported cases combined with the necessity of protecting witnesses can lead human rights workers to resort to categorized abuses and accounts of abstract suffering (Binford 1996). But, as a former health rights activist, I would argue that this becomes a different kind of "body count" for evaluating war and, when combined with personal stories, carries moral power as an alternative to dominant narratives of state militarism in transnational discourse, lending voice to those living in Agamben's "state of exception." Even though calls for intervention may go unheeded for years, this critical sanction assists struggles to designate violators as outside the moral community of nations. Such a stigma endangers vital trade and political alliances, thereby undermining the effectiveness of politicians.

U.S. Intervention: A "Two-Track" Strategy on Human Rights

It would be a mistake to see the United States as the main arbiter of these discourses. Just as Guantanamo and the Iraq War have undermined American moral authority in the present, during the 1980s, the poor human rights record of the Salvadoran government influenced policy in Europe and the rest of the world to a much greater degree than in Washington (Porpora 1990). Mexico and France, for example, had official diplomatic relations with the FMLN during the 1980s and extended aid to the insurgency. European humanitarian relief offices dotted the capital and clandestine European doctors were linchpins in the FMLN's medical units.

Unfortunately, manipulation of human rights data became a regular aspect of policymaking by the Reagan administration throughout the decade. When the U.S. government boosted military aid to El Salvador in early 1981, the Democrat-controlled Congress, alarmed by the death squad accounts, required the administration to demonstrate that the Salvadorans were making progress on respect for human rights prior to granting new aid requests. The semiannual "dog-and-pony" show of hearings, some of which I attended, made a great deal of noise but often had little substance. The effect was almost tragicomic as State Department spokespersons pointed to slides of Salvadoran student protests as evidence of new army tolerance, and Sen. John McCain red-baited Aryeh Neier, the director of Human Rights Watch, while waving a copy of Chairman Mao's *Little Red Book* in the air.

Reagan's policy in the early 1980s was effectively a "two-track" strategy on human rights. Whereas under the Carter administration military aid had been coupled to pressure for economic reforms, under the conservative ideology of the Reagan administration key redistributory efforts such as the land reform plan were reduced to window dressing. On the one hand, policymakers made public appeals for democracy, respect for human rights, and a "clean counterinsurgency." But behind the scenes officials helped cover up evidence linking high-level Salvadoran authorities to well-publicized atrocities (see Krauss 1993) while exerting pressure for legal reforms that would give the army more leeway to imprison civilian supporters of the FMLN (Montgomery 1995).[10] This duality reflected the Pentagon's desperate need to shake off the ghost of Vietnam and laid important ideological groundwork for the two Bush administrations' policies in the Middle East.

A book-length sympathetic account of the U.S. LIC project in El Salvador quoted a military intelligence specialist explaining that "the [need for] improvement in human rights was presented to the Salvadorans as a way of getting more military aid, which they needed. It was a reasonable proposition and they accepted it" (Manwaring and Prisk 1988). And so in the capital both death squads and official security forces began to limit their targets to leaders of organizations, to bury the bodies instead of leaving them on roadsides, and to torture with less detectable' methods such as forced calisthenics, captives forced to stand or kneel for hours, and more reliance on psychological torture.[11] By the mid-1980s military aid had increased tenfold and U.S. personnel were intimately involved—training troops, orchestrating military strategy, and providing intelligence for selection of air raid targets (MacLean 1987; Montgomery 1995; and Rosa 1993). At the same time the contra war next door was escalating as Reagan vowed to overthrow the Nicaraguan revolution while drawing the line against communism in El Salvador. This shifted the terms of the policy debate. In the words of political scientist Lars Schoultz, "The original question was: Is the instability in Central America caused by poverty or by Communist adventurism? Over time the question became: How much Communist adventurism exists? Poverty became irrelevant" (Schoultz 1987, 63).

In a classic analysis of the views of U.S. policymakers on Central America, Schoultz found no evidence that Reagan policy was motivated by strategic trade issues, or vital security interests, or Soviet involvement. He concluded that much of the Reagan-era obsession with Central America was related to how the region became cast as a "symbol of U.S. power and resolve." Political instability in the region became a showdown for the United States because of the challenge it presented to longstanding U.S. military and economic domination hegemony in Latin America. Despite Reagan's persistent failure to produce evidence of Cuban or Soviet adventurism, the belligerent Cold War accusations continued as the popular justification for intervention to the point where the rhetoric actually "creat[ed] a vital interest" in itself (Schoultz 1987, 279)—justifying military strategies of "showing the flag" or "projecting U.S. power" in the region.

Col. John Wagelstein, former head of the U.S. military team in El Salvador, referred to intervention as a "laboratory" for development of a post-Vietnam LIC strategy, which he predicted would "be useful to the next generation of security and advisory practitioners in the Third World." Writing in *Military Review*, he warned that "low-intensity" was a misleading term because it reflected the level of violence only from a military viewpoint. Instead, he called LIC warfare "total war at the grassroots," involving "political, economic, and psychological warfare," with the military having the least important role.[12]

In press statements, U.S military spokesmen emphasized the nonmilitary "nation-building" aspects of LIC policy—for example, land reform and U.S. AID funds for campaign ads—but their rhetoric was belied by the growing scale of U.S. military involvement. Development, like human rights, took a back seat to the war effort, and funding was allocated accordingly. A congressional study of U.S. economic aid to El Salvador concluded that a full three quarters of aid to El Salvador served military and military-related programs, and USAID spent more than 40 percent of funds on loans and guarantees for businesses rather than basic needs or long-term development (Hatfield, Leach, and Miller 1987).

That human rights reporting was influential in reducing the carnage in El Salvador is without question. The frequent visits by U.S. civilian delegations, combined with reporting by Americas Watch and other human rights organizations, frequently put the Reagan administration on the defensive about the war, and by mid decade the executive branch realized it could not sustain military aid flows without demonstrating that death squad murders had been reduced. While the killing machine was racheted down in the cities, funding and military strategy shifted to take advantage of new U.S.-supplied Vietnam-vintage air power such as A-37 ground attack jets, A-47 gunships, reconnaissance aircraft, and helicopter gunships (Nelson 1985; and Stanley 1996). The air war became the new focus in human rights and antiwar efforts, and this criticism led to cut-backs in plans to send more A-47 aircraft to El Salvador in 1984 (Cody 1984).[13] In general, however, given the restrictions on travel in rural El Salvador, establishing visibility in contested rural areas remained a major challenge for human rights monitoring and relief work.

Psychological Warfare . . . or Low-Visibility Conflict?

The usual explanation from the military for turning back aid shipments to conflicted areas was to deprive the FMLN of food or medical resources. However, the sweeping (and violent) nature of interference with health work in marginalized areas make this justification incomplete, except in the most paranoid reading of National Security Doctrine (a view that prevailed during the first two to three years of the war) in which every citizen was potentially a guerrilla. In a 1988 interview, Col. Mauricio Vargas, then chief of military operations, responded to my questions about army attacks on medical facilities by claiming that any medical operation not registered with the Ministry of Health was "illegal," whether civilian or guerrilla-run. He argued that Geneva Conventions protections did not apply to the Salvadoran civil war, which he dubbed "an illegal Marxist-Leninist insurgency." This view was out of line with positions of most nations, which have increasingly recognized humanitarian law as applying to civil wars (Ferrell 2005). (But in the post-9/11 world, Colonel Vargas's words sound eerily reminiscent of Bush administration claims about Islamic terrorism.)

Health services for combatants, as well as civilians, are in theory protected under the Geneva Conventions, although international law states that clinics should clearly identify themselves. In El Salvador, FMLN medical personnel argued that to display white flags or Red Cross emblems would invite attack. Indeed, on several occasions the air force used information from the International Red Cross about planned deliveries of medical aid or evacuation of guerrilla wounded to stage air attacks on rendezvous sites (Clements 1984; and Stanley 1996). Aware of these practices, even relief workers in "safe" (nonconflicted areas) learned to maintain low profiles. Pablo, a German physician with the FPL, ventured two reasons why the army attacked guerrilla hospitals:

> Number one, a hospital doesn't put up much resistance, and the army needs successes. There were only a few security people guarding them.

Even when our sanitarios were armed, the girls didn't know how to use the guns. They'd never had to fight. So if you want to report a lot of guerrilla dead, it's the easiest way. Number two, was for strategic reasons: they knew the attacks had a psychological impact on our troops. I think this was more important than the rationale of taking out the hospital because it was a resource for the guerrillas. One of the worst fears of a compa was to be in the hospital without a means to defend himself. To attack the hospital damaged morale. Compas became more afraid of what would happen if they were wounded [and the hospital was destroyed].

In 1995 I asked Felipe, the popular health organizer, why he thought NGO health work in rural areas was viewed with such suspicion by the army. He grew very thoughtful, then replied:

The truth is that during the war, those who opposed the struggle for social justice took health work as supportive of the left. Even after the peace, the work of the popular organizations is always taken as the work of the left, because it is regarded in a prestigious way by communities that have organized themselves. But the work of health is not political so much as a response to need. On the other hand, it is political in a sense, in that our work is based on the premise that communities have a right to take care of themselves, when they can't rely on the state.

Ramon Flores, the medical student imprisoned for aiding displaced persons in Guazapa, interpreted the army's interference with relief work as a way of keeping the nature of the war in the countryside under wraps.

If foreigners documented what is happening with refugees, it would be a problem for the government. It would be evidence of how they are fighting, and who they are harming in their war of extermination against the people. They wouldn't be able to say they are killing communists, because testimony and photographs would show that they are attacking children and elderly. . . . They captured . . . those who coordinate the work in the camps . . . [and] "disappeared" people to create terror. Because of this many people left, including priests, catechists, members of the Red Cross and the Green Cross.

In 1983 the government began a campaign against health workers. They claimed that we had defamed the government to the foreign press, damaging the country's image. . . . Many people were imprisoned. About 18 people were accused of being "doctors collaborating with the rebel forces." They seized me and my entire family. We [were] "disappeared" for 22 days, after which my wife and children were freed and I was taken to prison. I spent one year there. (Frieden 1985)

Lily Hoffman (1989) lends insight here, noting that possession of medical credentials translates into a license for exploitation of scarce and valued resources. Thus, medical practice carries a "symbolic power" (as well as power in the conventional sense) through its control of services and funds. In a similar vein, Ruth Stark (1985) observed that their role as healers enabled lay health workers to gain social status and power. Because health care delivery involves issues of social control, she concluded that political leaders in a community would be very sensitive to the health worker's power, particularly in a situation of civil unrest. Perhaps it is the threat of this credibility that explains why eight of the eleven of the Salvadoran physicians who formed a National Committee for the Defense of Patients, Workers, and Health Institutions in the early 1980s were disappeared or murdered (Lundgren and Lang 1989). Similarly, writing about South Africa, Alex Butchart and colleagues (1998) traced the influence of professionals and humanitarian ideas in Steve Biko's promotion of "Black Consciousness," which helped legitimize the struggle against apartheid. In the post-apartheid era, mental health professionals drew on ideals of primary health care to delegitimize state propaganda that sought to pathologize violence by black males. Such professional and humanitarian voices would have high credibility and would compete with official accounts in the international arena. The elite discourses of LIC strategy and the euphemisms used in military propaganda are treated in more detail in chapter 5.

Toward a Transnational Anthropology of State Terror

Although concepts of human rights are often posed in opposition to local culture in anthropology, the prevalence of human rights discourse in El Salvador became a rich field of cultural innovation. One day in 1987 when I asked a Salvadoran friend if he had seen my friend Lisa, he replied by creating a new verb form: "Creo que ella fue al campo—esta derecho-humanizando" ["I think she went to the countryside—she's 'human right-zing' "]. An American physician working in the Mesa Grande refugee camp told me he had seen refugees practicing their "testimonios" about the violence (thus supporting anthropological interpretations of testimonials as socially shaped, e.g., see Stephen 1994). As someone who participated in documenting political crimes, I was particularly interested in the wider-scale political "instrument-effects" of human rights reporting in a low-intensity war. Just as occurred during the recent Iraq War, spokespersons in the U.S. Embassy in San Salvador often dismissed inconvenient crimes attributed to their military allies as the product of a "violent culture"—deflecting attention away from transnational contributions to political repression. Anthropology during the 1980s was complicit in casting culture as predominately near and intimate. Taussig (1992) famously called for a "refunctioning of anthropology" to turn ethnography's "resolute gaze away from the poor and powerless to the rich and powerful—to current military strategies of "low-intensity warfare" . . . [and] the role of memory in the cultural construction of the authority of the modern state" (51).[14] Philippe Bourgois issued his own challenge to the discipline when he testified before Congress about fleeing a scorched-earth army operation with hundreds of civilians while conducting fieldwork in Chalatenango (1982, 1991). Elaine Messer (1993); Carolyn Nordstrom (1992, 1997); Carol Greenhouse, Elizabeth Mertz, and Kay Warren (2002); and Diane Nelson (2002) have been among those who have incorporated state and paramilitary violence into transnational ethnographic analyses, shaping new approaches to structural power and broadening the purview of culture.

There is no denying the interested nature of state terror. Events documented in this chapter involved machineries of terror that were imprecise in their functioning and targeted victims by vilifying whole social and political categories, allowing officials plausible deniability. When the social education of a soldier includes messages that "those who organize meetings are selling out the country to foreign communists," there is little need to give precise orders, and the risk to officers remains low. In order to "fix" certain social categories as threatening, successful LIC warfare depends on maintaining a high degree of political polarization, fear, and distrust.

Likewise, human rights protests have consequences. They contributed to ending the Salvadoran war. International outrage over the 1989 army murders of the six Jesuit priests prompted Congress to make deep cuts in military aid, which compelled the army to cooperate with peace negotiations. Norms of international law are now embedded in national laws, constitutions, or penal codes in most nations and are the basis for the International Criminal Court. The North Atlantic Treaty Organization (NATO) bombing of Kosovo to prevent Serbian abuses against ethnic Albanians helped establish a precedent for international coalitions to undertake moral interventions to mitigate greater civilian bloodshed (Ferrell 2005).[15]

This chapter emphasizes the productivity or generative aspect of a humanist discourse based on suffering bodies, which could be regarded as a transnational moral orthopedics that affects the perceived legitimacy of nation-states. Once the premises of humanism become accepted and written into international codes and national ideals, it becomes reasonable for both citizens and those shunted into "spaces of exception" such as refugee camps and war zones to demand that offending states recognize standards of dignity. Conventional human rights discourses, however, may be interpreted in ways that serve hegemonic interests. And documentation of abuses depends on access by credible witness to scenes of crimes. Successful LIC warfare depends on control of visibility. The necessity to keep the real nature of LIC warfare invisible in El Salvador had to do not only with public relations in El Salvador but also with minimizing opposition to the war in the United States. Doctors, nurses, and other professionals who documented abuses, spoke to the press, and testified before Congress played important roles in making the practices of the state visible to citizens and to the international body politic.

Of course, knowledge and agency at high levels of a military and foreign policy apparatus are never sufficient explanation of genocide-like events. Recent work on state terror tends to confirm Hannah Arendt's "banality of evil" thesis, which argues that genocidal policies cannot be blamed in any simple way on moral depravity or psychological deviance. These practices are aided by silent complicity and moral indifference on the part of ordinary people who make up bureaucracies, write news stories, and vote in elections. Americans feel removed from foreign interventions that do not put large numbers of U.S. soldiers at risk, and, as the Iraq War has shown, in the absence of a draft, most citizens fail to engage with the destructive nature of a foreign war, allowing the imperial presidency great leeway in pursuing militaristic goals. Increasingly corporate control of the media and cuts in foreign news bureaus worsen that isolationism (Arendt 1963; Fein 1979; Kuper 1981; and Porpora 1990).

Explaining foreign wars to U.S. citizens requires more than human rights discourses. Such narratives must have accompanying sociocultural and political analysis to put abuses in a context that helps answer "Why" questions, and to place the war in historical perspective. For example, those who looked primarily to human rights as criteria for evaluating U.S. intervention faced the quandary after 1985 of determining whether the drop-off from one thousand political murders per month in the early 1980s to only one hundred murders per month five years later should be interpreted as political reform (when no significant reduction in military control had occurred).[16] When terror becomes an everyday event, there is a desensitizing effect. Stanley (1996, 230) observed that while violence levels in the capital stabilized at lower levels in the late 1980s, the actual numbers of political murders remained higher than in the last half of 1979, which at the time was regarded as an extremely bloody period. (Likewise, El Salvador today has one of the highest homicide rates in Latin America, but since causation for common crime is more complex than that for political abuses, this is seldom treated as the same international "emergency" that human rights crimes evoke.)

In addition, the peace process is incomplete. Despite the UN Truth Commission in 1992 that attributed 85 percent of human rights abuses to government forces—impunity remains intact. Relatively few of the Salvadoran officers named by the commission were purged. Nor have the U.S. military trainers and suppliers of weaponry to the Salvadoran army been called to account. The only criminal convictions have involved two Salvadoran officers and lower-level troops tried for high-profile cases that involved murders of Americans or internationally known individuals (e.g., the six Jesuit priests in 1989), and several of those convicted were later released from prison.

In 2002 two former Salvadoran officers living in the United States were convicted of crimes against civil rights for orders that led to the torture of individuals (who are today U.S. citizens). The case provided insight into the enormous scale of atrocities that remain alive in the memories of victims and families while mass murderers still walk the streets and contemplate comfortable retirement in gated communities. This is a living history that should inform U.S. foreign policy—given the extraordinary number of Iraqi dead from both Desert Storm and the 2003 Iraq War (a far larger number than any human rights atrocities laid at the feet of Saddam Hussein). Would such policies prevail if the United States recognized the International Criminal Court, and its officials could be prosecuted under similar standards to those that the Bush administration so frequently cited to condemn foreign leaders like Mahmoud Ahmadinejad or Kim Jung Il?

As Inhorn (2008) points out, "when it comes to war there are trails of human misery that take generations to overcome. War is bad for human health and well-being on multiple levels. . . . [and] precludes the possibility of the Alma Ata's Declaration's goal of 'Health for All'" (422). But war has the awful legacy of being both an "in-your-face" affront and a horror that we simultaneously repress. All the more so when we are citizens of a country that boasts a larger military than all others combined. Anthropologists are well positioned to elucidate these connections. To see and yet not speak out is another kind of violence.

5

<hr>

Pacification

Psychological Warfare and the Uses of Medicine

pacify: 1a: to allay anger or agitation: placate, soothe. b: to make benign or amicable: appease, propitiate. 2a: to restore to a tranquil state: quiet, settle. b: to reduce to a submissive state, especially by force of arms: subdue "U.S. Marines . . . went in as early as 1910 to pacify the country."—*Time*.

—*Webster's Third International Dictionary*

Before we can appreciate (the subversive form) we need first to work through the form it butts against, namely the romance . . . the catharses of the fantasy of order by which the conquest of the New World has been so constantly rendered.

—Taussig (1987, 288)

Military literature is replete with references to the fact that a properly fought low-intensity conflict (LIC) cannot stand public scrutiny and therefore must entail what U.S. general John Galvin (1990) calls a "war of information." The problems of public scrutiny go far beyond security considerations; they result from LIC strategy of muddying the criteria dividing military combatants from civilians—the same vital distinction that forms the basis for international humanitarian laws on conduct in wars.

Military analyst and LIC promoter Sam Sarkesian was particularly frank in warning of the difficulty in establishing a national consensus for unconventional conflicts, which he called "a direct contradiction of the American way of war" (1993, 8–9). Taking the offensive in LIC, he noted, may involve covert operations "that are particularly uncomfortable for a democratic system" (20). The end of the Cold War did not change this fact. After 2003, a series of U.S.-financed counterinsurgency tactics in Iraq were undertaken with similar apparent disregard for humanitarian goals. Nation-building served as crude public relations for the civilian human rights debacle that emerged from the American invasion and occupation (Chatterjee 2004).

In testimony before Congress during the Iran-Contra affair hearings of the late 1980s, Oliver North said, "There is great deceit [and] deception practiced in conduct of covert operations. They are in essence a lie" (Klare and Kornbluh 1988, 16). LIC advocate William Yarborough wrote, "Since Americans believe in the right to legitimate protest, it falls to the lot of U.S. counter-insurgency doctrine to sort out the differences between legitimate protest and subversion. Sometimes the line between these two becomes very thin indeed" (1989, 113).

U.S. general Fred Woerner described counterinsurgency war in Latin America as "provid[ing] a security shield" behind which democracy and development could be achieved (Woerner 1990). Yet, far from the "hearts and minds" images often associated with LIC, this form of warfare is not primarily a "soft" conflict that relies on persuasion and nation-building; rather, as data presented in chapter 4 demonstrates, it is a particularly dirty warfare, the details of which must remain hidden. In El Salvador, it was a war fought on two fronts with two faces—the visible urban face, with surgical strikes on terrorists and humanitarian aid for civilians caught up in the (terrorist-caused) violence, and the invisible, rural face in which terror was directed at civilian supporters and even "potential supporters" of movements seeking political reform. Both faces were always present.

Taking this more dialectical view, a better term for LIC might be "low-visibility conflict" (Nelson-Pallmeyer 1990). The human rights record in El Salvador forces us to question interpretations that paint nation-building and pacification as rectifications of former repressive policies. Rather, policies to "humanize" the war (for consumption by international observers) were often carried out by the same officers who were overseeing terror tactics in the countryside. The goal was to keep both aid and international observers away from insurgents, to "remove the category of the civilian" in areas where guerrillas were active, and in less remote areas where this was not possible (usually because of high visibility), tactics had to be made to appear to pacify or co-opt, rather than coerce.

In this chapter I present a series of vignettes on the ways that medicine functioned as a key signifier in the Salvadoran government's "war against health"—a term that I use to refer to both systemic violence and counterinsurgency campaigns. My attempts to gain in-depth interviews with state authorities, or to "study up" (both during and after the war), were often countered with an invitation to a formal social event or a carefully orchestrated group interview. Some of these accounts are based on such encounters. I show the use of the medical promise as pacification—medicine's "sheep's clothing" to disguise the wolves of state terror. These awkward martial demonstrations of compassion had their counterparts in the urban "fantasy of order" that the Ministry of

Health presented to inquiring publics, most of whom were fortunate enough not to have to depend on its services.

Public Health as a Gift Relationship

Foucault described power as "tolerable only on condition that it mask a substantial part of itself. Its success is proportional to its ability to hide its mechanisms" (1980, 86). In Benedict Anderson's study of nationalism, he equated the preferred vocabulary of the nation-state with the rhetoric of kinship and home—both representing natural ties, which are unchosen and therefore blessed with the "halo of disinterestedness" (1983). Only such a benign, disinterested nation that has its people's welfare at heart can ask for sacrifices. Healing, with its association with family and unconditional love, serves as an especially convincing façade.

Symbols of the medical "cure" as charm or fetish were prominent features of the Salvadoran state's self-representations. The following account traces the medical fetish to the origins of the ORDEN network of rural vigilantes and anticommunist death squads.

Don Lito (a pseudonym) was an elderly campesino from rural Chalatenango who spoke at length about the origins of the civil war with writer María López Vigil. This was his tale of the military's promise of aid when a general came to town soliciting members for ORDEN. Here he cites Gen. José Alberto Medrano giving a speech to residents:

> Here in ORDEN we're learning to be good brothers who help each other out mutually. If in this cantón there is no clinic, all together, without exception, we're going to unite to work together on that. We're going to form a directiva. The PCN, our party, is here to guide us so that we can learn to work as a community. And here we will build a clinic so that you don't have to go to Suchitoto, you won't have to go to Ilobasco, and you won't have to go to San Salvador (for medical care). There'll be a doctor right here, and a nurse, and medicines! That's how we'll solve our problems! Do you agree?

Don Lito described rural citizens as enthusiastic about Medrano's promises: "People responded with applause, saying 'cachimbón!' He made so many promises—a new highway, a school, a priest, [he was going to resolve] all the needs of the cantón. He gave an identification card to all those willing to collaborate." But the reforms never materialized: "ORDEN? Shit! ORDEN never did any of that stuff. This ORDEN never did one thing! I remember that the only thing they did in my town was the clinic. But that work wasn't done by ORDEN, but by the people. It was just a little cantón, and we put in 100 days of work, each man, to construct that clinic. It wasn't ORDEN. . . . ORDEN has never done anything good" (López Vigil 1987, 26–28).

WHILE STUDYING THE Ministry of Health clinic in San Pedro del Lago, Chalatenango, in 1993 (see chapter 6) I heard stories of a local Salvadoran army program to recruit teenage boys to participate in a forty-member Red Cross youth organization. The local nurse described the program as similar to a Boy Scout troop—just a bunch of good-natured boys trying to be good citizens. But Marco, a local vendor I met, said there was a lot more to the story. The attraction of membership for the local boys, Marco said, was the army's promise (similar to that of ORDEN) of an identification card so that if they happened to be on a bus stopped by soldiers in one of their forced recruitment drives, the boys with ID cards for the youth group would be let go.

"That's why so many joined up," explained "They were organized like soldiers, each team had a commander, and subcommander, and everyone had someone they had to answer to." In addition to doing some health tasks like talks on cholera and planting trees for reforestation, the youth received training in civil defense and the army issued them guns. Some of them had duties of staying up each night and guarding the town. "Mostly they stared at the stars and smoked marijuana," said Marco. But he told a story of one night when the boys were playing around, "and taking drugs," and two of them shot at each other. One was killed, and the other was wounded. But when local people took the wounded boy to the San Salvador military hospital for treatment, the hospital authorities said he was not eligible for treatment there.

"Can you believe that?" he asked me, "They said the injury wasn't their responsibility."

IN THE LATE 1980S THE Armed Forces press office issued constant invitations to reporters to attend one-day "civic–military actions," essentially state-sponsored giveaways, with clowns, entertainment, and medical consults in rural towns to help the government build influence near areas where the FMLN had an active following. People would come from miles around to get the free food and medicines. In 1986, Col. James J. Steele, the commander of the U.S. Military Group in El Salvador, remarked on the high interest in psychological operations and civic action in the Salvadoran army, which he described as "far greater than anything we saw in Vietnam. It's an integral part of what they're doing. . . . They are training Psy-Op experts for every unit. We've played a role in that process, and I think it's one of the things we can be really proud of. They're putting out a lot of leaflets. They're using loudspeakers. They're using radio spots very effectively" (Manwaring and Prisk 1988, 321).

Martín-Baró (1990) observed that such pacification strategies were designed to work through "key communicators" (113) or people who are social role models, and worked their effects through a form of psychological "transference," in which the prestige attached to good works becomes associated with the government and the military, enhancing the reputation of authorities with local people. There are hardly better candidates than doctors and healing for this civic–military hat trick.

I asked a church worker with long experience in the country if she thought this was effective. She opined that it probably was in areas where the government had remained in control. "But why would the army giving out gifts make people patriotic," I asked? She replied: "It's easy, and it makes you feel special to have that powerful person, the doctor, smile at you and pay attention to you. It must mean you're pretty special, and that's something to people who've been devalued."

In fact, pacification programs did not always achieve their ends. The first such effort in El Salvador was a massive project called the National Plan in 1983, a combination military and civic-action project designed by U.S. military advisors to reassert government influence in the economically important provinces of San Vicente and Usulután where the FMLN had been operating freely.[1] As in the Vietnam War, the plan "placed emphasis on civic action and developmental projects behind a security screen" (Manwaring and Prisk 1988, 224). It involved the Salvadoran government's agricultural, economic, health, and education ministries as well as the armed forces. A central component was the U.S. advisors' training of thirty-six mobile *cazador* (hunter) companies of thirty soldiers each, who were to remain in the area long term. Although the program seemed to be working in its early months, it began to fall apart due to faltering government commitment and a guerrilla counteroffensive. The FMLN conducted its own program of political education (called consientización) to counter the government propaganda. They broke up large concentrations of combatants into small groups to interact more with civilians living in local villages. Months later, when government trucks arrived with goods, the peasants in the area gave the appearance of cooperation, but after benefiting from the aid, they refused to cooperate with the army's efforts to organize civil patrols. In effect, the gift was received but not reciprocated (Montgomery 1995).

Because of organized resistance from the peasants who had been previously victimized by the government army, the government's civic–military actions were also poorly received in towns in conflicted areas that had been repopulated by refugees. In 1989 a woman who lived in Guarjila told me,

> If the army enters here, we never invite them inside to sit down because we don't accept the things they do. They are assassins of children and of the people. There is no official relationship between the community and the army. We reject their overtures. They've come here offering medicines and "protection," whatever that means. But we don't need their help. We can take care of ourselves. I told one of them, "Without that gun you're like one of us." I said that because they're also born of poor mothers like us.

A man who lived in the same village told me, "The soldiers know we give food to the guerrillas. When the compas pass through, they get a plate of food, not just a tortilla to eat on the run, which is what the people give a soldier who asks for food. That's why [the soldiers] hate us."

Despite the chilly relations, the army made several efforts to stage civic–military actions in the repopulated communities even after the cease-fire. In July 1993 I was at a popular health meeting in San José Las Flores when Michaela, the FMLN doctor, arrived with an urgent message for the town's directiva. Earlier that day near the city of Chalatenango she'd seen a caravan of twenty military trucks full of sacks of food and boxes with banners on the side that read "Health for La Laguna" (a military-controlled town in an area with strong FMLN influence). Two of the trucks had pulled up in front of a union office affiliated with the repopulations where Michaela was meeting with other workers. She recounted:

> They wanted to deliver the aid to the repopulations. We told them no military trucks could enter the zone because we couldn't guarantee the security of soldiers. People won't stand for soldiers entering. They [the soldiers] might be okay in a large group, but [they know that] if they come in small groups "something might happen. . . ." We offered to let them leave the food and we would take it in, or we said they could put it in other trucks, but they refused. They wanted signatures from the directivas for each village. We said we could arrange that, but they weren't interested. I don't know where they went after that.

We piled into the back of her pickup and drove to Guarjila. The rumors had preceded us, and villagers had already held an emergency assembly. Several cars and a crowd of people mobilized to ambush (*emboscar*) the trucks if they arrived at a nearby crossroad. The plan was to bar passage and unload things onto a civilian truck if possible. They waited, but the trucks never showed up. It turned out they took another route to La Laguna.

The Militarization of Health

The medical effectiveness of the physical examinations offered in one-day civil–military programs has been widely questioned by community health advocates. U.S. physicians Paul Epstein and Steven Gloyd, who attended a U.S.-sponsored "Medcaps" civic action in rural Honduras, called the program "insensitive to the particular health care needs of Hondurans." They reported that most treatments given out were inappropriate, and that benefits may have been actually offset by side effects of the medicines. Dr. Gloyd was especially critical of the military doctors prescribing Kaopectate, an antidiarrheal, and the antibiotic ampicillin for infants with diarrhea (instead of oral rehydration therapy, the approach recommended by the World Health Organization). He said Kaopectate was of no use and potentially harmful, and ampicillin would be helpful only in 5 percent of cases. He also charged that the military doctors prescribed the wrong antiparasitic drug for hookworm. Dentistry services, the U.S. physicians noted, was limited to pulling teeth, noting that one military dentist told them as many as 30 percent of the extractions done were unnecessary. The program did not reflect a real government commitment to health, they argued, since the Honduran Ministry of Health budget had been cut by more than a third in 1984 while, at the Reagan administration's urging, the Honduran government had spent $35 million on fuel for military exercises and on U.S.-Honduran military bases which supported the contra war (Danby 1984).

Likewise, U.S. public health specialists, writing in a *New York Times* editorial, criticized the sending of twenty-five military medical specialists to help "in the regeneration of medical infrastructure" with a new USAID health initiative in El Salvador.[2] They argued that "in light of the Salvadoran government's extensive history of human rights abuses against health workers and patients, the program must be condemned as contributing to further militarization and politicization of the health sector" (Chopoorian and Messinger 1983).

When I worked as a reporter in El Salvador, I initially thought of army civic–military actions as little more than propaganda and threw invitations to attend them in the trash. One day I ran into a colleague who had attended one held in the town of San Martin. She described how the local kids ran to hide when an army helicopter flew over. Then a loudspeaker proclaimed: "Come out. We are your friends," and the pilot flew over again and dropped candies attached to toy soldiers. My friend laughed at the absurdity of finding American neckties in the bags of used clothes handed out to campesinos. She had noticed a boy leaving a medical consult with an entire bottle of cough syrup, and asked him, "Are you sick?" "No, but you never know," he said to her with a smile and a wink.

I attended my first civic–military action in the town of Tejutepeque in 1989. I walked among the small crowd milling about under the trees. A group of kids were shouting as they hit at a piñata that a soldier dressed like a clown held up on a stick. A uniformed man gave a speech at a microphone. A peasant couple sat in the grass nearby. The man appeared to be a farmer, gaunt with sunburned skin and a straw hat. His wife was fussing over a squalling two-month-old baby. He told me they lived about a kilometer outside of town where he had a milpa (cornfield). I asked him about effects of the war on the town. He said violent encounters were rare, except for occasional FMLN attacks on the National Guard. "Are there still guerrillas here?" I asked. "Oh yes," he said, "they come into town every day and buy food from stores as civilians, only to become combatants at night." A municipal policeman had just told me things were calmer since the National Guard had arrived. I asked if that was true. "No, nothing has changed," he said.

His wife had gotten a tooth pulled, and the government doctors had given her little bags of pills and vitamins. She also showed off a bag of used clothes for the children and sweets. I had noticed a Ministry of Health clinic on the way into town, so I asked her if she had gone to seek care there. "There's no point," she said, "They're always out of medicines, and the doctor never comes." We were interrupted by a speech about the new initiatives of the Ministry of Health to develop public health goals jointly with the community. "In the future, we must think of health," the speaker emphasized, "as responsibility of both the government and the individual."

The crowd then gathered around a stage for a dramatic performance. It was a kind of counterinsurgency morality play. A man had a disobedient son who defied his father's orders, hanging out with delinquent types who gave him a gun and incorporated him into the guerrillas. The boy hid the gun in the house. A policeman came over and asked the father if he had seen anyone with a gun. He said no but kindly invited the policeman to search the house. The policeman found the son in the back room wearing a ski-mask and holding a gun. He arrested him. The father scolded the son and disowned him. "Lock the boy up," he angrily told the policeman.

IN JUNE 1992 I ARRANGED an interview with Col. Bautizar López Hernandez, chief of the Armed Forces press office. He received me in his large, dark carpeted office, and we sat facing on two sofas divided by a glass coffee table. His secretary brought us sweet black coffee. I asked him about the army's civic–military actions.

LÓPEZ: Civic–military actions are as old as the conflict, and they are still going on during the peace process. They are a way that the army can help the people minimize the damage to their lives from the war. The FMLN had a strategy of trying to destroy the economy by blowing up bridges, sabotaging electrical plants and the coffee harvest—this was a very bad idea which hurt poor people the most.

SS: Are civic–military actions part of the army's new initiative to promote respect for human rights within the ranks?

LÓPEZ: Civic–military actions correspond with the press office's interest in projecting a new understanding of the army. (He gestured to an army public relation's poster on his wall of a smiling soldier assisting an elderly campesino woman while holding a rifle in one hand and a hoe in the other.) Soldiers now have a new consciousness about human rights, and they get special training in this area. One of the most outstanding points of this training I believe is teaching respect for life in the countryside. We now have programs in agriculture, literacy, and reforestation. Each cuartel [barracks] connects with the local civilian population through local authorities, especially the mayor—traditionally here the three most important persons in any small town are the priest, the mayor, and the colonel.

ss: What was the role of civic–military actions in the war?

LÓPEZ: They are not part of the war. They are a service mission. Constitutionally the armed forces have the duty to defend the people against interior and exterior threats, and to serve the people. Our civic affairs division is set up to prevent the loss of civilian lives and property.

ss: How do they do this?

LÓPEZ: You see, what the terrorists want is to get close to people and destroy them.

ss: But don't they need the population's support to build their revolution?

LÓPEZ: You have to understand their Marxism: the guerrillas see the people as the water for the guerrilla fish to swim in; but what they want the people for is to give them logistical support. The FMLN arrives at the camps of returned refugees and indoctrinates them in Marxism. And campesinos are very susceptible; they're ignorant. The FMLN tells them they have control of the area, but what I want to say is they don't. And they are rejecting government aid.

ss: What does the army see as the main objective of civic–military actions?

LÓPEZ: To keep the FMLN from gaining the support of the people, and to show that the army supports the democratic process.

ss: How does the army plan these actions? Are they part and parcel of military operations? How do you choose the sites?

LÓPEZ: Many times civic–military actions are planned with military operations, but not always. We also plan them where they are most needed, whether there is military activity planned for that area or not. We've just carried out several in the areas around the Morazán conflicted area.

[There is a pause, as Col. Lopez introduces me to a lieutenant who joins us.]

ss: Can you tell me about health programs in civic–military actions?

LÓPEZ: We send out doctors to vaccinate and give consults, dentists to pull teeth, and medicines which are given out to those who come for consults. We do some operations jointly with the Ministry of Health. And we do a census.

ss: What is the purpose of the census?

LÓPEZ: The reason we do that is to assess the needs of the population. For vaccinations, things like that.

ss: I understand that in low-intensity conflict, civic–military actions play an important role in political strategy. Could you talk about that?

LÓPEZ: Civic–military actions don't have anything to do with counterinsurgency, although they may have been used in psychological operations. For example, psy-ops may hold a speech or other event at the same time when a civic–military action is held in an area where the FMLN has influence, but this has nothing to do with the humanitarian aid.

SS: If they have no role in low-intensity conflict, then why is the army involved? Why not leave it up to the Ministry of Health to carry them out?

LÓPEZ: Because the Ministry of Health didn't assume the role.

SS: Do you build clinics or give courses?

LÓPEZ: No, we don't stay long enough for that.

The lieutenant: There is only so much we can do in a civic–military action. It's not really comprehensive, but more to relieve some of the people's suffering, and this has a psychological effect on them . . .

LÓPEZ: [cutting him off] But they are not psychological operations.

[The lieutenant clams up.]

Colonel López invited me to view videos of four civic–military actions carried out jointly by the army and the National Commission for Restoration of Areas (CONARA), a military-run civilian aid program, in 1988. Each began with the raising of the national flag. Then the commander made a speech (in one case with his M-16 dangled conspicuously across his chest). Next, a scratchy recording of the national anthem was played on a loudspeaker as officials stood in a line saluting. The local peasants usually stood in front of them in a small crowd, faces blank. At some events an army social worker in a camouflage uniform led everyone in prayer. Then people formed long lines for medical consults at a row of tables under a tent. One table, covered with bottles of medicines, would serve as the pharmacy; a dentist pulled teeth to one side. Medical consults were brief and impersonal. The patient described the problem—a stomachache, diarrhea— to an army doctor across a table and he asked two or three questions, then handed out pills or liquid medicines to nearly every patient, in tiny plastic bags. There was no privacy, no physical examinations.

The camera panned food giveaways as sacks of beans, rice, and corn and cans of oil and powdered milk were handed off the back of pickup trucks to crowds of waiting campesinos. There were scenes of soldiers giving haircuts, handing out used clothes or toys, and a clown doing magic tricks. All the while, a loudspeaker blared propaganda: "The FMLN destroy our countryside. They will fool you; they want to exploit your children. Don't fall into the trap of the Marxist-Leninist delinquents. They destroy the electrical towers and buses. Collaborate with the armed forces, your friends. Terrorists just go around robbing people. Don't listen to them. Don't help them."

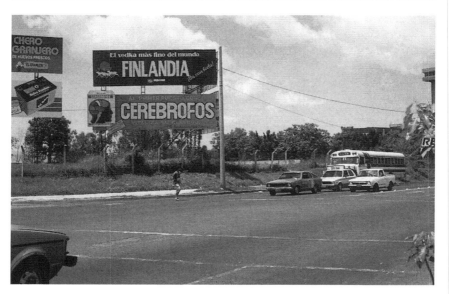

"Cerebrofos: Boost your brain power." Ad that towered over entrance to the University of El Salvador in the late 1980s. Regulation of pharmaceuticals was lacking; both prescription drugs and poor quality knock-offs were sold over the counter at corner pharmacies. Photograph by Sandy Smith-Nonini.

War Is Health

In November 1992, I obtained a rare appointment with Col. Nelson I. Saldaña, chief of Conjunto Five, which oversaw civic–military actions (and, incidentally, psychological operations). I waited for an hour outside his office then was told he could not see me and I should come back another day. On the second try, he spoke with me across his large desk in a dark office with leather-padded chairs and a conspicuous display of electronics, including a stereo system, three-foot-high speakers, a shortwave radio, and three phones. One wall was full of plaques. Colonel Saldaña seemed impatient at my initial questions, so I adopted a passive mode and listened.

He explained that in planning civic–military actions, the army studied a rural town's health and environmental needs and prioritized villages where the conflict had caused the most damages. He said the presence of the FMLN in an area was not a factor in planning. He told me the army had started leaving medical equipment and medicines at rural clinics to help with shortages in the Ministry of Health supply chain. Since the cease-fire, he said, the army had delivered 10 million colones (US$1.25 million) of surplus medical supplies and equipment this way, some from foreign donations.

He described how that very afternoon a woman with kidney failure would be flying to the United States for a transplant, thanks to army intervention, and said that the army's Second Brigade gave out temporary prostheses to amputees. He handed me the latest issue of the military newspaper, *El Nuevo Heróico*, which carried four articles on army medical assistance.

IN LATE 1992 I LEARNED that U.S. Marines planned a series of civic–military actions the following spring along the shores of the Cerrón Grande reservoir that separated Chalatenango from Guazapa. The plans involved four trips of fifteen to thirty days each with American soldiers moving from site to site in boats and staying a maximum of three days in one place. They would build schools and roads, and help communities with preventive health and veterinary medicine. Spanish-speaking ability was not a requirement for soldiers' participation, according to Josúe Ramón, of the Batallón de Sanidad Militar, who was based out of the U.S. Embassy in the capital. Ramón told me the project was part of the U.S. Southern Command Health Project under the "Foreign Internal Defense" program. I asked how planners decided where to carry out the actions.

"What we look for is a population with many problems that has been very abandoned by the government and has no other resources. But we want at least three thousand people in a place, so sometimes we have to compromise on the level of need." He said they tried to avoid FMLN-occupied areas because of the danger. He reported that doctors from the Ministry of Health and the Salvadoran army would assist. Interestingly, among the sites chosen were San Francisco Lempa, which had a well-stocked Ministry of Health clinic visited by a physician once a week, and Suchitoto, a town with an *unidad de salud*, a larger public clinic that in 1993 had permanent doctors. I asked Lt. Col. Júlio Rivera, the operations and administration officer in the U.S. Embassy, why Marines were doing civic actions in areas with relatively good medical coverage. He told me that it was actually the Ministry of Health that chose the sites for the U.S. Marines' civic actions. "They initially chose a site in Chalatenango, and they did a site survey, and everyone was agreed on it. Then someone higher up in the military had a fit, because they wanted to go to an area loyal to the army."

IN JULY 1993 I ATTENDED a two-day civic–military action planned by the U.S. Navy and Special Forces in the town of Sesori, in the department of San Miguel. U.S. Army colonel David Stockand, who worked with the U.S. Military Group in El Salvador, offered me a ride to Sesori. The American soldiers planned the event in which Salvadoran Army and Ministry of Health personnel took part. Sesori was a formerly FMLN-controlled town, now governed by an ARENA mayor. I asked Colonel Stockand why they included medical consults in civic–military actions.

STOCKAND: I don't imagine they [civic–military actions] can do much good from a medical point of view. We mainly do them for the propaganda value. And they are useful in training U.S. soldiers—that's more important to us than showing the Salvadoran army how to do them. The medical part is probably the most valued component of civic–military actions. Salvadorans may not have a lot of education, but these people know the value of the dollar. And when they hear American doctors and free medicines are coming, they take advantage of that.

SS: Do you think that so many come because they believe they will get a higher quality of care from foreign doctors?

STOCKAND: Well the fact is that two out of three [coming for consults] end up seeing the Salvadoran doctors—so it's more of an issue of the civic–military action being associated with the United States.

SS: Are any actions like this planned for Chalatenango?

STOCKAND: We can't do uninvited civic–military actions in FMLN-controlled areas because of the peace accords.

During our drive from San Salvador to Sesori, Colonel Stockand commented on the Salvadoran Army's weak noncommissioned officer corps (there are no sergeants; only higher ranking officers), which he said impeded the ability of ground troops to function well in the field and maintain good discipline. He said the civic–military actions helped the Salvadoran soldiers model on U.S soldiers' behavior. He noted that in recent years Salvadoran officers were less likely to treat their soldiers badly, compared to the early years of the war. The approach to Sesori was a dusty dirt road. We drove up to a squad of men in U.S. camou-flage uniforms gathered in front of a school. Colonel Stockand introduced me to Sergeant Suarez, a U.S. Special Forces advisor, who had followed in the other jeep. A Salvadoran soldier ran up to Suarez to tell him there was a problem—the local kids were still attending classes, and the agreement was that the school would be available. The sergeant shrugged, telling them, "Well, get 'em out of there."

A squad of Navy SEALs milled about in front of the school—huge muscular men who made the Salvadorans seem like munchkins. They horsed around as if on a beach trip—one wore an Atlanta Braves cap and white sunscreen on his nose, another sported a brush cut and sunglasses with day-glow orange frames. The Salvadoran kids couldn't take their eyes off them, but the soldiers seemed oblivious to where they were; no one made an effort to talk to the cluster of kids. The soldiers formed a semicircle between a large truck and a schoolroom and began unloading large boxes of medical supplies by throwing them from one to another with great macho style. The kids and I scrambled back, to give the flying

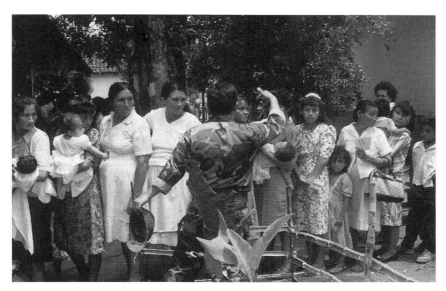

A soldier directs women and children waiting in line to be seen by doctors at a joint civic–military action held by the U.S. Navy and Special Forces, the Salvadoran military, and the Ministry of Health in the town of Sesori, San Miguel, in 1995. Photograph by Sandy Smith-Nonini.

boxes a wide berth. The SEALs kept up a constant banter among themselves about rock musicians, Hollywood movies.

I helped set up the rooms. We hastily rearranged three of the small school-rooms with tables and benches so each could accommodate five patients in consultation with a doctor. Chairs were squeezed in for translators beside each doctor. Separate pharmacy tables held piles of pill bottles, cough syrup, and packaged drug samples. Yes, there was also Kaopectate. Three dental stations for pulling teeth were set up at one end of the building—one with a reclining chair and the other two using school desks.

While soldiers set up the makeshift clinic, a crowd gathered at the gate to the schoolyard, and two American soldiers took up guard duty. Soon scores of bodies pressed against the gate, and it became an ordeal to go in or out. Several vendors set up shop along the dusty road to sell drinks. A system of triage was used: women and children first. Those who had squeezed to the front of the crowd were let in. Each group of new patients passed through several stations, with waits of about forty-five minutes to an hour. First they were herded in groups into a classroom for preventive health education where mothers squeezed into child-sized desks. Children, many sniffling and sneezing, filled the corners of the room and sat on the floor. The campesinas waited patiently with blank expressions while a uniformed Ministry of Health nurse, pointer in hand, instructed them on germ theory and basic hygiene using a flip chart.

"Who can tell me what you do to prevent the spread of disease?" she asked the group. The bedlam from the children made her lecture hard to hear, and only two or three women responded to her questions. The no-nonsense nurse, in her starched white dress, navy heels, and red lipstick, made a stark contrast with the weary-looking peasants, wearing cheap polyester dresses, their dusty feet in rubber flip-flops. Their eyes glazed as she droned on about boiling water and burying trash.

After the lecture, the Salvadorans and their children moved as instructed from one school desk to another in the schoolyard, waiting their turn to see the doctor. I sat by a woman with a tiny sleeping baby in her arms that was the size of a three-month-old, but she said he had been born eight months ago. Juanita said she had walked five kilometers to bring the baby, which had a cold and fever. She held a bottle and a half-eaten package of Oreos in one hand. I noticed dark crumbs on the baby's cheek, and realized the cookies were breakfast. Juanita told me she had two other children at home with their grandmother. "And your compañero?" I asked.

"He died in the war," she said. The family lived in a small resettlement community with other families who had come returned to their original homes in 1990.

"Why do so many people come to these civic–military actions?" I asked her.

"For the medicines," she said.

I asked if she thought people formed better opinions of the army when they come to these events and go home with free medicines. She did not reply, but rolled her eyes up and smiled, shaking her head from side to side.

In the schoolrooms there was no space for physical exams; a consultation consisted of a short description of symptoms, perhaps a listen with a stethoscope or an otoscope in the ears for children, and, most important, a small plastic bag of pills or cough syrup—this was the magic gift that the peasants had walked to town and waited in the hot sun for.

Sergeant Suarez complained that there were not enough translators and asked me to fill in. "What's the word for 'month?'" a uniformed U.S Navy doctor asked me. He was trying to ask a pregnant woman how far along she was. I suddenly begin to worry about the men's inability to communicate with their patients—one commonly used antiparasitic drug should never be prescribed to a pregnant woman because of risks it would pose to the fetus. I was called to another table to help an American doctor tell a woman how to take her pill (his Salvadoran translator could not understand his English). Behind me another U.S. doctor, abandoned by his translator, was pointing alternately at his tummy and his head trying to explain to a campesina what the pills he'd prescribed her were for. Colonel Stockand looked over at me and shook his head with a smile and a look of resignation.

"It's always disorganized the first day," he said.

Fantasies of Order in a Ministry of Ill-being

In 1988 a photographer friend and I toured several public hospitals. I had heard complaints from lower-level government health workers of inadequate resources, but it surprised me to hear the director of the mental hospital (not some disgruntled underling, but the director) fill my ear with tales of patients with no follow-up and erratic supplies of drugs, which precluded long-term medical management. I still have photographs of the ward with two women to a bed in the maternity hospital, and photos from Rosales, the main public hospital, of flies crawling on a patients' bandaged arm and a humorous snapshot of two surgeons posing in their operating room with grim expressions on their faces as they held up for the camera not scalpels and instruments of their trade but fly swatters. "Tell people in your country the conditions we work under," one of the surgeons told me.

In the two years that followed, I began to get more of a picture of this. On a trip with other reporters to San Vicente, part of our group fell behind, so our driver pulled over to wait on the outskirts of a town right in front of a Ministry of Health clinic. A little boy of perhaps seven or eight, naked except for a pair of underwear, sat in front of the clinic on a concrete slab bawling. His torso and legs were covered with a bright red rash. Measles, I wondered? He held out his hands to me, pleading for help. Where was his mother? I went inside the dingy building. There were no other patients; perhaps the hour for consults had passed. I asked to talk to the nurse who said the boy had a skin rash. "Can't you help him?" I asked, "He's miserable."

"I don't have anything to give him," she said with a shrug. She took me into the pharmacy and gestured at the almost empty shelves. We're out of the skin cream he needs. We haven't had any in months."[3]

In 1989 I was preparing a newspaper article on a new measles epidemic that killed at least one hundred children and swamped the medical system with five thousand cases of sick (and contagious) children during the first four months of the year. Reading the ominous headlines in local papers, I became concerned for my own one-year-old son, who had only recently received his measles shot. I interviewed several health specialists with foreign NGOs and got warnings from them against quoting the ministry's statistics, charging that the government was understating the death toll and downplaying the seriousness of the problem. Some of my informants estimated that several hundred children had died. UNICEF officials said the epidemic was most serious in government-controlled areas, particularly in the western provinces, where vaccination coverage had been low (57 percent). Doctors at the Bloom Pediatric Hospital in the capital told me that most of the sick children being brought in had never been vaccinated.

I was thinking about this experience several years later during my 1995 fieldwork while I stood in the Chalatenango Ministry of Health headquarters staring at a large framed map of the province which had dozens of multicolored pie charts laid over municipal health zones. The odd map hung on the wall of the director's office. Our interview done, the administrator had directed me to the extravagant (and confusing) graphics display as he left for another appointment. The figures reported steady progress in vaccination coverage since the 1992 cease-fire in repopulated communities where the ministry had begun placing its medical teams beginning in late 1993. I knew that the popular health promoters in these resettlement sites actually carried out the rural vaccination drives. But the statistics seemed unusually good for an area with such inaccessible terrain—they reported coverage at 95 to 99 percent at some sites.

A senior nurse passed by the door and noticed me perusing the complex charts. She came over and whispered, "Don't pay too much attention to those figures." She took me to her desk and pulled out a sheet of census data, explaining that the population counts that the ministry uses as the denominator to calculate vaccination coverage were far too low for many rural areas, which had seen massive returns of refugees and displaced people since the war ended. In addition, the 1992 government census takers, who began their work right after the cease-fire, weren't welcome in formerly FMLN-controlled areas, many of which were never counted.

"And there were many errors! They even put a sticker on the Ministry of Health door that said '*casa censada*' [household counted], and we're an office!" she said with a laugh.

I was reminded of James Ferguson's concept of a self-perpetuating aid bureaucracy that he dubbed the antipolitics machine (1994). Similarly, in Taussig's (1978) study of USAID development programs and malnutrition in Colombia, where he described "a misplaced and mishandled emphasis on quantification as if this in itself guarantees scientific knowledge" (110). In El Salvador, as in Colombia, it seemed that "the problem of human numbers" had come to substitute for, and even mystify, the problematic social relations of rural health. Sayer (1994) made a similar allusion to the parallels between exigencies of scientific discourse (tales of coherence, predictability, control, logical causality) and the technologies of domination, noting that both logics of control often successfully marshal things and people based on claims to truth that rest on precarious abstractions (373).

As these cases illustrate, complaints about meaningless statistics and poorly supplied and managed systems came as much from staff within the Ministry of Health as from outsiders. Under ARENA administration, these charges of mismanagement and internal corruption continued well beyond the war years. In 2007 interviews, for example, I heard claims of supplies being misdirected both at rural clinics and at urban hospitals, and a newly formed union of public hospital employees charged that withholding of key medicines and supplies had become a tactic of the government to justify privatization of the health system. Lower-level staff said that the rigidity of the ministry's bureaucracy made it useless to file formal complaints, and they feared their jobs would be endangered if they persisted. When I succeeded in efforts to obtain interviews with higher-level administrators, I always asked about the charges of an overcentralized administration that failed to heed feedback from lower levels. The notion that there was a systemic problem was always dismissed as grumblings of leftists or disgruntled individuals. In 1995 the physician director of Chalatenango's regional public hospital told me, "We have some politicized groups of workers who complain about everything." [He rummaged in a drawer and pulled out three thick manuals]. "See this," he said angrily, waving one in the air, "This is Direction—the authority. And this [he held up the five-year-plan] is the National Plan—how we resolve health problems. And this Memoria," he said, waving a third book in my face, "is where workers within the ministry give feedback and report what they have accomplished."

The more dubious statistics during the civil war were sometimes clothed in spectacle. In the late 1980s, I took advantage of a visiting U.S. delegation of health workers to sit in on a rare meeting with the physician/army colonel who served as Minister of Health. On the wall of his office hung a large, framed renaissance-style etching of three figures: a white-coated medical doctor with his arms extended, struggling to rescue a birthing woman. Behind the woman stood a skeletal figure of death who reached out to seize her. Another frame over his desk enclosed a two-foot-square of velvet on which twenty or thirty scalpels had been arranged in a starburst pattern.

The minister ushered us inside a dark conference room where we sat around a long table. He stood at the head of the table and spoke woodenly of government objectives and five-year plans. Then he took questions. "How is the Ministry dealing with the problem of delivering services in rural areas affected by the war?" a visitor asked. The questioner knew, as I did, that more than thirty rural health posts remained closed at the time in conflicted areas that made up close to a quarter of the country's territory, and that many other government-controlled areas depended on a handful of irregular mobile medical units because the ministry had cut back rural staffing.[4]

But the minister did not flinch at this question. He rose, reached for a wall switch to dim the lights, and turned to a large wall-mounted map of El Salvador, where he flipped a series of switches one at a time. Each switch in turn lit up dozens of tiny color-coded bulbs pinpointing the geographic locations of the four levels of care—from rural health posts, to clinics, regional health centers, and finally hospitals—each of which he called out as he flipped the appropriate switch. The tiny glowing yellow, red, blue, and green dots filled up the country's borders. The minister turned to us with a triumphant smile: "As you can see, we have the country well covered."

These vignettes juxtapose cases replete with Orwellian cynicism alongside routine performances of modernist humanitarian concern as a means of illustrating the rhetoric and contradictory practices that described official policies on health in wartime and postwar El Salvador. The most well-known abuses of medicine occur when health professionals violate medical ethics for a political cause, such as aiding in torture or collaborating with a repressive regime by classifying political prisoners as mentally ill. But in a study of political abuses of medicine, Anthony Zwi included two other types of violations, including the use of health services as a political weapon to reward supporters (or withdrawing them to punish opponents) of a regime or political party, and ideological practices that perpetuate inequalities in access to health and social services (1987).

The uses of health services as a form of pacification in low-intensity conflict certainly fits the former description. The political manipulation of a health bureaucracy—whether to generate phantom statistics for foreign development banks or to reward political patronage with plum positions or contracts—must also be seen as an abuse of basic rights.

The crass lack of subtlety or professionalism in many of these efforts at public relations is not unrelated to the longstanding absence of public accountability in a militarized state. The international attention brought by the war coincided with enormous influxes of USAID funding of social programs (see chapter 9), including health, which maximized opportunities for graft, and the need to close ranks around administrative privilege—a process that exacerbated the administrative morass from the viewpoint of the health workers who staff hospitals and clinics.

White Flags, Innocent Civilians, and Wounded Bodies

International relief organizations also attempted to shape public perceptions with medical symbolism and propaganda. One of the most successful efforts to intervene in the civil war was the effort led by UNICEF and PAHO to coordinate a one-day cease-fire in El Salvador (as well as other Central American conflicts) each year between 1985 and 1991 so that health workers of all stripes could vaccinate children against polio, diphtheria, whooping cough, tetanus, and measles. UNICEF was motivated to act by epidemiological surveys showing that one hundred thousand children per year were dying in the region due to preventable infections, far more than the death toll attributed directly to violence, although without doubt, the regional conflicts had deepened suffering and impeded health services in much of the countryside.[5]

During the cease-fire days, and in the weeks leading up to them, more than twenty thousand Salvadorans were mobilized countrywide to coordinate the immunization, according to Ciro de Quadros and Daniel Epstein (2002), who speculated that coordination of the events likely contributed to achievement of

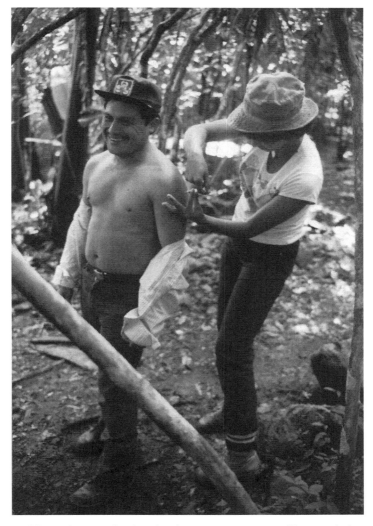

FMLN health worker vaccinating in the war zones. Guerrilla-occupied areas of Chalatenango and Morazán had higher rates of civilian coverage for immunizations than government-controlled areas in the late 1980s. Photograph courtesy of El Museo de la Palabra y la Imagen.

a level of trust between the guerrillas and the government, which helped pave the way for peace negotiations. The Catholic Archdiocesan Health Commission (CAPS), which coordinated the church's health relief work nationwide, had begun rural vaccination efforts in 1984 with a focus on rural areas no longer served by the Ministry of Health. That year Archbishop Arturo Rivera Damas and Bishop Gregorio Rosa Chávez led efforts to bring representatives of the

FMLN and the government together at a convent outside the country to coordinate the cease-fire plan, which was the first time since the war began that leaders of the two sides had sat at a table together (Blair and Siebert 1999). While the cease-fire was not unproblematic, it nevertheless offers a real example of the power that can be wielded when parties to a conflict find common cause around the white flag of medical neutrality.

The FMLN highly valued the immunization cease-fires because they provided opportunities for the guerrillas to gain international visibility for their popular health work in rural areas where the military had blocked access to outsiders. This relative openness to international visitors was a characteristic of the FMLN during the war. Once vetted by a trusted colleague, reporters or aid workers were often able to secure assistance from the FMLN or their supporters to travel in rural areas they controlled. This assistance often entailed considerable risk for both parties since guides who accompanied visitors on overland hikes usually had to pass through army-controlled territory on the way to a destination.

The most common symbolism used by the FMLN and the repopulated communities (after 1987) was that of white flags and wounded bodies—that is, images of the civilian face of the rebellion and of innocent victims of government violence. It was a strategy that seemed especially directed at foreign observers, designed to counter the faceless boogeyman of communist terrorism (which shares similarities to the Islamic terrorist images that haunt public airwaves today). As Brauman (1993) noted, in media accounts the symbolic status of "victim" is only granted in cases of unjustified or innocent suffering. The goal of leftist propaganda was to humanize the rebellion while propaganda of the right sought to tar dissidents with accusations of criminality and chaos. The human rights record for the war speaks for itself in answering the question of which side's propaganda most resembled reality (see chapter 4).

Just as the government sought to use medical relief to project itself as a humanitarian actor, so did the FMLN, particularly after 1983 as part of its shift to mobile tactics (in response, in part, to the air war that was forcing civilians to flee rearguard areas). Dubbed "expansion work" the campaign called on FMLN medical units to do more outreach in rural villages, including areas where the guerrillas previously stayed underground. This took the form of medical consults, usually announced a day in advance, combined with informal talks to those who attended about sanitation and preventive health practices. Former FMLN physicians said a key goal was to expand training of health promoters in new settings. Unlike past interaction with "well-organized" communities where Christian base groups had existed prior to the war, the campaign took medical teams into some communities where people feared association with the rebel army.

Some FMLN physicians such as Leo, and Isabél, a Salvadoran doctor who rose through the political ranks of the FPL, were enthusiastic about expansion work. In explaining the logic of health outreach in the revolution, Isabél ranked the Frente's priorities: The "number one priority" was military training and supplies, she said, followed closely by security and logistics. After this, she said "political work" was also vital, and she classified health as a component of political work. But Octávia and Ernesto, both internationalist physicians, expressed reservations about whether the health organizing was effective in new villages when there was no follow-up, a common outcome due to the demands of the war.

Another medical campaign that the FPL undertook in the last two years of the war had the goal of "legalizing [FMLN] wounded and disabled people," in Michaela's terms, or making it more difficult for the government to violate international human rights laws by killing them. During this period, dozens of wounded guerrillas were in fact killed in cold blood during military attacks on tatús and mobile clinics in remote areas (see chapter 4).

Such a language of bodies in political discourse is well established in Latin America, where suffering, sacrifice, and martyrdom on behalf of imagined nations and liberation movements resonate with both Christian and political traditions. Veritable cults over human remains of saints and political heroes dot the landscape (Johnson 2004). In the early years of my fieldwork, a political meeting led by FMLN veterans often ended with a revolutionary tribute, followed by a *consigna* (signal) from someone in the crowd who shouted the name of a dead comrade. All would respond, "Presente!" Another name would sound, with the same response, often mixing religious martyrs such as Archbishop Oscar Romero with dead comandantes.

The various Mothers of the Disappeared groups in the capital succeeded in tapping this sacred vein of public anger and sympathy during their silent vigils denouncing political murders of civilians. The FMLN's campaign for the wounded sought to capitalize on this well of sentiment as a way to humanize guerrilla fighters, whom the government had long tagged as terrorists and criminals. But in the repopulated villages, this posed a potential threat in that the returned refugees relied on the military's willingness to respect the neutrality of these sites based on their distinction as civilian population centers. A steady stream of international visitors to the sites helped to provide a level of scrutiny of respect for this neutral zone that had not existed prior to the mass repopulation.

Like the expansion work, Leo explained, the campaign for recognition of the wounded was part of a wider initiative that the FMLN had dubbed "*doble poder*," in which the Frente engaged in political work with civilian groups around issues of economic, social, and political rights. In addition, he noted, as prospects improved for a negotiated end to the conflict, the FPL medical teams became concerned about integrating compas with disabilities back into civilian communities where they would eventually live.

The project began in the most remote resettlement, Arcatao where residents were known for a high solidarity with the FPL and had a reputation for rebelliousness with state authorities. Michaela and local health promoters (most of them former sanitarios) told me hair-raising accounts of their (successful) efforts to keep various wounded combatants out of sight during a surprise army helicopter landing in the town during which soldiers rounded up and harassed civilians.

"When we first [hid wounded] in Guarjila in 1989, only the directiva [and promoters] knew the plan." Octávia recalled, "Then we learned there was a military operation coming and we thought we'd better get them out quickly. But [in moving them] we really surprised a lot of families! So we scheduled a meeting with the directiva [afterward] to discuss the issue, and Ana [the Catholic pediatrician and nun based there] was so pissed off. She said we were burning [*quemando*] her" (ruining her political reputation with authorities, since the international and Church support for the repopulations hinged on their self-description as "civilian" centers).

But Ana went on to become close friends with Michaela and other internationalist physicians during the last four years of the war, and she continued to work in Guarjila after the war. According to a diary that she left with colleagues before her untimely death from cancer in 1993, Ana frequently assisted FMLN physicians in responding to emergencies of wounded civilians and guerrillas. Besides army skirmishes with guerrillas, usually in more remote settings, government soldiers also made frequent incursions into the resettled communities looking for collaborators. Margarita, the sanitaria who went to Mesa Grande to give birth (chapter 3), moved to Guarjila in 1988 and worked closely with Ana in the makeshift clinic. She said the FMLN quietly moved surgical supplies into town, and on several occasions she and other promoters assisted Michaela and Leo when they came into town in civilian dress to operate on patients under a huge mango tree next to the clinic.

Both Ana and Michaela separately told me the story of the day that wounded compas arrived in Guarjila during planning for a celebration of the fourth anniversary of the town's resettlement. The spacious new cinderblock clinic and *hospitalito* had just been completed, and Ana and the promoters were moving supplies into it prior to its official inauguration by a visiting bishop who, along with international visitors, was slated to attend the festivities. That morning Michaela suddenly showed up at Ana's house out of breath, shouting "Where are the wounded?"

"What wounded?" asked Ana.

"We got a message that wounded were being brought to Guarjila," said Michaela. So Ana and the promoters joined her in gathering supplies and prepping for surgery. The clean new "little hospital" was in fact far nicer than any FMLN field hospital and had an "appropriate technology" operating room that must have seemed completely luxurious to Michaela. Sure enough in mid-afternoon three wounded combatants were brought into town, including Pablo, a member of a local family, who was in shock with a severe abdominal wound. Ana's diary entry recounted the events:

> Carmen ended up taking care of the young man with the shoulder injury, and Lucia tried to get blood for both, while Michaela operated on Pablo with me assisting. His stomach had a huge hole in it, and his liver and small intestines were nicked as well. We were operating with a light that ran on a battery. . . . But it got darker and darker, so we lit a Coleman lantern. Luke [an American doctor working with a Catholic health NGO], who had arrived for the celebration, ended up holding the lantern on a pole for the last couple of hours [until about nine P.M.] while Michaela and I finished operating. The next morning it fell to me to explain to the bishop why we had three guerrillas in the new clinic which he had come to inaugurate.[6]

The first time I heard the story from Michaela, she gave a deep throaty chuckle at this point, saying, "Can you imagine the bishop's surprise, finding wounded combatants in the new 'civilian' clinic?"

"What did he do?" I entreated her.

"He blessed them."

PART THREE

Health against War

6

The Anatomy of "Popular Health"
in the Repopulated Villages

They [resettled refugees] have hope . . . that's what makes them dangerous. If God is not here, He is nowhere.

—Padre Jon Cortina (on why the Salvadoran army harassed resettlements in
northeast Chalatenango)

Saving Rosita: Replacing the State in El Salvador

Four months after the 1992 cease-fire, I began a study of the popular community
health system that had developed (with assistance from the Salvadoran Catholic
Church) in repopulated communities of northeast Chalatenango. Sometime
after midnight on August 31, while sleeping in the back room of the clinic in
Guarjila, I was startled awake by a baby's shrill cries. In the examining room
I found Esperanza, a peasant woman who had arrived the previous afternoon,
wringing her hands while three health workers bent over a tiny infant. Tears
coursed down Esperanza's cheeks as Dr. Ana Manganaro, a Catholic sister and
pediatrician, and two community health promoters, attempted to start an intravenous line. Ana tried repeatedly to slip the needle into a tiny vein on the
infant's foot. Each time the baby squalled and twisted in the hands of the promoters, jerking the needle out again in a trickle of blood. The promoters, Elsa
and Lucia, yawned and blinked in the glare of the generator-driven light bulb.

They were exhausted. They had been up for hours taking turns trying to
spoon-feed suero (oral rehydration fluid) to this dangerously dehydrated baby.
The feverish infant, far too small for her age of nine months, had swallowed less
and less of the life-saving fluid, letting it drool down her chin onto her mother's
soiled apron. When the effort began to seem hopeless, Lucia had reached for her
flashlight and struck out into the darkness to awaken Dr. Manganaro.

In a few weeks of fieldwork in these repopulated villages, I'd already seen
about a dozen severely dehydrated babies like this one brought to popular clinics, their mothers desperate because they lacked money for transport and medicines, and they feared their country's overcrowded and underequipped urban
public hospitals. They feared all government institutions.

Three attempts and thirty minutes later, the IV line was established. I returned to my bedroll, leaving the exhausted mother with Elsa to monitor the baby. At 6 a.m. I found them both slumped over the gurney, the baby between them peacefully asleep, as was Elsa, her head on her arm. The groggy mother looked grateful for the quiet.

That afternoon Esperanza told me her story, which was similar to others I had heard. Rosita, her first child, had become feverish, with diarrhea and vomiting, two days earlier. Mother and baby had hitched a ride on the back of a pickup to the popular clinic, a forty-minute ride on a rocky mountain road. A trip to the public hospital in Chalatenango city would have taken twice as long; Esperanza did not even consider it. "They ask 10 colones for a consult," she exclaimed when I asked. She expressed doubt that a government doctor would have seen Rosita on a weekend night. The tears welled up again as she recounted the tale. Esperanza was aware that her daughter came close to dying. Only a few years before, when she and her neighbors repopulated their old village, near San José Las Flores, sixteen children had died in a diarrhea epidemic caused by the contaminated water supply. The death toll probably would have been larger except for the local promoters' swift reaction. Lacking commercial oral rehydration therapy packets, the Las Flores promoters turned to *Donde No Hay Doctor* and followed instructions for making dozens of homemade packets of suero using common ingredients—salt, sugar, and sterile water—packaging them in the same plastic bags used for refrescos (fruit drinks). They went door to door teaching local mothers how to use it. After that, no more children died.[1]

Assessing Popular Health: A Focus on Process

This chapter describes rural health services offered by the popular system and contrasts them with rural services of the Ministry of Health. My goal in Chalatenango was to document the politics of health in a civil war—that is the relationship between health policies and practices and relationships of social and political power, both at the local level and in interactions between the opposition movement and the state. I sought to identify the factors that made the Chalatenango system "popular"—that is, how the system resembled and how it contrasted with ministry-run rural health, and, more generally, what challenges the system posed for the dominant model of public health in settings where capitalism and the biomedical model are hegemonic.

I spent eight months in 1992 and 1993 studying day-to-day operations of the popular health system in the months following the peace agreement. In three additional months in 1995, I concentrated primarily on the Ministry of Health's orientation toward the popular system (and community health in general). Most data for this chapter was collected during participant observation in Guarjila and San José Las Flores. I also spent a week observing a Ministry of Health clinic in a government-controlled town for comparison of daily practices.

I did not attempt to study the epidemiology of the popular system per se although I tried to track down what data existed, and I studied five years of clinic records of preventable disease diagnoses at one site (see chapter 7).[2] I asked many questions about rationales for health practices and the correspondence of policies with findings in the literature on community development in health as well as patients' perspectives, since cultural studies of beliefs about health in Africa and Mexico suggest that peasants' perceptions about effectiveness of health services is related to real effectiveness (Finkler 2001; and Pearce 1993). This chapter lays the groundwork for chapter 7, which focuses on the popular system's efforts to develop community participation in health, and chapter 8, on postwar negotiations between the popular system and the government, a process that led to the ministry's gradual reentry and assertion of control over the ex–war zone's health services, beginning in mid-1993, which was resisted by popular health workers.

The health division of the Catholic diocese trained promoters in Chalatenango and supplied basic medicines to a growing network of clinics and health posts. The diocese also supported a small technical team (*equipo técnica*) of health professionals made up of international volunteers and Salvadorans who assisted in organizing and training, oversight of the promoters, and medical backup for patients with serious conditions. After 1992 the Church promoter-training program expanded its reach throughout Chalatenango. At the end of my fieldwork in 1995 the Church was assisting three hundred lay promoters who worked in health posts in eighty-six rural villages.

Guarjila and San José Las Flores were considered by the diocese technical team to be well-organized towns with competent promoters, and I chose to study them for that reason. My goal was to study the popular health system where it was best established to better understand the potential for the model. My overall focus was the politics of health, so over time my field site expanded from local practices to regional planning meetings, and negotiations with the ministry.[3]

Just as I studied the popular system's best organized sites, I chose to observe a Ministry of Health clinic that was operating under somewhat "ideal" conditions in San Pedro del Lago (a pseudonym), which had been a government-controlled town during the war that had drawn considerable state funding in part because it was the hometown of an important Salvadoran army colonel and in part because of its strategic location near a lake that separated two formerly rebel-controlled "fronts." Conscious that the town was adjacent to rebel supply routes, the government had invested in a number of community improvement projects in an effort to win the loyalty of citizens.

Although the popular health system had some similarities with large-scale state-supported health projects in developing countries, it diverges from such models in important ways. Importantly, the program in Chalatenango grew out of a clandestine wartime health network in response to local necessity and in an environment that stressed social justice and development of alternatives to capitalist social forms. Perhaps the most appropriate models for comparison would be primary health initiatives associated with social reform movements or revolutions. Segall cautioned against the tendency to too quickly assign a "socialist" label to health systems in revolutionary societies (1983). For systems moving in a socialist direction, he suggested several empirical indicators: (a) an emphasis on the social etiology of disease and on more equal access to food and services, (b) priority given to formation of participatory organizations, and (c) empowerment of local people to take economic and political control of the health system as a balance against professional dominance of planning at the national level.

In what follows I look specifically for such empirical indicators of social change. Following John Donahue (1991), I also undertook a process-oriented analysis, in contrast to a structural analysis, which focuses on identifying points of change in a social system with a dualistic "before and after" orientation. Citing Raymond Firth, Donahue points out that structural analysis alone cannot interpret social change. A process-oriented approach puts the social change aspects of popular health into historical context and focuses on choices of actors within social settings, looking at the outcomes of decisions, struggles within and between groups, and institutional realignments within the health system. A process-oriented approach is particularly appropriate because, as popular health workers pointed out to me repeatedly, their system was evolving in "the struggle for a better life." And "struggle" (*lucha*) in the ex-refugee communities referred to a permanent social process, not only the military conflict.

Campesino Experiences with the Ministry of Health

Before the war, medical facilities in Chalatenango were the poorest of any department. In 1971 only 51 percent of the population had access to health services, compared to 93 percent in the coffee-growing department of Santa Ana. One of fourteen departments, Chalatenango received only 2 percent of the health budget that year, compared with 12 percent for Santa Ana. Two-thirds of the Chalatenango households were rural. In a 1978 health survey of San Miguel de Mercedes, a rural town of three thousand, only one-fifth of the houses had electricity, half lacked potable water, and 90 percent lacked latrines or toilets. Only a third of the rural population was literate, and few children stayed in school for more than two or three years (Pearce 1986, 50–54).

Chalatecos in rural hamlets had to walk, sometimes for several hours, to reach the ministry clinics based in towns. Each was staffed only by an auxiliary nurse, and doctor visits were irregular. More clinics were constructed in the late 1970s, but funds were never allocated for the necessary additional staff positions, and staffing actually worsened in the early 1980s, resulting in further declines in services (and scarcities of medicines) (Fiedler 1987; and Zwi and Ugalde 1989). Peasants' memories of ministry clinics with bare shelves no doubt colored their opinion of government services. The only urban-based hospital in the department was built in 1973 and has remained chronically underfunded and ill equipped, a situation that two succeeding regional directors of the ministry who spoke with me openly conceded but claimed was out of their control.

The situation of the rural population in government-controlled areas was little changed during my fieldwork compared with before the war. The Central American office of PRODERE, the United Nations Development Program for Refugees, Displaced, and Repatriated Persons, estimated the department's infant mortality rate in 1990 at ninety per one thousand live births, compared to a national rate of sixty-seven per one thousand. Sixty percent of the morbidity of children under one year of age was attributed to infectious diseases and parasites, problems that usually manifested as diarrhea. Malnutrition affected about half of the children in this age group. Surveys by PRODERE and the University of El Salvador showed that half of children under five had suffered diarrhea in the previous year (PRODERE 1992).

In 1993 the ministry maintained thirty-four health posts and clinics in rural municipalities of the department accessible by poorly maintained dirt roads. A year after the war ended, most were only visited by physicians irregularly, since there were too few physicians to cover the rural areas. The Ministry of Health continued wartime practices of sending caravans of physicians and nurses to rural areas, but these were very irregular and poorly advertised. Residents of cantónes who got sick sometimes hiked to see the doctor only to be disappointed when he failed to show on the appointed day. Beginning in mid-1993 additional funding from the ministry's central office allowed "permanent" doctors to be assigned at some of these clinics, which meant that doctors were expected to spend two to three days per week at the clinic.

Nurses at ministry clinics dealt with a small number of basic medicines, but antibiotics or antiparasitics for diarrhea or for respiratory infections—the two largest killers of children in El Salvador—could only be handed out by (frequently unavailable) government doctors. In interviews with residents of repopulated communities, a common refrain emerged about government services. Don Manuel, a fifty-three-year-old man, said, "Before the war . . . the ministry doctor came every eight to fifteen days. And there was a nurse, but she had bourgeois ideas. They treated people like themselves best. They only gave pills to the poor and pushed them out the door. We have a better health service now. There's more brotherhood. These promoters are poor like us." Juana, a sixty-six-year-old patient, said: "The [ministry] clinic closed in 1980. The doctor only came now and then. He gave away a few medicines, but if it was something expensive he'd just give you a prescription. Sometimes you couldn't afford to buy it. The nurse couldn't handle serious illnesses like measles or a fever. For things like that you'd have to walk to Chalatenango [city]."

Residents of the resettlements maintained that the hospital in Chalatenango (city) discriminated against them. This was undoubtedly related to the general fear the ex-refugees had of government institutions, during the war years. Just living in or coming from an area where rebels were active was enough to warrant detention by police. For someone in San José Las Flores, going to the hospital during the war involved walking four or five hours, passing through a hostile army roadblock, a long wait, having to answer questions about where she is from, being asked for a ID card that Salvadorans are required to have but that ex-refugees often didn't, and being asked for a "voluntary" contribution to the hospital's "Patronato," or benefactor fund (which most campesinos interpreted as required payment for treatment).[4] If the appointment was not completed before midafternoon, the patient would need to pay for lodging in the city.

Once, Karen, a new nurse-practitioner volunteering at the Guarjila clinic, and I accompanied a man with a broken leg to the Chalatenango hospital in the back of a pickup truck. A campesino by the side of the road flagged the driver down requesting a ride and jumped on the back. He saw the injured man and asked where we were going.

"To the hospital," Karen replied.

"No," cried the hitchhiker speaking to the injured man, "you don't want to go there. They'll mess you up at that hospital." Karen hastened to cut him off, then leaned over to the hitchhiker to whisper, "Now is not the time to discuss this."

I interviewed a fifty-seven-year-old ex-refugee who shared these sentiments. She said, "Sometimes they treat you bad at that hospital. One time I went and as soon as they learned I was from Las Flores, they were rude to me. But they did treat me. In 1989 I took my little girl there for an ear infection and they asked me for a 25 colones [US$5 at 1989 exchange rates] donation to the Patronato del Hospital. But I only had money for transportation."

The chorus of criticism was no doubt colored by residents' experiences of losing friends or family to repression by army soldiers and their years of living in a community that literally defined itself by its antigovernment stance. A decade of isolation from the rest of the country meant that many young people viewed anything associated with the government in a negative light.

During my week observing the ministry clinic in San Pedro del Lago, a mid-sized government-controlled town, I found some of these observations to be valid. Because of its strategic location and its native-son army colonel, San Pedro had reaped the benefits of government and USAID largess through many public improvement projects. Compared with most rural towns, San Pedro seemed prosperous, which probably was reflected in the health of citizens. Even some outlying barrios enjoyed potable water and a sewage system, and urban houses were well constructed with cement floors.

The town's Ministry of Health clinic was conveniently located, clean, and open every day. Its full-time staff included Consuelo, an auxiliary nurse (graduate of a one-year ministry training program), and her aide, who washed glassware and cleaned floors. The walls of the waiting room were decorated with WHO posters and graphs about the government vaccination programs. Consuelo, a local resident who had been a nurse for ten years, had a congenial demeanor and was cooperative with my efforts to learn about her work.[5] This clinic contrasted greatly with poorly supplied and understaffed rural clinics in other areas that I had visited.

Despite this impressive exterior, however, I learned that very few patients (only eight to ten per day) came to see the nurse. Mostly Consuelo and the aide sat around talking all day in the empty clinic. The services she performed were limited to injections of vitamins, penicillin, and vaccines (for small children) and handing out aspirins and skin cream. It was a striking contrast with clinics in repopulated communities that served two to three times as many patients in a day, even though the villages were smaller than this town. However, the lack of traffic may have partially reflected a healthier population in San Pedro del Lago.

Consuelo referred most patients with medical problems to the hospital in the city of Chalatenango or suggested they come back on Thursday, the day for physician consults. For three mornings in a row I watched the nurse give aspirin and finally an antibiotic injection to a little girl with a high fever and a badly inflamed and swollen knee, all the while counseling the mother to bring the girl back on Thursday to see the physician. The mother worried that she would have to take her daughter all the way to the pediatric hospital in San Salvador to get her treated. On a trip to Chalatenango city on Tuesday, Consuelo ran into the doctor assigned to San Pedro and asked him to make a special trip to see the girl. But he said he was too busy. Finally on Wednesday the mother announced she could not wait any longer and took the little girl on a bus to the hospital.

From interviews with town residents I learned that one reason few residents visited the clinic was a perception that the nurse "couldn't do anything." I spent one day traveling with Padre Leonel, the local priest, to the town's outlying cantónes. In San Francisco, a village about twenty minutes' drive into the hills above town on a gravel road. Leonel introduced me to a parishioner named Blanca, who expounded on the town's clinic:

No one goes there except if they need to see the doctor on the day he comes for something serious. People don't have confidence in the nurse because they know she only has a year of training and her social service. She doesn't know anything. She refers almost every problem to the doctor. So why do I want to pay three colones to hear that? If I have a headache I'll go straight to the pharmacy and buy an aspirin. If I need an ointment, I go to the [herbal] clinic at the convent.

Compared with San Pedro del Lago, two of the outlying villages were very poor, with dirt-floored houses and undernourished children. In one, we dropped in on Doña Marta, a middle-aged woman who said she had been in pain for the previous three months from a bladder infection. The pills she was given at the ministry clinic did not work, and a doctor in Chalatenango city had only given her a prescription that she could not afford to fill.

This sense of being abandoned by the ministry fueled rapid expansion of the popular system after the end of the war. In two cantónes, Padre Leonel and I met parishioners who were planning to start popular health posts (puestos) Three girls had nearly completed the diocese's Basic Health Course, but the priest predicted a struggle with the Ministry of Health over setting up more popular health posts. "They don't like the competition," he said, explaining that the ministry tolerated local projects for eyeglasses and herbal medicines because those were services the government did not offer.

On Thursday, to my surprise, only twenty patients showed up to see the physician in San Pedro del Lago. The nurse and patients attributed the low turnout to the recent arrival of a new physician in the post who was not as well liked as his predecessor. Consults with the physician were short, lasting about five minutes, and were conducted in an impersonal mode from behind a desk. He performed no physical exams but did look at skin infections. While appearing confident in diagnoses, he seemed uncomfortable relating to the campesinos. While waiting to be called, two patients told me that they preferred a Knights of Malta clinic in a nearby town that "had more medicines and better trained foreign doctors."

An Overview of the Popular Health System

In the former war zone where I did most of my research, about 100 health promoters served a population of about 11,000 residents after the 1992 cease-fire. The six largest resettled villages had populations ranging from 750 to 1,200 in 1992; these villages doubled in size by mid decade and have continued to grow. Most villages had outlying cantónes, many reachable only by hiking. In 1995 cash incomes of families ranged from 200–1,000 colones (US$25–$125) per month, with the more well-to-do families living in the center of town and the poorest in remote areas. Most relied on subsistence farming of corn, beans, and a few vegetables. A wealthier family might farm ten manzanas of land and hold two to three head of cattle, while a poorer family would get by with one to two manzanas and only one cow. Many ex-refugees squatted on land previously owned by wealthier families who abandoned the area in the early 1980s. Richer peasants often sold part of their crop for income or had a second source of income such as a small store or eatery (cafetín) (see Bergmans 1995; also based on my interviews and diocese statistics).

After the repopulation, local governments were elected by direct vote for a directiva, consisting of a president, a vice president, and secretaries for health, education, finances, communal works, women's concerns, and lands. Decisions of the directiva were made in consultation with the general assembly of the community, which had veto power over elected representatives. In addition to popular clinics, there was a popular education system for primary grades with classes taught by lay educators (see Hammond 1998), which gained recognition in 1995 from the Ministry of Education after its teachers passed a national exam.

Other collective projects that helped offset costs of living for participating members include cattle and crop cooperatives and childcare facilities. Some village-based projects sold subsidized goods to the entire region, including a chicken farm, a shoemaking cooperative, a carpentry cooperative, and crafts cooperatives. Some cooperatives functioned well, and others poorly. Shortages of funds, poor accounting or management skills, and petty corruption contributed to the difficulties. Some residents opted out of collective activities to take advantage of private sector options after the war, but even as late as my last visit in 2007, many co-ops continued operations in the zone.

The popular health promoters worked out of six general health clinics (each in a community of 750–1,200 people), three dental clinics, and about a dozen health posts in outlying hamlets. During 1992 the system was backed up by two full-time physicians, (one ex-FMLN and one from the Church). Ana Manganaro, the Church physician, was based at the new clinic-hospital complex in Guarjila, built from $20,000 in funds raised in U.S. churches. In addition to three examining and treatment rooms, the cement-block clinic had a pharmacy and a small laboratory. With its tile floors, high roof, and bright interior (due to skylights), it was easily the finest structure in town.

The adjacent hospitalito had a low-technology operating room and three rooms for in-patients, one with hospital beds and the others with canvas sling cots. One room was equipped for gynecological exams; another held a stack of ex-FMLN medical supplies recovered from secret underground tatús since the cease-fire. The hospital was used rarely, and mainly for short-term stays because the promoters and Ana had decided they lacked enough staff for daily care and feeding of inpatients. Consequently, after the cease-fire, most seriously ill patients were sent to the dreaded public hospital in Chalatenango city. An exception was made during a cholera epidemic in spring 1992 when the hospital housed several cholera patients.[6] Special canvas sling cots were used with holes under the patients' buttocks, where a bucket was placed on the floor for the watery diarrhea.

Since the repopulated villages had no electricity in the early 1990s, a kerosene generator was used for lights at night, but only during emergencies. Skylights sufficed in the daytime. Ana, lived and worked full time in Guarjila, and the clinic served as a referral center for all the repopulated villages in

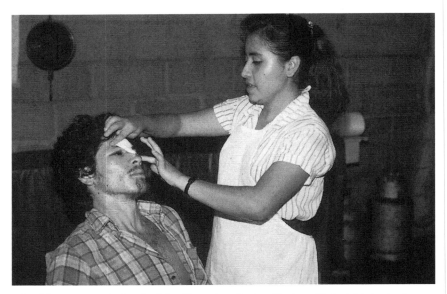

A health promoter in San José Las Flores treating a villager with facial injuries from a fall, 1995. Photograph by Sandy Smith-Nonini.

northeast Chalatenango.[7] A popular system physician visited the other clinics once a week. Promoters made two- to three-hour hikes once a week to see patients in rural cantónes. Most of these hamlets eventually sent a local person for health training and set up a first aid botequín in that promoter's house.

Eight lay promoters rotated shifts at the Guarjila clinic, at least two on duty at a time, twenty-four hours a day. They also rotated responsibilities for record-keeping, pharmacy, lab work, and cleaning duties. The physician saw patients for four hours each morning Monday through Saturday, except when she was away teaching health classes or aiding with vaccination drives. All the promoters had at least three years' experience, and one had worked in health eight years. From twenty to forty patients per day came to the clinic, many referred by promoters in other villages.

The clinic in San José Las Flores was smaller, located in a former telephone office.[8] It had a cement floor, with the main room divided into two sides, one for patient interviews and one equipped with a bed (strung with a rope-mesh covered by a woven mat) for exams. A new birthing room had been added. The clinic was open five days a week and was staffed by five promoters (two with extensive experience) who rotated between clinical work, maintenance tasks, and home visits. Most days the promoters saw fifteen to twenty-five patients.

The most common medical problems treated at popular clinics were diarrhea (especially in infants), respiratory illnesses, and skin infections, which between them accounted for roughly half of diagnoses. Other complaints included muscular pain, headaches, anemia, earaches (in children), asthma, urinary tract infections, and gastrointestinal problems. A few patients in each village had chronic problems requiring medical maintenance such as high blood pressure, epilepsy, chronic depression, and heart disease. Unlike the ministry's community health promoters (CHPs), who were trained under a new USAID-funded program and had very limited training in curative medicine, the popular promoters in the former war zone were essentially "barefoot doctors." In addition to preventive tasks, they were trained to prescribe about thirty-five medicines, including antiparasitic drugs, antibiotics, and antispasmodics, and they did minor surgical procedures such as debriding wounds, lancing abscesses, and suturing cuts.

Like government nurses and CHPs, the popular promoters vaccinated children for diphtheria, pertussis, tetanus (DPT); polio; and measles, but the diocese vaccination schedule was more frequent, with a two- to three-day campaign every four months.

On monthly prenatal days, pregnant women came for checkups by a female promoter trained in obstetrics and gynecology. Like other patient exams, these were privately done and in a casual atmosphere with mother and promoter exchanging local gossip. The promoters took blood pressures and did hemoglobin analyses for anemia using a handheld device. Pregnant women got vitamins for the first three months and iron supplements for the entire gestation. Most gave birth at home with local midwives, many of whom attended diocese training on birthing. But a growing number were choosing to give birth at the clinic attended by a midwife or promoter with birthing training. The popular system workers had congenial relations with local midwives, although privately they considered some to be more competent than others.

Once military roadblocks were lifted in early 1992, the Church was able to keep clinics' pharmacies well stocked with basic medicines. During the war, a medical visit and medicines were free, but the diocese began encouraging the clinics to ask patients for small donations to offset the cost of medicines. The San José Las Flores clinic requested a donation of one colón (12 U.S. cents at 1992 exchange rates), which most patients offered, but if they did not, promoters did not ask. Some patients brought fruit or firewood instead of money.[9]

Popular Dental Health

Dental health clinics were based in three repopulated communities, and these had their own complement of promoters. This project grew out of the efforts (during and after the war) of an international NGO based in San Salvador that stressed appropriate technology, community-based dental care. The dental promoters handed out toothbrushes, gave talks in schools, and taught campesinos to make toothpaste from ashes and bicarbonate of soda. The promoters not only pulled rotten teeth (the only dental service offered by the Ministry of Health in rural areas) but also drilled out cavities and filled them, and in the region's small dental laboratory based in Las Flores, several more highly trained promoters made bridges and crowns at affordable prices. Each clinic had its own generator to power drills and lights, and an ingenious gravity-driven system with plastic water barrels in the rafters and long plastic tubes was used to operate hand-held water sprays.

Dental health workers, who lacked the direct support of the diocese, were encouraged to achieve self-sufficiency in financing. Their small salaries depended on profits being generated by their clinic, which charged nominal fees for services. Each newly trained promoter was given a cow with the hope it would generate ongoing family revenue. This worked for some, but in other cases the cow got sick or died, and dental promoters often complained because of their low incomes. There were few funds to fix broken generators, so sometimes clinics closed for lack of electricity. Nevertheless, the project struggled along. The oral health system sent representatives to popular health planning meetings until 1995 when its NGO support faltered. Leo, an FPL physician, took a special interest in promoting dental work and advocating for more support for it from the diocese. In meetings he pointed out that tooth decay, an extremely common problem in corn-eating peasant populations, introduced bacteria into the body and was a large contributor to systemic infections in undernourished people.

The Popular Health Promoters

The San José Las Flores promoters helped me design a survey with quantitative and qualitative questions that I administered to forty-one promoters at regional meetings. Thirty-nine surveys were completed. About half the respondents (nineteen) worked inside the formerly FMLN-controlled zone and the other half (twenty) were based in areas that had long been under government control. (Between 1992 and 1995 about two hundred promoters trained in diocese health programs worked outside the former war zone, and these areas represented the most rapidly growing part of the popular system.) About half of respondents were under age thirty. All lived where they worked, and two-thirds were based in remote areas. About three-quarters of promoters in the FMLN-controlled territory were female, compared to half in government-controlled areas. Church workers attributed this to women being more restricted in their activities in areas not influenced by the FMLN. Both male and female promoters said that in rural areas, fathers (and husbands) frowned on young women traveling because this took them away from their domestic responsibilities. Health promoters needed to be able to travel to attend health classes, and to hike to more remote villages.

Most promoters in the former war zone had been recruited by community leaders or church workers for health training. Reina, a promoter in San José Las Flores, described how she came to work in health:

> It was in February 1988. I was seventeen and still single. I was in the third grade at school. Cristina and Maya [more experienced promoters] came to ask me if I wanted to work in health. You see, many couldn't take on the commitment because of family responsibilities, but I didn't have any children. And some couldn't because they didn't know how to read and write. At first I didn't want to do it because I wanted to continue in school. But I decided to enter the course. They presented me to the [village] assembly [for approval]. They always look for someone with initiative, so the assembly rarely says no. There were eight of us in the course. The idea was to see who did best; some dropped out because they didn't like it, especially working with injuries. Only Inez and I stayed.

Reina said that the large need for health work due to the war was one reason she stuck with it, but she also found that the more she learned about health work, the more it interested her.

One survey question asked if promoters' health work caused problems with their families. Seven promoters from government-controlled areas cited problems with child care or a father or husband opposing their work, compared with only two from the former war zone. Women in the repopulations encountered fewer problems because each village had a collectively run child care facility. Also, men were more accustomed to women working outside the home because women were drafted into a wide variety of tasks from food production to military duty during the war. Once when I expressed surprise at the lack of family strife over health work, a promoter in Guarjila shrugged and said, "Our husbands are *consiente* [politically conscious]."

Nevertheless, a similar number of promoters from both regions complained that they had trouble finding time for health work, given other household demands such as grinding corn for tortillas and farming. About half worked part time in health, and half (primarily in the former war zone) worked full time. Another "family problem" cited by four promoters in the government-controlled area was lack of economic resources, a problem mentioned by only one promoter in the former war zone. Promoters in the repopulations received small stipends (from a fund raised by Dr. Ana in U.S. churches), whereas promoters in formerly government-controlled areas were volunteers.

Three-fourths of those surveyed had worked in health more than three years. In the former war zone, where public schools closed during the conflict, slightly more than half had three years or less of formal education, whereas promoters in government-controlled areas averaged five or more years of schooling. Three-quarters of the promoters had completed the Diocese's basic health course (six sessions of two to three days each spread over several months) and over half were enrolled in the seven-session advanced course. Many also reported completion of specialty courses in natural medicines, oral health, anesthesia, laboratory science, mental health, or midwifery.

Daily Work at the Clinic

Patient visits with promoters tended to be informal, often taking place on benches in the common area of the clinic. Those with serious problems were given a physical exam in a private room. Promoters saw patients first, referring more serious cases to the physician. Patients were accustomed to this "gate-keeping" role on the part of promoters, but occasionally someone asked specifically to see the physician, and promoters usually tried to comply. Most patients I interviewed expressed respect and admiration for the promoters. Several pointed out that they served the community for years with little or no pay.

Unlike ministry nurses, promoters wore no uniforms and neither the physician nor the promoters used makeup. When Dr. Ana examined a patient in the examining room, a promoter always stood by. As a learning device, the physician would defer to the promoter first to see if she could do the diagnosis alone. She then would explain, in simple language, to the patient (and promoter) what the diagnosis meant and how to treat it. Because peasant women tend to be very modest, patients were not routinely asked to disrobe, except as necessary for the exam.

The clinics were run in a collective style. Although Dr. Ana helped coordinate the clinic in Guarjila, she never gave orders, and promoters shared decision making. One concern the staff had about the return of the Ministry of Health to the area was the government's tradition of hierarchical structures in which a rural clinic answers to a distant, often unresponsive central administration, and the doctor assigned to a clinic is the supervisor of all other personnel. As Ana put it succinctly, "We would not like to work that way."

The collective approach worked well most of the time in San José Las Flores and Guarjila; its main drawback was that it was easy to bow out of responsibility when a group of promoters lacked enthusiasm about a task or project. In two other repopulation communities, more poorly organized promoters teams sometimes failed to follow through well with community campaigns. Conversely, the collective approach protected promoters from pressure to serve as assistants to every professional passing through. For example, Leo periodically used the operating room at Guarjila to do elective surgeries such as repairing hernias and removing pterygial growths from eyes (a common local affliction). This service was not a priority of the popular health system, but Leo insisted it was important because peasants often waited months for elective surgery at a public hospital. But his use of the operating room meant more work for the Guarjila promoters.

One day he asked them to clean and set up the room for him for an upcoming surgery day, but his request was conveniently neglected. When I ran into Leo later at the Guarjila cafetín, he was fuming because nothing had been cleaned or sterilized in advance when he arrived with the patient, causing a two-hour delay in the operation. He complained: "The problem is no one is in charge. They work in shifts here, so when I complained, the promoters just told me, 'I wasn't on duty' or 'It wasn't my responsibility.'" But from the perspective of the Guarjila promoters (and Dr. Ana), they had too many other demands on their time to be also serving as Leo's surgical assistants.

In interviews with me, Ana, described herself as a technical resource for the promoters and the repopulations. She saw her teaching as equal in importance to clinical work, and she was looking forward to turning over some clinic responsibilities to a newly arrived nurse practitioner from the United States so she could spend more time preparing her advanced health class. Like other members of the diocese technical team, Dr. Ana was a long-term volunteer with a minimal stipend for living expenses and transportation. Two or three professionals on the team drove four-wheel vehicles owned by the Church while others used their own vehicles. The technical team typically consisted of two or three physicians, two or three people with nursing or allied health degrees, and two or three experienced promoters. Most professionals were "internationalists" in 1992, but gradually the team replaced foreign volunteers who left with Salvadorans and recruited more promoters. Three ex-FMLN physicians from the former war zone helped set up a new (FPL-affiliated) health NGO after the cease-fire to support health development. They obtained funding through the NGO for office space, modest stipends, and access to four-wheel drive vehicles or motorcycles, but their grant-writing efforts for health projects in the repopulated communities were not very successful, in part due to a decline in the endowments of a European foundation that had supported them.

Because most volunteer physicians managed to secure (NGO-provided) access to vehicles after the cease-fire, they faced fewer transportation problems than promoters did. One result was that the physicians spent a lot of time on the long "four-wheel-drive" excursions taxiing promoters home after meetings or transporting patients (there were no ambulances in the repopulations). I sometimes spent nights at their houses in the villages, (most built of the same bajareque construction as peasant houses and lacking plumbing).

Although most technical team members downplayed their importance as leaders, deferring to the promoters, these professionals were clearly in the habit of serving in a wider role. They often complained about the constant demands on their time; typical nonclinical tasks involved planning and attending endless meetings, representing the health system to community leaders and visitors, grant writing, and teaching promoters. Because they had vehicles, advanced education, cultural capital, and bilingual ability in some cases, they were the natural ambassadors to the outside world. While their frequently stated goal was to prepare health promoters for such organizing tasks—and indeed, a number of promoters stepped into these roles—during the three years of my fieldwork, there never seemed to be enough promoters willing to take on the myriad of leadership roles that materialized.

One day around dusk after a frustrating meeting on this topic in Arcatao, Leo offered me a ride home on the back of his "moto." As we slid around trying to gain traction on the muddy hillsides, we talked about the meeting, shouting to be heard above the roar of the engines. He groused about the dilemma. "Sometimes it seems like what we've done is turn these girls [bichas] into doctors, and the doctors into organizers!" I laughed out loud; it was a fairly accurate description of the situation.

From the promoters' perspectives, there were serious downsides to taking on leadership jobs. A big one was transport, which at that time meant piling into the back of whatever pickup was going your way. Hours passed between vehicles in more remote towns. Another problem was money for bus fares and meals on the road.

Popular Health Organizing and "Participation"

The sine qua non for keeping the popular system going was participation. Promoters were encouraged to take initiative at meetings and in community outreach work to promote practices and policies aimed at preventing disease. One example of preventive health work was promoting the building and use of latrines. Since 1987 the Catholic Church had invested international relief funds in potable water projects and latrine construction in the repopulations, but often the labor to build them had to be coordinated locally. A 1995 household survey of one large village (including nearby barrios) showed latrines had been built for 7 percent of the 236 households, however, only 3 of 59 households in the more remote hamlets had latrines (Bergmans 1995).[10] Other campaigns included vaccination drives, education about protecting children from parasitic infections, and workshops on making and using herbal medicines.

One of my favorite events during my fieldwork was monthly retreats of representatives of health teams from villages across the department. These were held at one of several training centers that had been established by the Church for training of rural catechists at the height of liberation theology organizing. The two-day events included reports from villages, educational classes, interactive group activities such as role-playing or short dramas, and roundtables on problem solving or strategic planning. The sessions were put together by technical team members and were very loosely structured and participatory. When policy changes were proposed, the problem was discussed and voted on in these sessions. Promoters often returned to their village health committees to discuss options or proposals aired at these meetings. Finding ways to implement new policies fell to the technical team, but this was a slow process because of all the consultation.

If the system had an ideology (beyond general social justice goals) it was an ethic of participatory democracy. An individual who was seen as too egotistical or who was lazy and failed to follow through on group commitments risked becoming a subject of gossip. The most frequently cited explanation for failed initiatives was poor participation, either by an individual or by the community.

Members of the technical team or experienced promoters tended to criticize less experienced promoters for being too focused on curative care at the expense of community education work. For their part, campesinos living in the villages valued the curative services more than preventive ones. For example, a young woman from San José Las Flores told me, "Sometimes [the promoters] tell us they don't have the medicines we need or they tell us that medicines won't help. We need someone who has a better understanding." Dr. Ana argued that the main challenge facing community-based health was the degree to which a system could balance epidemiological priorities with the "felt needs" of the population. Residents of the repopulated villages tended to talk about health in terms of personal experiences with illness. Most patients left the clinic with some kind of pills, and the most common complaints came from people who had been told the clinic did not have the medicines they needed (or wanted).

In teaching promoters, the technical team health workers actively discouraged overmedicating, which was seen as a chronic problem in the country given the lack of regulation and abundance of street-corner pharmacists. Rural Salvadorans frequently asked for vitamin injections to "boost their energy" and firmly maintained that injections were more powerful than pills. An elderly woman told me, "I knew a woman about to die in her bed, but she wouldn't go to the [popular] clinic because they wouldn't give her an injection." In contrast to the Ministry of Health, which offered vitamin B injections, the popular system discouraged this practice.[11]

The complaints, however, seemed to come from a minority. Most reported satisfaction with the promoters. A middle-aged woman from Las Flores told me, "The promoters are well trained. Sometimes we need a doctor, but that is not essential much of the time. With the ministry we'll have to pay for consults. And if we don't have the money, then what?" A few elderly residents, expressed a preference for doctors, but always with the qualifier of a doctor "who you can trust," using the term "confianza"—a synonym for someone with revolutionary politics.

In addition to Dr. Ana, three ex-FMLN internationalist physicians, Michaela, Octávia, and Leo, remained active with the system after the cease-fire. The physicians expressed a strong sense of camaraderie with the campesino population likely born out of shared experiences of adversity, which seemed qualitatively different from the respect born of awe or subjugation that I later saw peasants accord to urban-based ministry physicians when they came to the area in 1993. The campesinos' faith in doctors, and particularly in foreign doctors, was a constant challenge for the popular system. One elderly woman from Guarjila told me, "I usually wait until the doctor is in before I go to the clinic. Sometimes the promoters don't know what to do. But it's good to have them when she's not here." One Church physician who floated between multiple popular clinics said he had decided his greatest contribution would be to stick with administrative and organizing duties and to stop seeing patients. "When I go to a remote community people still line up to see me. But am I helping the local promoters by seeing thirty patients with headaches and colds—things they can treat? The only benefit I see in that is teaching. It's better to see just the serious cases they can't handle."

I asked a foreign volunteer why she no longer saw patients in the town where she worked as a coordinator in popular health. She said, "I am only going to work here for a short while. What will people do if they learn to depend on me instead of their local promoters and then I leave?" This concern about not deepening dependency on experts in rural areas contrasted starkly with ministry doctors who had been taught that only doctors could cure most diseases.

To the ex-refugees, the existence of a popular health system run by local people was one of the concrete gains from the war. The health system's importance lay in the imminent and visible practicality of the work as a way of making some level of health services available in an area where there was none. Like the collective cattle herds, the carpentry shop, and the childcare cooperatives, popular health was a visible gain over the prewar years when campesino families lived precarious existences with men migrating to distant plantations for day labor. People referred to popular health as part of their lucha (struggle). Wall murals and posters about the repopulations nearly always showed a health clinic in the middle of town.

What Makes Popular Health "Popular"?

Chalatenango's popular health system challenged the professional dominance and hierarchical structures that characterized the Ministry of Health. The issues of contention involved how health services were conceptualized and resources prioritized, how medicine was practiced, and who was authorized to practice it. The Catholic diocese's orientation to health planning had been shaped by the "primary health care" promoted by the World Health Organization, as opposed to the more dominant biomedical model, which treats the distribution of disease as "an aggregate of individual phenomena" (Navarro 1988). Church-trained health promoters were encouraged to place clinical therapeutics in the context of the social, political, and environmental causes of disease, which involve a broad spectrum from personal attitudes to unemployment and the productivity of a farmer's soil.

There were sacred cows—for example, the Church did not address family planning, although more secular members of the health teams often found ways to aid residents seeking contraceptives, if only by referring them to a sympathetic ex-FMLN health worker who did not work directly under the diocese. Also, promoters in remote areas sometimes found themselves in awkward positions negotiating with mothers of children with diarrhea who preferred to seek out one of the few reclusive native healers, who performed spiritual healing rituals. This was officially discouraged in the popular system because it delayed families from bringing the child to a clinic until babies had become dangerously dehydrated. But balancing respect for cultural beliefs against concern that a baby should receive rapid rehydration required touchy diplomacy. A set of tense negotiations of this kind took place over the course of a morning while I was visiting in Arcatao, but it was a relatively rare problem in part because faith in biomedical cures had deeply penetrated rural El Salvador.

Community participation—for example, the health assemblies, home visits during campaigns, and the physical and social accessibility of local promoters—enhances possibilities for citizens to learn about health issues and to give feedback to those who provide services (Gilson et al. 1989). It also builds a sense of self-reliance and personal responsibility for health instead of treating such services as commodities provided by outside specialists (Werner and Bower 1982).

Although the ministry, under increasing influence from bilateral funders (especially USAID) after 1985, belatedly expressed interest in public health, its programs and funding did not reflect its mission statements (Hanania de Varela 1990). The Ministry continued to devote more than 60 percent of its budget to hospital-based curative care in urban centers while neglecting staffing and supplies in rural clinics (Fiedler 1987; and APSISA 1991). In the early-to-mid 1990s, the ministry's most effective nationwide preventive programs were the vaccination drives it had carried out with UNICEF since the mid-1980s, but even with USAID and UNICEF assistance, this program could not shine in rural areas where the ministry had little or no infrastructure or ties to the peasant population (García Jiménez 2001).

Other ministry programs such as latrine projects addressed environmental causes of disease but in practice fell far short of projections. One reason was the ministry's policy that families should purchase the materials for their latrines. Since latrines had not traditionally been used by many campesinos in rural areas, they were seldom considered a priority in a poor household. The problem is that wind-blown fecal matter contaminates water and food for the entire community, so from a public health perspective, lack of sanitation is a community concern, not a private matter. (In contrast, diocese policy was to donate latrines but solicit labor to dig holes for them from community members.) This problem was acknowledged in a study by FUSADES, a San Salvador–based (USAID-funded) think tank that concluded that, despite large infusions of U.S.

funds, the ministry lacked sufficient funds of "political will" to promote preventive practices in rural areas (Hanania de Varela 1990).

The fundamental differences between grassroots-oriented and biomedical health models lay not so much in medical methodology as in the sociopolitical paradigms within which decision making occurs. In Chalatenango, analyses of the causes of most disease was sociopolitical as well as medical, and the popular health leaders saw fundamental social change as the key to improving health. The commitment of promoters was directly tied to their belief that they were playing a role in a movement for social change. Also, unlike the Ministry in Health, the popular system emphasized community participation and expanding services to remote areas. The most central piece of this plan was reliance on health promoters who were native to their communities.

Studies of community health workers globally have concluded that living in the place they work is vital to workers' gaining rapport with patients (Bender and Pitkin 1987; and Woelk 1992). The Alma Ata era was presaged by community-based health work in the 1960s such as Catholic Action projects and the Behrhorst health promoter project in Guatemala (Green 1989). But popular health traditions have older roots. Steven Palmer documents how local Costa Rican health activism, which incorporated popular medical concepts with the new science of public health, laid the groundwork for the Rockefeller Foundation's hookworm campaign in the early 1900s (2003). There has been much debate over who makes an effective lay health worker, and most researchers now stress the importance of adapting programs to cultural norms in specific settings. For example, Dr. Ana regarded the ideal lay worker in rural El Salvador to be a mature female, given that adult women with children made up so much of the patient population.

While it might seem ironic given the emphasis on prevention in the Chalatenango popular system, the popular promoters actually spent more time doing curative care than did ministry CHPs. From observing divisions of duties and time use in the former war zone, I estimated the promoters devoted about 60 percent of their time to curative work in San José Las Flores and about 80 percent in Guarjila. (The tertiary care role of the Guarjila clinic, compared to other clinics in the area, accounted in part for this difference.) Dr. Ana described curative care as the "felt need" of impoverished people. The lay promoters' competence as health providers offered a strong challenge to the ministry's "doctor-centered" system. Chapter 7 addresses the issue of promoter competence in more detail.

Despite the appeal of curative work, the popular promoters engaged in a large number of preventive health and community education activities. Health assemblies were held two or three times a year in each village, and promoters were consulted by local governments considering latrine or water projects. For example, during a cholera epidemic in spring 1992, the popular system conducted a cholera prevention campaign, and that fall they undertook a campaign to reinforce mothers' knowledge how to make and use oral rehydration fluid for infants with diarrhea.

One of the striking differences between ministry health services and the popular system lay in the orientations of the physicians. Professionals in the ministry placed a high value on being based in cities and associated rural work with low status. In fact, the ministry was known for punishing troublesome employees by transferring them to remote rural clinics. Popular system members, in contrast, placed the highest value on rural work and close interaction with campesinos, and put a premium on stretching resources to permit treatment cases of chronically ill patients in remote places. Some of foreign volunteers saw their commitment in El Salvador as temporary—for example, two years—while other's had literally "thrown in their lot" with the "struggle." But in both cases, the prevailing ideal was to, in Paulo Freire's words, "enter into communion" with the population (1982). As a consequence of long-term association with peasants who were actively promoting a communal ideal, many who had worked in rural areas during the war appeared to have revalued their own identities, denigrating to some degree the individualistic, technocentric, and hierarchical aspects of medical practice and reinforcing service-oriented aspects of health care delivery.

In interviews, the professionals and promoters of the popular system were frank in discussing the problems and failures of the popular system in community health education, which included cultural differences in attitudes toward health, practical difficulties that the campesinos had putting public health knowledge into practice, and problems posed by the lack of resources. In contrast, administrators in the Ministry of Health, who seemed unaccustomed to critical evaluation, and often described public health programs as successful by definition while offering little evidence (anecdotal or statistical) to back up abstract claims. Over time I came to see the traditions of critical discussion and evaluation of practices in popular health meetings and community assemblies as the strongest evidence of the system's promise—even where (as usually was the case) there was insufficient epidemiological evidence to judge whether a given approach to public health was succeeding.

The energy level of popular systems workers in 1992 was boosted by optimism over the end of the war. For the first time in memory for many young people, the guns had quieted; with the murderous elite army battalions restricted to barracks, it was possible to grow crops, walk the roads, and take a bus without fear. Everything seemed possible. This was an almost palpable thing. I asked one San José Las Flores promoter, "Do you think the war was worth all the suffering?" She replied, "Look at all we've gained! I think its beautiful living like this in an organized community. We have a good directiva. It's very different from before the war. People look out for each other now."

Over the next two years this optimism diminished somewhat as the peace accords were delayed or fell short of expectations, and as the popular system leaders confronted the intransigence of the Ministry of Health to offer support for the community-based model (see chapter 8). The ingredients of "community participation" in health and the contrast between the popular system and government in this regard are examined in the next chapter.

7

The Elusive Goal of Community Participation

No, No . . .	No, No . . .
No basta rezar	No, it's not enough to pray
Hay que pasa muchas cosas	There is much to be done
Para conseguir la paz	Before we'll achieve peace

–Verses of song sung by promoters at a monthly retreat
of the popular health system

The famous 1978 Alma Ata international health conference, which elevated primary health care (PHC) to the level of international policy, established the year 2000 as the target year for achieving "Health for All." As the millennium turned over, the failure to meet the goal received little fanfare in the media. For health development specialists, it was a failure long anticipated. By the 1990s the focus had shifted to neoliberal health reforms that placed emphasis on efficiency and individual responsibility for health and downplayed state involvement in primary care. By then a growing literature attested to failures of large-scale PHC programs based on lay health workers to impact local health problems in poor nations (see Matomora 1989; and Walt, Perera, and Heggenhougen 1989). Although comparative studies verified that well-trained community health workers could expand access to care at low cost, many national programs built in the 1980s had been hobbled by poor training and inadequate support for lay providers (Berman, Gwatkin, and Burger 1987). Many scholars and development planners blamed a lack of "political will" on the part of governments to carry out true reforms in public health (Bender and Pitkin 1987; and Chen 1989). The seeds of the dilemma were tied to the Alma Ata consensus that public health indices reflected not only available health services but also prevailing socioeconomic conditions such as family income, access to potable water, education, and so on (Poteliakoff 1987). PHC's emphasis on prevention and community education was a corrective for the biomedical model's myopic curative orientation in health development work, and its effectiveness was to hinge on shock troops of informally trained community-based providers. These controversial, heavily mythologized lay workers constituted a tactical end run around the shortfall of physicians in rural areas.

A key aspect of PHC as initially conceived was "community participation," to involve citizens in understanding the causes of disease and motivate them to engage in solving common problems. The idea was for recipients of aid to become agents of their own development instead of passive beneficiaries. WHO recommended that projects involve local residents in assessment, definition of problems, setting of priorities, and planning activities (Foster 1982). Health promoters were to be the intermediaries in this outreach work, acting as social change agents—not only educating their neighbors about oral rehydration therapy but also organizing villagers to lobby local authorities for a better water system. Yet by the 1990s, despite two decades of experiments in PHC, community participation remained a rhetorical staple of government health development proposals that often had little reality in practice (Woelk 1992; Wayland and Crowder 2002). The problem was in part political. Alarmed by the potential costs and the implications of hundreds of "social change agents" in rural areas, some governments reacted with skepticism to the Alma Ata plan. Backed by the Rockefeller and Ford foundations and USAID, more conservative health development experts sought to scale back comprehensive PHC to what became known as "selective PHC" (SPHC)—emphasizing a few vertical programs aimed at reducing mortality from a handful of preventable diseases (Unger and Killingsworth 1986). The lay provider under this new SPHC conception had strictly defined duties, often confined to preventive health education. In practice these "mass-produced" village health workers were usually trained in the capital city, were not always native to the towns they served, and often ended up more closely tied to a distant, centralized Ministry of Health than to their village (Gilson et al. 1989; and Matomora 1989).

In their landmark endorsement of SPHC, Walsh and Warren argued that comprehensive PHC was idealistic and too costly (1979). Instead of a focus on community participation and equity, SPHC advocates convinced the United Nations to back a few top-down (or vertically designed and controlled) programs targeting a handful of preventable high mortality illnesses (Unger and Killingsworth 1986). So, instead of locally based initiatives, WHO and UNICEF endorsed the well-known "GOBI" programs to reduce child mortality—consisting of growth monitoring, oral rehydration therapy (ORT), breast-feeding promotion, and immunization. International finance institutions aided ministries of health in setting up urban-based training of lay health workers, although the effectiveness of many programs that "mass produced" lay health workers has been questioned (e.g., Matomora 1989; and Walt, Perera, and Heggenhougen 1989). In a review of six large-scale PHC programs, Berman and colleagues found that due to poor training and low support for lay workers, the quality of services they offered was often poor (1987). They found no measurable health impact but noted that there was a paucity of data on effectiveness for any rural health program, whether PHC or clinic-based services.

Neither did the vertically implemented GOBI technologies by themselves prove to be the "magic bullets" they were touted to be. One review of international health literature showed GOBI approaches to be compromised by inattention to local cultural and social factors (Rifkin and Walt 1986). Also, continued inattention to basic sanitary infrastructure in many countries led to patterns in which a child saved through immunization or ORT ended up dying of another illness. Others challenged the accounting methodology in the handful of studies showing SPHC to be cost effective and pointed out that by focusing so exclusively on child mortality, SPHC ignored the health of other age groups and the bulk of conditions that caused pain and suffering in marginalized populations (Unger and Killingsworth 1989). Researchers Susan Rifkin and Gill Walt concluded, "To the advocates of SPHC, community involvement is only significant in terms of getting large groups of people to accept the medical intervention the professionals have selected to use" (1986, 562).

The popular health system in Chalatenango aspired to a form of community participation more closely aligned with the Alma Ata ideal. This orientation became a chief stumbling block in negotiations with the Ministry of Health, a topic treated in more detail in chapter 9. This chapter evaluates community participation in the popular system, comparing it with El Salvador's USAID-designed community health promoter (CHP) program operated by the Ministry of Health. The findings challenge the prevailing pessimism about the potential for lay providers and participatory approaches in international development.

Components of Community Participation in the Popular System

Understandings of health in the popular system were strongly influenced by Paulo Freire's participatory pedagogy. Educational materials written by international church volunteers relied heavily on David Werner's rural health guides, with adaptation to Salvadoran peasant culture.[1] Teachers revised lessons as they learned what worked best, eventually generating a course manual. The texts used simple explanations and colloquial expressions, drawing on local terms for illness and illustrated with humorous cartoons of peasant characters drawn by a local artist. The focus was on common illnesses, combining preventive and curative information. In classes there were few lectures but many participatory exercises, games, and hands-on workshops where promoters could practice new techniques.

In one workshop I observed, promoters learned the structures of the respiratory system in a game. After dividing into groups, the students had the task of arranging colored cards to show all the parts of the body that air passes through on the way to the lungs. Each group posted their solution, and they debated about which was right. During the discussion, an older male student said he had drawn on his knowledge of chicken anatomy in ordering the parts.

Besides learning to prescribe about thirty-five medicines for common problems, in one module promoters learned to prepare and use local medicinal plants that the church had found to have therapeutic value—knowledge that their grandmothers had but that had been dying out. A course was developed on health rights, partly in response to repression against health work and other civilian services in conflicted areas during the war. By August 1993, 189 promoters throughout the province had completed the basic course and fifty-one had completed the advanced course.

Barbara Jordan has commented on the culturally inappropriate use of abstract reasoning in lay health training courses instead of the empirical experience that is more meaningful to people who lack a formal education (1993). At first glance, the Salvadoran Ministry of Health's CHP promoter-training manual appeared similar to materials of Chalatenango's popular system, with simple drawings and step-by-step treatment guides. But when I compared a section on diarrhea in the two manuals, I was struck by the ministry's use of abstract, professional terminology. Diarrhea was defined as "an increase in volume, fluid and frequency of evacuations of an individual in relation to his normal habit of defecation, caused by viruses, bacteria, parasites and other vectors . . ." compared with the popular system manual's description, which used the colloquial term "pupu" and drew attention to empirical signs: "diarrhea is pupu that is liquidy and frequent. It has other characteristics that can help you determine the cause. For example its color and consistency, whether there is fever, or vomiting, how many times a day. . . ." Interestingly, I discovered that because it is a common household concern, peasant women were often more knowledgeable about symptoms and types of children's diarrhea than North American citizens, although their terminology and "explanatory models" differed.

Popular system promoters who took a Ministry of Health promoter training course in 1994 were frustrated and intimidated by its abstract materials and by the formal, didactic teaching methods used. Maya, a San José Las Flores promoter, described the ministry course: "There was a lot of theory. And they taught too many themes in a day. The teachers were very concerned about how the students presented themselves. They demanded that they come to class well dressed, with nice shoes. That's difficult for someone from a cantón. Sometimes I think the ministry did this just to make the popular promoters drop out. But the promoters did the best they could." By 1993 experienced Salvadoran promoters were training as instructors in the Church course, and on my last visit in 1995 local Salvadorans taught large sections of both the Basic and Advanced courses.

Another characteristic of popular promoter education was an effort to situate health in political realities. In a workshop I attended on pesticide poisoning, diagnosis and treatment were only part of the lesson. The heart of the class was small group work on how to alert the community to the problem and prevent further exposure, followed by a discussion. Interventions proposed by the promoters ranged from worker education to meetings with the landowner and the Ministry of Health.

In another popular education module, the promoters read and discussed a story of a girl who died of tetanus. They then participated in a discussion to identify the "chain of causes," which ranged from the biological (becoming infected after she stepped on a sharp object), to the social (the child being barefoot due to poverty, the father being uneducated and not having her vaccinated), and to the political (a poorly run vaccination program on the part of the Ministry of Health).

Locally Based Lay Health Promoters

Even opponents of comprehensive PHC do not dispute that in rural areas of developing countries, equity in access to health services depends on training lay workers due to the shortage of rural health professionals in most settings. Nevertheless, professional dominance has been a persistent barrier to acceptance of lay health workers. Many national programs, including El Salvador's, placated physicians by casting promoters as health aides with extremely limited duties who were tied to regional clinics rather than working in the community where they live.

In the Chalatenango popular system, lay health promoters were the linchpins. They were the main providers of services, organizers of village campaigns, liaisons to provide feedback on community concerns to the NGOs, and spokespersons for the system. The strong rapport I witnessed between promoters and community members in the repopulations was in part due to the promoters' competence in curative care—their ability to solve people's everyday medical problems. Studies have shown that when lay health workers fail to respond to community members' "felt needs"—usually defined as treatment of acute illness and injuries—they rarely achieve the status and rapport necessary to promote preventive health practices (Bender and Pitkin 1987).

Health promoters in Chalatenango were volunteers, so motivation was an important factor shaping their work. As noted previously, promoters in the repopulated communities tended to cite community service as the most important reason they entered health work, and in the former war zone, women promoters told me their husbands and fathers seldom complained about their work, noting that they were "consiente"—that is, they understood the importance to the community (and to the political struggle) of the health work. But as Cristina, a promoter in San José Las Flores, explained, the issues went beyond any simple conception of gender relations. During the war, she said, all understood that there was a sacrifice involved if a family member worked in health:

> There are tensions. Issues of children who go without care. Meals fixed
> late. And sometimes I have to go away on weekends. We have the child

care facility, but it costs one colón a day, which is a small amount but still significant. My father never told me not to work in health, but I felt I was taking advantage of (my family) since they did all the work in the house. In a sense I was working for everyone, but this wasn't directly helpful for my family. My compañero works hard all day in the milpa, and he deserves to eat when he comes home.

To recruit people as health promoters, the training had to be accessible and affordable. The popular system conducted classes in rural education centers of the Catholic Diocese, and courses were divided into two-day modules spread over several months to minimize disruption of promoters' farming and household duties. In contrast, when a group of popular promoters (hoping for official accreditation) took the Ministry of Health's CHP promoter course in 1995, they had to travel to the capital; pay for lodging, meals, and supplies; and spend weeks away from their families. Because of their teacher's emphasis on appearance, some had to buy expensive leather shoes. Since ministry travel stipends were too low to cover costs, many had to borrow money or sell things to complete the course.

Although the popular promoters began as volunteers, beginning in 1992 promoters in the repopulated communities received nominal stipends equivalent to US$15–40 per month (depending on hours per week worked) from a small fund administered by the Coordinadora de las Comunidades Repobladores (CCR), a regional repopulation council. This fund, initially raised in U.S. churches, remained in danger of running out, and the regional representatives for the resettled villages were hesitant to commit to long-term support of promoters, particularly since national health services were gradually being resumed since the cease-fire.[2] This was a source of constant insecurity to the promoters. Despite the nominal levels of the stipends, most promoters regarded them as critical support.

The issue of remuneration was passed off lightly by the Ministry of Health when, in negotiations with the government after the cease-fire, leaders of the popular system asked the government to pay minimal stipends to those popular promoters who passed the ministry's CHP course. The ministry's Chalatenango health director told me, "They've served as volunteers all this time, so why are they complaining. Why don't they just keep volunteering?"

In contrast, the salaried CHP promoters of the ministry tended to function more like employees than community members, according to official evaluations of the program carried out in 1995.[3] The study revealed that the approximately fourteen hundred ministry CHP promoters trained since 1990 were frequently transferred from one community to another, and they lacked adequate training or supplies to resolve most routine health problems they encountered in rural areas.

After mid-1993, a negotiated agreement between the two systems allowed the Ministry of Health to place physicians (during their social service year) in repopulation clinics, where they worked alongside popular promoters, as discussed in chapter 8. The popular promoters played a central role in these negotiations, but few were pleased with the outcomes. In several sites ministry physicians effectively sidelined promoters by taking over "high status" medical consults, relegating promoters to support tasks and rural vaccination campaigns. This hurt promoters' local reputations and created discontent within their ranks, particularly after 1994 when the ministry reneged on a negotiated plan to hire twenty-two repopulation promoters who completed the ministry's CHP training course.[4]

Another major difference between popular promoters and ministry CHP promoters was participation in management. Within the ministry, promoters had only one option for advancement, which was to become a CHP program supervisor. And plans were under way to eliminate most supervisor positions as part of a quiet downsizing effort in 1995. In contrast, in 1995 the Chalatenango Catholic diocese was expanding promoter opportunities and hired a team of promoters to do regional outreach to spur the building of community-based health committees that would work (with local promoters) to solve health problems in remote areas. Plans were also under way to bring more promoters onto the diocese's technical support team, replacing foreign volunteers. These were not unproblematic efforts but involved a myriad of logistical and social discussions. Despite new promoter members on the technical team, I noticed that foreign volunteers still tended to dominate discussions and decision making. Furthermore, even with the lure of better pay, not many promoters were lining up for these promotions because many preferred staying in their community to traveling.

The Preventive/Curative Debate

The concept of PHC evolved as a corrective to urban-based, hospital- and physician-centered services. Many developing countries are like El Salvador in that most of the health budget is earmarked for hospitals while the vast majority of mortality and morbidity is tied to preventable, poverty-related conditions (Fiedler 1987). Based on an analysis of inpatient care staffing requirements, Fiedler and colleagues (1998) found that El Salvador's hospitals continued to receive funding "far in excess of what case-mix and case-load considerations would warrant" (296). Supporters of "intersectoral" PHC in the Alma Ata years underestimated the degree to which professionals, politicians, and development agencies had vested interests in curative care. They also mistakenly assumed health planners would be able to influence aspects of rural infrastructure such as roads and water systems, which have often turned out to be in the jealously guarded turf of other government ministries.

In addition, there are few immediate visible gains from preventive efforts, and most politicians, development agencies, and poor people themselves like to see results that can be demonstrated in a few months or years, not decades. Thus preventive health has remained the unimportant, underfunded stepchild of curative medicine. This was true in Chalatenango's popular system as well as in the ministry CHP program. Both faced similar pressures but while the popular system struggled to keep prevention and community education as central components, the ministry's mechanisms adhered to the curative model. Moments of innovation repeatedly degenerated as if caught in a gravity well of bureaucratic hysteresis.

A one-week course on community education was added in the popular system in response to a survey showing that promoters spent four to five times as many hours in curative care as in community-education work (Capps and Crane 1989). During fieldwork in San José Las Flores, I witnessed promoter involvement in home visits including a health campaign on cholera (during a regional epidemic) and discussion of health in village meetings. Arcatao, Las Vueltas, and Guarjila had similar levels of community health activity. However, promoters in three other repopulations appeared less active in local education.

In my own survey of promoters, 33 percent of them reported participating in three or more community-wide health campaigns during 1992, 28 percent said they participated in two campaigns, 18 percent in only one, and 15 percent in none. Three-quarters reported that they had given three or more educational talks to community groups that year, and 20 percent reported giving two or more talks.

I studied community education activities noted on promoter monthly reports for a popular health region containing three villages and seven small hamlets. In a twelve-month period from 1993 to 1994, promoters reported a total of forty-eight educational talks (some in village assemblies), twenty health campaigns (several involving house-to-house visits), and eight meetings with community health support committees.

I also followed a community campaign to convince residents to corral their pigs so they would not enter (and defecate in) houses. The promoters made humorous posters and towns held assemblies to discuss what to do. One village passed a rule that pigs caught running wild would be confiscated until the owner paid a small fine, but this was not enforced because it made some townspeople angry. Over the next two years I noted that pig sties slowly got built next to many homes, but some pigs also continued to run free. Many poorer and older residents felt their pigs should run free because the residents did not have enough food in their households to feed a fenced-in pig. The popular health workers were unable to find solutions that satisfied everyone. Nevertheless, through the village assemblies, it grew to be general knowledge that pigs inside houses were associated with disease—a first step, some might say, in education. The problem was eventually solved when more houses were built, each one surrounded by a fence, with gates to keep animals out of the house, but this took several years.

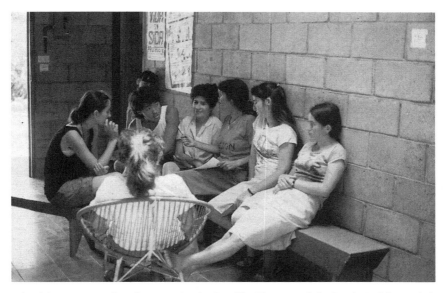

A health promoter planning meeting in Guarjila. Photograph by Sandy Smith-Nonini.

No member of the popular system's technical team felt the amount of preventive work was adequate, and the level varied greatly from site to site. Promoters said they found curative work more enjoyable, and they sensed a high community demand for it. Interestingly, in 1992 I noted that in Guarjila, where there was a locally based physician and a clinic/hospital that served as a referral center for the other resettled villages, promoters spent considerably less time in community education than did promoters in San José Las Flores, where there had never been a permanent physician. The promoters with the most resources were reaching out the least, instead emulating their physician role model and her prestigious curative work.

A key contradiction that emerged in popular system negotiations with the Ministry of Health centered on promoter competence to prescribe antibiotics. While this had long been common practice in the popular system, it was in the eyes of the ministry not only irresponsible but also illegal. Given campesinos' constant requests for medicines and the impossibility of doing tests for every probable bacterial infection in rural areas, physicians in the popular system suspected that many promoters overprescribed antibiotics. But Tomás, a Venezuelan physician working with the Church, insisted it was not a problem of promoters specifically: "This concern ought to apply as much to doctors as to promoters. Doctors do it too in rural areas, for fear that the patient will get worse after they go home, and won't be brought back to the clinic. I've done it myself. And it is beneficial for that patient being treated."

Due to these concerns, members of the diocese technical team designed a teaching module about the problem of overprescribing. From my observations, and interviews with popular physicians, this problem seemed most prevalent among less experienced promoters. Guarjila's clinic records for September 1992 were typical. They indicated that promoters had treated twenty-one patients with colds and sore throats that month but had only prescribed antibiotics for three of those cases. The more typical treatment for a cold was acetaminophen and sometimes onion and honey cough syrup made locally by promoters trained in herbal medicine.[5]

Popular teaching materials specifically warned against prescribing ampicillin (the most commonly used antibiotic in the popular system) for simple colds. Marlene, who had three years' experience as a health promoter, described her criteria for prescribing antibiotics.

> I only prescribe them when someone has been sick for a long period of time, like fifteen days, and hasn't recovered. I always check their throat, and listen to their lungs, and look for fever. But if they come in after three or four days with a cold asking for antibiotics, we don't give them out. Only Tylenol. But they always ask, they say, "No this won't work. I want those little capsules, they're the only things that will cure it." But we have to tell them no. They think it's magic.

In 1995 this issue also became a major disagreement between the ministry and USAID. Community health development experts hired by USAID to advise the ministry CHP program pointed to studies showing that lives were saved when lay health workers were permitted to give sulfa drugs or antibiotics to infants with acute pneumonia in situations when physician referral was impractical. Nevertheless, high-level ministry officials declined to permit this question to be debated in in-house evaluations of the CHP program carried out by the medical and nursing staffs.

In a barrio outside the capital, I attended a community meeting held to evaluate the role of the local CHP promoter. Several mothers asked why the ministry did not train their promoters to use thermometers so they could evaluate feverish infants. Another complained that promoters were not even able to treat cuts or minor infections but instead told people with injuries to go to the ministry clinic. The complaints were quelled by a ministry physician who chided participants, "You're asking for a miracle. [The promoter's] role is very limited. If she intervenes too much she can make sickness worse. She's not a doctor!" It appeared that "felt needs" were not a ministry priority if they implied lay workers doing even minimal curative care.

Because so many promoters in the repopulations gained hands-on experience in curative care during the war, competence was less of a problem in this setting. In standardized interviews with promoters from San José Las Flores and

Guarjila, I asked them how they dealt with a child with diarrhea. Nearly all displayed detailed empirical knowledge of how to diagnose diarrhea due to multiple causes (including viral, bacterial, "worms," giardia, amoebas, and eating "bad food"). All routinely made and used oral rehydration fluids with dehydrated infants. Most of the time they made diagnoses based on visual examinations of stool combined with mothers' reports of symptoms, although the Guarjila clinic had a small lab for microscopic exams of feces, which they used for difficult cases.

Visiting physicians and ministry physicians who observed promoters at work reported favorably on most promoters' abilities to treat common illnesses. There is little doubt that the prestige that promoters had gained as caregivers enhanced their credibility with rural peasants. Outside the former war zone, however, physicians in the popular system reported greater variability in promoter competence, especially for new promoters in remote areas who had had little clinical supervision. The shortage of popular system professionals to oversee promoters and consult on serious cases in remote areas was a chief complaint of promoters.

Neither the popular system nor the government's PHC programs had conducted evaluations of effectiveness in terms of health benefits to populations from services. In fact, such data are rare in any international PHC program (Berman, Gwatkin, and Burger 1987). I compiled several preliminary observations and findings that suggested the popular system did impact health status in areas it served. For example, in 1992 Catholic NGO health workers reported they were finding much less infectious disease in repopulated villages in formerly FMLN-controlled areas than in areas of Chalatenango that had always been under government control. They attributed the improvements in the former war zone to NGO relief funds being directed into water projects, latrines, and support of health promoters. As a result, in 1993 the diocese health division began redirecting their resources to more needy areas outside the former war zone.

UNICEF surveys showed higher vaccination coverage in zones of war than in government-controlled areas. In 1988–1989 coverage for DPT and polio was 85 percent in northeast Chalatenango where Church-trained promoters and FMLN paramedics worked, compared with 58–68 percent in three of the country's five health regions that were predominantly government-controlled, including the capital. UNICEF personnel attributed the high coverage in war zones to the close ties between health promoters and the rural population, noting that the ministry had a poor record of working in marginalized areas (see Smith 1989b).

A short epidemiological survey in a repopulation village carried out by Boston public health researchers in 1988 reported that, despite ongoing problems with undernutrition, most local mothers knew how to feed and rehydrate

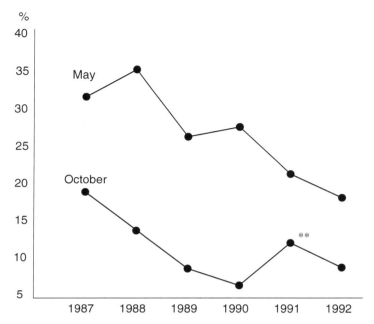

* Including diarrhea from multiple causes, eg. viral, bacterial, amoebas
   and intestinal parasites.
** Only 1st 22 days of month recorded.

FIGURE 7.1 Cases of Diarrhea as a Proportion of All Diagnoses, San José Las Flores
Clinic, Wet and Dry Season Months.

infants with diarrhea, and most made frequent use of the promoter-run health
clinic (Meyers, Epstein, and Burford 1989).

In a survey of five years of clinic records in San José Las Flores, I found consistent drops in percentages of patients coming to the clinic with diarrhea and
skin infections between 1987 and 1992 (see figures 7.1 and 7.2). There was also a
steady drop in patients each year diagnosed with malaria and conjunctivitis, but
the total number of cases for these illnesses was smaller. This declining incidence of infectious diseases in the clinic population occurred during a period
when the local population and monthly clinic visits were growing.[6]

Participation: Revolutionary versus
Christian Styles of Leadership

There were two extremes in soliciting participation—one was the militant
ex-FMLN style, exemplified by Carmen, the first promoter elected coordinator of
popular health in the repopulation. Trained by European FPL physicians,

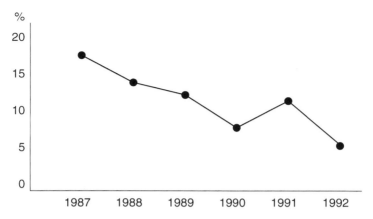

* Including scabies, fungus, dermatitis, abseceses, infections, impetigo.

FIGURE 7.2 Cases of Skin Infections as a Proportion of All Diagnoses, San José Las Flores Clinic, May 1987 to 1992.

Carmen had grown into a highly organized if sometimes impatient leader. When she spread her arms and asked promoters at a meeting to "participate," it was a revolutionary exhortation, a moral demand—"This is your struggle, so play your part!" A few seemed intimidated by this style, but most admired her, and she was elected president of the first national promoter union in 1993.

The other extreme was exemplified by Laura, an American church volunteer on the technical team who strongly believed in pastoral work at the grass roots. She saw her work as "accompanying" campesinos in their struggle, facilitating—but not leading—their efforts to organize and become more self-sufficient. Laura was as patient as Carmen was driven. When she spread her arms at a meeting to solicit promoter "participation," it was a comforting, nonthreatening gesture like Saint Francis of Assisi feeding his birds.

Both Carmen and Laura were successful leaders. But most leaders in the popular health system were somewhere in between these extremes, alternating passive and active approaches to leadership. The most serious offense of a health professional in the popular health system was behaving arrogantly or with a lack of deference to campesinos. It was bad manners for foreign visitors or new volunteers to lapse into their native language with a compatriot in front of Salvadorans, and long-term volunteers chastised those who did. Likewise, the majority frowned on a leader who monopolized discussions at meetings, thereby discouraging promoters' participation. Leo, who, like Carmen, had fought in the guerrilla army, was a frequent offender. His behavior was constantly (and rather openly) criticized by other leaders but to little avail. Promoters from the repopulated villages who worked with him, however, were not intimidated. Leo had married into a family in Arcatao and continued to practice medicine in the former warzone, so his dedication to the popular system more than made up for his garrulous style.

Community Participation in Decision Making

When I arrived in 1992, an elected health representative (responsable) and the lay promoters were the extent of community health committees in San José Las Flores and Guarjila; despite elaborate plans on paper to expand, two years later most village committees had not expanded beyond this model. My survey of community education activities described earlier showed a conspicuously low number of reported meetings between promoters and community health committees (eight in a twelve-month period for a region with eleven communities). Even allowing for the underreporting expected in promoter-prepared monthly reports, my field data suggests that this level of activity was not atypical in the repopulations.[7] The health representative on village councils was supposed to coordinate with but not administer health workers, and to serve as a liaison between them and community members or local politicians. But even in the most well-organized communities, health representatives were often negligent at their duties and left the initiative up to promoters. The town council in San José Las Flores was one of the few that took an active role in health, but even there leadership came from a health promoter who happened to also serve as an elected member of the town council.

More representative feedback was sought through periodic village-wide health assemblies. Promoters sometimes led community "self-diagnostics" in which villagers were asked to identify the town's most pressing health needs. In addition to providing a forum for complaints and feedback to the promoters, these exercises also served to help people draw connections between their poor health and socioeconomic conditions. But as Sjaak van der Geest and colleagues observed, poor peasants are often already well aware of their deplorable living conditions, and health per se is seldom their greatest concern (1990). Such village self-diagnostics sometimes challenged the boundaries of health workers' concepts of public health. In one Guarjila assembly, villagers identified the town's primary health concern as the poor drainage around a residential area where houses were surrounded by mud. It was not a concern that ordinarily falls under the realm of "health," yet the promoters could not deny the obvious health consequences of living in mud. They committed to work with the directiva to seek funds for a housing project to relocate affected homes (which got under way two years later).

In another assembly, village mothers asked the physician and promoters why they were weighing infants. The health team had been trying to determine how widespread malnutrition was in Guarjila, so they weighed 150 children. They found that 53 percent had first degree or mild malnutrition, 27 percent were second degree, and 6 percent were third degree. Only 13 percent had normal weights.

"What good does it do to know our infants are underweight when there's no nutrition program for them?" the mothers asked. The assembly agreed this should be a priority, so the promoters worked out an arrangement with the village council and the community cattle cooperative to obtain milk for the underweight children. Because the chicken farm did not produce enough eggs, they sold a bull and used the proceeds to buy eggs. After that children with mild malnutrition got a daily glass of milk, and those with more severe malnutrition received a daily supplement of milk and eggs. However, by mid-1993 that program was discontinued due to production problems, and mothers were again anxious about food for their children. Neither the popular system nor the Ministry of Health were able to offer long-term solutions to malnutrition and the shortage of vegetables in the diets of rural Chalatecos.

The popular health system continued to struggle with the problem of how to build local leadership and promote a higher level of consciousness about health in rural areas. Marlene, a health organizer in western Chalatenango, was a member of the diocese's new efforts in 1995 to organize more health committees in rural areas. She described her work and how it was received in different areas:

> We always start with Bible classes, and health needs. There are many passages in the Bible that one can relate to social life. We try to establish a common ground. Some communities respond rapidly and form a health support group; in others people have other ideas of what's needed. There are many projects we can help them undertake. But the main problem is people say they don't have enough time. They're busy with their work.
>
> There are some areas where people suffered a great deal during the war, and they have a fear of even talking about the Bible. Some have told me, "We lived through times so hard, when we went on guindas, that we came to question whether God existed." I had never thought about this sort of thing. But if people are interested in working with the community, it's the same thing, because in the Bible helping others is the most important thing. Most of the communities I know like that are engaged in health work.
>
> In communities that did not experience the war, people ask us, "Is this work of the Church, or is it work of the guerrillas?" And in areas with lots of evangelical activity, people talk of community and many beautiful things, but they don't actually do anything; they just spend their time criticizing their neighbors instead of building community.

Marlene and the other members of the organizing team faced formidable transportation problems in remote areas that required them to work long hours for relatively low pay. In addition, their work received a hostile reception in towns where evangelicals had aligned with conservative politicians and the work of Catholics was seen as subversive. At a health planning meeting I attended late in 1995, many expressed concern about their slow progress.

Community Responsibility for Health

By attending a health assembly, community residents enhanced their understandings of causes of disease, but they also came face to face with the limits of a health system's resources. Confronted with such limits, I noticed that health workers (in both the popular and government systems) often attempted to shift the focus to the public's responsibility for their health. For the government (and USAID) this was usually defined as patients' individual financial responsibility. In the popular system, where health promoters were all too aware of their neighbors' almost nonexistent cash flow, this meant local campaigns, such as better trash disposal and fencing in free-roaming pigs as well as "self-financing." Understandably, poor peasants become less interested in participation when the topic became what they would commit in terms of time or payment for basic health services.

After years of free care, "self-financing" became a central dilemma for the popular system in 1993, when the Church, anticipating drop-offs in foreign relief funds in the postwar period, recommended that communities develop schemes to share costs. A variety of plans emerged in different communities, from nominal fees for consults to family insurance plans. In 1994 the popular clinics began paying 25 percent of the diocese's costs of medical supplies. In 1995 that share was to go up to 40 percent, but it became clear that promoters in more remote (and economically marginal) hamlets hesitated to insist on payment from their poorer patients. The technical team delayed moving ahead with the plan until promoters had discussed how to solve the problems. This spurred the decision to focus on outreach by hiring a team of promoters (like Marlene) to visit remote sites and confer with (or help organize) community health committees.

In contrast with the popular health system, promoters in the Ministry of Health CHP program were not encouraged to become involved in organizing, beyond calling on local community leaders to address common concerns, such as latrine projects. (And even with latrines, the issue was individualized since families were asked to pay for the necessary materials.) In a community meeting I attended to evaluate the CHP program, residents requested more help from their local CHP promoter to organize their neighbors and respond to individual problems such as inadequate emergency medical transport and malaria control. But a ministry physician attending the meeting told the residents that such tasks were not central to promoters' duties. A health development consultant who had advised the ministry on the CHP program informed me that high-level ministry officials "don't want promoters organizing people, because they see that as a suspicious and dangerous activity."

Evaluating Community Participation

Interestingly, while rhetoric about participation abounds, concrete studies of programs are rare. Despite the laudable efforts of some scholars to develop measures of participation (Muller 1989; and Rifkin, Muller, and Bichmann 1988), comprehensive efforts by large agencies and government Ministries of Health to apply these measures in evaluating existing program are rare (see Ugalde 1985). A short time after returning from the field, I evaluated the Chalatenango popular system's approach to community participation in the repopulated villages, drawing on Susan Rifkin and colleagues' (1988) "process indicators," including measures of leadership, organization, resource mobilization, management, and needs assessment (Smith-Nonini 1997b). I found leadership indicators to be high but ranging widely, depending on the village. In most cases the health workers themselves dominated health committees, whereas a more ideal model would be greater civilian participation. I gave the system high scores for community organization, however, because village health committees were always interacting in this setting with municipal and regional political structures, and there was democratic selection of regional health representatives, who answered to the resettled villages coordinating committee as well as the NGOs supporting the popular health system (Smith-Nonini 1997b).

One vulnerability of the system by these criteria was resource mobilization, since the system had only limited ability to raise funds locally. Nevertheless, participation in financial decisions was high, with self-financing being discussed in village assemblies by late 1995. Guarjila and San José Las Flores ranked relatively high on "management" for their efforts to balance professional control with community-level control over the health system. But in many villages, communities were less involved. Supervision of promoters was also low in remote areas due to the shortage of physicians. Compared with the clinic-based biomedical model, the popular system was far more tuned into both felt needs and preventive and educational needs in these villages. A key factor in this was their reliance on promoters native to and responsible to the organized villages.

The government's CHP program did not fare as well by the Rifkin criteria for participation because rural communities had little control over organization of health work or its use of resources. The primary activities developed by CHP promoters were house visits for preventive education, and prenatal and infant follow-up care, but their ability to assist patients in need of treatment was limited to referrals to often-unresponsive ministry clinics. Nominal "*patronato*" donations, seen by campesinos as required fees, had long been charged for doctor visits by the ministry, which poorer rural residents saw as a barrier to care. There was little qualitative data available on the CHP program, and USAID-funded evaluations only involved short field visits and relied heavily on interviews rather than observation (Smith-Nonini 1997b).

A second approach to evaluating community participation emphasizes a focus on the social etiology of disease, the building of participatory organizations, and empowerment of local people (Segall 1983). By these criteria, the popular system also ranked well due to its socially conscious pedagogy, attention to equity, community assemblies, participatory modes of decision making, and the linchpin role played by promoters. This was not because the system had succeeded in all areas (for example, community health committees were clearly weak) but because its systems of feedback were reflexive enough to allow the system to adapt to local needs and changing conditions.

John Donahue argues for more attentiveness to process in evaluation as an alternative to analyses that overemphasize programmatic factors or bog down over the difficulties of measuring health outcomes (notoriously difficult to assess for preventive health work except in rarely done longitudinal case studies) (1991). A focus on process sets up a hermeneutic bias, forcing the researcher to confront the fact that critical reflexivity does not reside in a program but rather in the interaction between local residents and specialists.

The high degree of participation in the popular system made the process of decision making less efficient. Problems became discussed at multiple levels, sometimes generating open dissent. As was demonstrated in the "self-financing" project, in order to accommodate dissent, organizers sometimes elected to tolerate more inconsistency in programs than a large development agency would find acceptable. This degree of openness contrasted greatly with the Ministry of Health where many employees expressed fear of sharing their opinions openly. Those who confided in me turned out to be extremely alienated with what they saw as inadequate services and seemingly arbitrary decisions from the top of the institutional hierarchy. Traditions of rigid centralized control and advancement that depend on patronage instead of merit date to the colonial era and are common in Latin American health systems (Fleury 2001; and Iunes 2001).

Consideration of larger historical and cultural traditions brings us to a caveat: The popular model that evolved in Chalatenango cannot be easily lifted out of this setting. The successes realized in community participation in this system were in part due to a new social ethic and new local organizational forms that developed as a means of surviving military conflict. New political and economic tensions created by the end of the war challenged many of these social forms, prompting widespread reassessments of viable goals and strategies.

The harsh conditions in rebel-occupied areas forced peasants to organize themselves to survive, and it was the absence of government institutions that created the political space for this creativity. The FMLN encouraged this "us against them" mindset, so popular health work was nestled in a social setting favorable to new ideas. The new emerging popular leadership had a far higher legitimacy than the distant and hostile national government. In such a setting it was more feasible to risk airing problems and publicly face up to the limits of the system's resources. Conversely, for the government of El Salvador, given its reputation for favoring elites, the peace process negotiations presented a serious risk in that real community participation encourages airing of dissenting views.

Many contemporary communities in the Global South lack the unity and ethic of participatory democracy that existed in the Chalatenango resettlements. Furthermore, definitions of community in primary care models vary greatly (Wayland and Crowder 2002). Benjamin Paul and William Demarest documented a Guatemalan case in which the best-laid community participation plans of PHC organizers crashed into the shoals of local political divisions (1984). This was also a problem in Chalatenango communities outside the war zone where populations were more heterogeneous. These cases illustrate how a community-based approach to health can threaten other bases of power that (sincerely or not) lay claim to having democratic support.

Why Community Participation in Health Fails

By the 1980s, many Latin American health ministries had adopted community participation as a goal, yet reviews of national programs often indicated that this rhetoric served more as window dressing in brochures than descriptions of actual practice (Ugalde 1985; and Werner 1981). Interestingly, community participation was often most successful in settings with low levels of social stratification (Ugalde 1985). Domination by medical professionals stifled community participation in many Asian programs (Rifkin 1986). A provocative experiment by Mark Nichter on participatory research in India found that nonprofessional local researchers (with minimal training) had more success than did professionals at interacting with rural communities and learning their felt needs (1984).

Antonio Ugalde charged that the form of community participation adopted by many Latin American Ministries of Health grew out of two false assumptions: the belief that traditional values of the poor were the main obstacles of development, and the idea that the poor were incapable of organizing themselves (1985). My ethnography of Chalatenango supports his claim that these assumptions were not valid. Most so-called cultural problems with health education and building community participation in Chalatenango were tied to pragmatic realities of poverty that characterized peasant life.

For example, in interviews with residents of the repopulations, most people said they did not boil water except for consumption by infants, even though they knew boiling made it safer to drink. But the reasons they gave also made sense; either they didn't have a pot big enough to boil water in or they didn't have enough firewood.[8] A household survey of attitudes toward health in one resettlement found that, even in hamlets at some distance from the village center, campesinos made use of the popular clinic and had knowledge of environmental causes of health. But the findings were consistent in both the town center and in cantónes that only more well-to-do peasant families felt they had the means to put many public health measures into practice (Bergmans 1995). For poorer peasants, what sometimes appeared to be against a group's interests by epidemiological criteria (for example, overreliance on curative care) was often very much in people's immediate interests. A mother whose child has diarrhea is not interested in hearing about latrines until her particular emergency is resolved. And rural poverty is a running series of such emergencies.

The myriad of community forms that grew out of the repopulation efforts is testimony that rural peasants are capable and creative organizers—when they have the political space to step out from under the paternalistic and institutional constraints of colonial and neocolonial economic systems. International human rights advocacies and NGOs that offer financial support to grassroots initiatives have played essential roles as allies to movements working for reforms in these settings. There have been many provocative examples of PHC success stories, especially in settings where national governments made major commitments to equity in health. Bender and Pitkin reviewed and compared the positive experiences of such programs in Costa Rica, Columbia, and Nicaragua with lay health providers (1987). Yet many such programs have been short-lived due to loss of political support at the state level or to rural security forces that were hostile to community organizing efforts (see also Lloyd-Sherlock 2000; and Nelson 2004).

There are few comprehensive reviews of participation in existing international PHC programs or qualitative studies of community participation that address process rather than programmatic results. Ethnographic approaches continue to be rare, perhaps because public health specialists are more accustomed to epidemiological measures of effectiveness while medical anthropologists have tended to focus on experiences of illness in individuals rather than the health of populations (Inhorn 1995).[9] In addition to (and related to) the lack of data, some planners in the past had unrealistic expectations about the timelines for community development.

Godfrey Woelk noted that some of the most effective programs of community participation have been in settings where people shared a common history of struggle against oppression (1992). As Frits Muller observed, participation is a form of power and is threatening to local elites (1989), so perhaps it should not be surprising that workers in some projects have fallen victim to violence (see Cliff and Noormahomed 1988; and Stark 1985). The post-1990s neoliberal period has been similarly rocky in terms of primary health gains as PHC programs juggled proposals for government cooperation juxtaposed with cuts in NGO funding.

My comparison of the Chalatenango popular health system and the Ministry of Health on community participation suggests that the reasons that large-scale, national-level PHC programs often prove disappointing may have more to do with limited resources and control of politics by antidemocratic forces than with traditional values of peasants or any inherent flaws in the concept of PHC and community-based lay providers. Vertical SPHC programs such as that of the Salvadoran government often belie their own rhetoric by discouraging participation when faced with the specter of local dissent or demands that cannot be met. The Ministry of Health's reluctance to collaborate with the popular system and recent cutbacks in the national CHP program provide another example of the decline in community participation that many PHC advocates have documented in countries of the developing world in the era of neoliberal structural adjustment (Abel and Lloyd-Sherlock 2000, Rao 1999).

Yet while "Health for All by 2000" turned out to be a pipe dream, the year 2000 in El Salvador heralded a new mobilization of popular health workers backed by unions as well as tens of thousands of other citizens who converged in downtown San Salvador to protest government plans to privatize health services. The build-up to this surge in health activism, treated in detail in chapters 9 and 10, spanned several years and united rural workers with urban organizers around a common humanitarian agenda; it changed both the landscapes for multilateral lending and for electoral politics. The mobilization raised hopes for a new era of democracy for activists who look to the day when it is no longer blasphemous to talk of ordinary people emerging as agents of health development rather than its objects.

PART FOUR

War by Other Means

8

Popular Health and the State

Reasserting Biomedical Hegemony

> The supernatural virtue of justice resides in behaving exactly as though there were equality, when one party is the stronger in an unequal relationship.
>
> —Simone Weil

Although most political analysts cited El Salvador's legacy of inequality as a central cause of the war, the social reform goals of the revolution were only partially met after the 1992 cease-fire. FMLN achievements in the pact included demilitarization of the country, creation of a new civilian-controlled National Police, and a program to transfer land to ex-combatants and some squatter settlements. But in the rush to achieve a peace accord by December 31, 1991 (the end of mediator Pérez de Cuéllar's term as UN secretary general), rebel leaders dropped demands for social welfare reforms. Details on many issues remained to be negotiated during an extended "peace process" overseen by the United Nations.

The accords called on the government and the FMLN to negotiate on future control of social services (including health) in the near one-quarter of the country under rebel control. Thus, questions of future control of health services in Chalatenango became a key focus of my study. In 1993 these negotiations brought advocates for popular health face to face with the Ministry of Health.

For months following the February cease-fire, however, the level of distrust was so high that the talks degenerated into mudslinging. The confrontations reflected a dialectic between the ministry's commitment to a centralized, biomedical model dominated by physicians and the popular system's commitment to a strong degree of community control over health and reliance on local lay health promoters.

The issues reflected similar debates on the international level over health development. Progress in international public health has often taken place in societies that have adopted strong government policies and public-sector investments in health services (Chen 1989). Canada, Costa Rica, Cuba, the state of Kerala (in southern India), and Nicaragua (under Sandinista rule) are examples

195

of such public health efforts. These success stories span a spectrum of economic systems, but in each case health was but one of a number of social reforms aimed at achieving greater economic equity.

As noted in chapter 7, such reformist interventions have often been short-lived due to political opposition in societies that have long-standing disparities in ownership and control of key resources. In many cases PHC projects that emphasized lay workers and community involvement have clashed with regional or state authorities. In an article titled "Will Primary Health Care Efforts Be Allowed to Succeed?" Heggenhougen (1984) reviewed the history of threats, harassment, and even assassinations of community health workers in Guatemala, predicting that in highly hierarchical societies, PHC initiatives "will be repressed when they begin to succeed, since success of necessity implies an attack on existing socio-political structures" (220). This implicit antagonism between grassroots-based health models and wider power structures is perhaps the reason so many promising PHC initiatives remain small projects in isolated rural settings (see Werner and Bower 1982; and Muller 1989). Even in national health system reforms, issues such as community control and lay participation sparked internal political struggles in Costa Rica (Morgan 1989) and Nicaragua (Scholl 1985).

Many critiques use the term "political will" as a nod to the contentious power politics behind health reforms. But Morgan cautioned that the concept of political will implies that commitment by national leaders is central and may obscure internal debates and struggles as well as the roles of international aid agencies, thus diverting attention away from the "global relations of dependency and institutionalized inequality that create and perpetuate poverty and ill health" (1989, 233).

In her study of Costa Rica, Morgan found that the government often backed paternalistic models of local health care that impeded the citizen participation that PHC was designed to encourage (1989, 1993). She documented inconsistent shifts in rhetoric and program goals as politicians adapted to party lines and international health trends while they continued to reap the political rewards of appearing to back public health. "A politician who deliberately promotes health places himself, by symbolic association, above the dirty business of politics. By . . . perpetuating the notion that health is above politics, political interest groups can and do manipulate . . . health to their own . . . advantage" (1989, 242).

The tendency of politicians to trade on the moral reputation of health is particularly blatant in Latin America, where post-colonial capitalist states have traditionally mediated the relationship between medical services and patients. Hence, Navarro's observation that, despite rhetoric of paternalistic concern for the common good, the public sector in much of Latin America has primarily served the employees of urban businesses (1977). He documented the concentration of curative medical services in urban centers throughout the region, juxtaposed with almost universal neglect of rural health and preventive approaches.

It is ironic that in rural Latin America the mystique of physicians and the bio- *worship of doctors* medical cure is, if anything, stronger than in the United States, thanks in part to unhindered advertising campaigns by pharmaceutical companies since the early 1960s. This tight historical relationship between the state and biomedicine in a setting in which most morbidity and mortality could theoretically be greatly reduced by public health and preventive measures is no less than tragic. In 1989, for example, UNICEF estimated that one hundred thousand children were dying *but no access* each year in Central America (twenty thousand of these deaths in El Salvador) from preventable infections—far more than the death toll from war. And yet, compared with the spectacle of war, this killing field was virtually invisible to the public and often ignored by national physician-administrators who designed health policy.

Public health–oriented evaluations of health projects often mention political problems of implementation as an aside, but it is rare for researchers to turn their gaze directly on the political process of health decision making. The political barriers in access to intra- and interinstitutional discourse make research of this kind difficult. Occasionally, however, health reforms emerge as issues in political struggles, thereby gaining public exposure. The Chalatenango negotiations in El Salvador offered a rare opportunity to contrast rhetoric and practice between advocates of two very different models of public health.

Authoritative Knowledge and Biomedical Dominance

The politics of health turns on the mechanisms whereby knowledge comes to weld social power. The reputation of medicine and health is based in part on scientific authority, which is grounded in claims to efficacy. Yet, practitioners of curative medicine and public health adopt very different models of efficacy. Although the individualistic efficacy of the biomedical cure is an analytical level removed from epidemiological control in a population, medicine's individualistic influence invades public health's domain. This is more than a mere division of labor; it is a paradigm breach that generates tension both in the heuristic sense and in practice (for example, see Gray 1992).

One result of medicine's professional dominance has been the reduction of *health for poor stigmatize* public health in the West to "a low-prestige specialty," often subsumed within the biomedical sphere (Hoffman 1989, 15). The gradual assertion of professional authority on the part of public health specialists in industrialized countries has been paralleled in the Global South, where urban-based physicians, frequently from elite classes, continue to dominate Ministries of Health in settings where the bulk of mortality and morbidity is directly linked to poor sanitary infrastructure and inadequate access to health services in barrios and rural areas where these professionals have little experience.

In evaluations of international health programs, efficacy continues to be defined primarily by statistics on mortality (especially infant mortality) and a relatively small number of communicable diseases. In fact, many health development programs make little effort to reduce morbidity or to monitor the health status of men, older children, and the elderly (Rifkin and Walt 1986; and Wisner 1988). El Salvador's national program is one such program. Furthermore, as Berman and colleagues point out, little data exists internationally on the large-scale health impact either of primary health care programs or of clinic-based health services (1987). Thus, scientific knowledge about health is often based on inappropriate science and inadequate knowledge—an ideal example of Brigitte Jordan's concept of "authoritative knowledge," referring to a knowledge system that becomes dominant or authoritative either because "it explains the world better for the purposes at hand ('efficacy'), or because (it is) associated with a stronger power base ('structural superiority'), and usually both" (Jordan 1993, 152).

One of the hopes of Chalatenango's popular health leaders was that the health efforts of the repopulated communities would serve as a model for international development. Yet the events depicted in this chapter illustrate how over a two-year period the Ministry of Health managed to reassert authority or co-opt many aspects of popular health in the repopulated villages. My analysis of the negotiation asks why popular health knowledge did not effectively counter authoritative biomedical knowledge in Chalatenango, or conversely, how it was that government professionals who had lost a monopoly on specialized knowledge in this area (which had been bereft of government services for twelve years), and who made no effort to demonstrate superior efficacy in health care delivery, nevertheless were able to reassert authority. In fact, a remarkable aspect of the negotiations over health in Chalatenango was the apparent unimportance of efficacy as an issue to government negotiators, although advocates for the popular system attempted on many occasions to introduce such criteria into the talks.

The Ministry of Health in this case had a structural advantage in its access to funds and supplies and its official status as a state service, but it was handicapped by association with an unpopular political regime (especially in this formerly rebel-controlled area) and a reputation for inefficient and inadequate rural services. Thus the negotiations and the confrontations between these two health systems provide insights into how knowledge gains authoritative status on the basis of structural superiority alone.

I sat in on regional peace process health negotiation sessions and followed interactions between the two health systems between June 1992 and December 1995. Early in this period I focused on operations of the popular system, and my access to the decision-making process within that system was always much greater than my access to the ministry. To get a more balanced perspective, during three months in 1995 I devoted most of my time to gathering information about the ministry's rural health practices, including activities of an USAID-funded evaluation of the ministry's health promoter program.

As with all aspects of Salvadoran life since the war began, the Chalatenango negotiations took place in a polarized atmosphere. Participants were suspicious of ulterior motives on the part of the opposing side, often speculating on motivations behind, and political implications of decisions. Such speculations were revealing, but in drawing conclusions about consequences of policies, I relied primarily on ethnographic observation supplemented by multiple accounts of events and meetings I was unable to observe and by documentation generated by participants about the process.

[handwritten margin note: Both sides suspicious of each other]

Negotiations and Boycotts: A Problematic Beginning

Both sides had compelling reasons to negotiate. Anticipating a drop-off in international donations in the postwar period, the popular system needed a permanent source for medicines and minimal salaries for promoters as well as backup from ministry physicians in remote rural areas where promoters were operating with little supervision. Most observers noted that the ministry needed to reassert government authority in former war zones for both epidemiologic and political reasons. The presence of the ministry helped qualify a town for international development assistance (allocated in unusually large amounts for reconstruction during the early post-cease-fire period), and under El Salvador's political patronage system, ministry physicians historically had served as both a form of political capital and as political allies for the governing ARENA party.

The initial meeting between the two sides in early spring 1992 was somewhat hostile, ending in a standoff. The popular health negotiating committee, made up of health promoters and physicians, asked that the government legalize the lay promoters (who technically violated the law by practicing without government recognition) and pay them minimal salaries. The ministry regional director replied that the ministry had no capacity for changing the law. Part of the problem lay with the ministry's very different concept of community-based health. Although the ministry had its own (USAID-designed and -funded) CHP promoter program in rural areas, in contrast to the popular system promoters, ministry promoters had far more restricted duties and almost no curative role. For the next five months, ministry officials repeatedly failed to attend scheduled negotiating sessions.

[handwritten margin note: Doctors wanted law change to be easier to practice medicine]

This problematic beginning occurred simultaneously with several confrontations between the two sides in repopulated villages as the ministry unilaterally sent caravans of mobile medical workers into the former war zone for one-day visits to villages. For the residents of repopulated villages, the caravans were reminiscent of army pacification programs, which typically featured medical services as a central component (see chapter 5). Since the ministry failed to coordinate these overtures with local political leaders (as they were required to do under the peace agreement), the ex-refugees in the villages called assemblies and decided to boycott the caravans. As a result, the arriving doctors and nurses were treated like unwelcome aliens when they pulled into town. They set up their tables, but no patients showed up for consults. In a group interview, three San José Las Flores promoters speaking in tandem gave this (almost gleeful) account of the caravan's visit:

> They [ministry employees] came to the clinic and asked to see the doctor. And we said, "No doctor works here. We work here." Then they asked if we could take them to people with serious illnesses. We said, "We treat all the illnesses here." Then we asked "Haven't you heard of the negotiation process?" They said no . . . so we told them, "Well, here you have to coordinate with the directiva if you want to work." Then they invited us outside to see their "beautiful" ambulance. So I said, "Well, our clinic is not beautiful from the outside, but at least we give care to people inside." Then they got angry. One physician said, "Look at all these malnourished children. It's clear that you need a ministry clinic here." So I said, "You can't cure malnutrition with a doctor. What we need are jobs and better food." Then they said, "Well, we'll just drive around so that people can see what a government ambulance looks like."

In an ironic twist, Arturo, a ministry nurse who had been riding in that 1992 caravan, was assigned two years later to work in San José Las Flores as part of a negotiated collaboration between the ministry and the popular system. In a 1995 interview he surprised me by evincing a quiet admiration for the villagers' boycott: "I didn't know anything about politics at the time. My boss just told us to come see patients. But the people knew we were coming . . . and blocked the road. The whole population! It was clear we didn't want to mess with them. . . . Now I admire them for that. They are a really humble people, and they all pulled together. It was true. We didn't have anything to offer them. In other areas we were well received, but in the repopulated areas, nothing."

On occasion such sparring by the two sides escalated to a showdown. For example, in August 1992 ministry officials, reportedly angered by villagers' boycott of the mobile caravans, broke with a long-standing agreement and refused to supply vaccines to the Chalatenango Catholic Diocese for an upcoming vaccination drive in the former war zone. In response, popular promoters staged a demonstration of several hundred people outside the ministry's Chalatenango headquarters, demanding the vaccines and a reopening of the stalled negotiations. Three days later the ministry delivered the vaccines, but two more months passed before the talks resumed.

Finally, after prodding by consultants from the United Nations Development Program (UNDP) and the Pan American Health Organization (PAHO), ministry officials agreed to a new round of negotiations in October 1992. At this long-awaited two-day session, a ministry official presented the ministry's new (PAHO-approved) model for "integrated local health systems." His presentation gave new meaning to the term "abstract theory:"

> We plan to have four multidisciplinary teams here in Chalate. Toward what end? To consolidate local health work through local programming with a development strategy, and the support to enable us to achieve the famous goal of "Health for All." The local programming will convert into an administrative instrument to allow development of primary health care. What is the administrative route for developing PHC? [It has to be] inside the community. Therefore, it has to be via a strategic operation that the ministry has accepted in response to the call of the whole world. With what end? To know the whole series of real conditions in the community, by means of a set of measuring instruments or a data base that will be generated to permit program planning and serve as a barometer, to allow us to proceed with a little more efficiency and a little more confidence in resolving the health problems that we're developing in the area. In this moment we're in this process of consolidation; I can't tell you a specific timetable for when we'll be able to carry out concrete local programs. Why? Because an important thing is missing and that is the participation of the community.

[handwritten margin note: If plans don't work, blame the people]

What the new ministry plan was exactly was not clear from his speech, but the knowledge behind it certainly sounded authoritative. This was followed by a presentation by an ex-FMLN physician on how the popular system functioned. Her talk, too, was jargony, larded with new acronyms and phantom levels of organization that had been invented that morning by the popular system negotiating team. But the description of the health work was clear enough. Afterward the PAHO representative spoke with great enthusiasm. He remarked to the group that the popular system had essentially put into practice what the ministry administrator had presented as theory. "What is beautiful here is that we have [an application of the model]. We have a community base—the most difficult thing to achieve. . . . It's a great opportunity for the ministry!"

And yet, as the course of events made clear, the ministry did not see things quite that way. Although relations were more congenial after this meeting, it became clear that popular system requests for recognition and minimal salaries for the promoters were not on the ministry's agenda.

One of the few appeals to public welfare made by the ministry in the *concertación* took place in a meeting held a month later when a government negotiator declared, "We have mobile teams standing by; we have physicians ready to go. All we need is your go-ahead and we can begin to bring medical care to the populations there who have gone without care so long." His appeal fell flat with the popular system advocates, who pointed out that no one in the repopulation communities had been "going without care." As we left the meeting, a

[handwritten margin note: Lack of gov't urgency]

diocese physician on the popular system's technical team took umbrage at the ministry overture, commenting, "What a lot of nerve, saying they had physicians standing by. Where are the ministry physicians in the rest of Chalatenango where there really is no care?" He named two towns he had just visited in government-controlled areas that hadn't seen a ministry physician in months. The ministry negotiator's humanitarian appeal also failed to impress foreign observers from the UNDP and PAHO, who had worked with the popular system since the cease-fire, and praised the promoters' accomplishments in meetings with the ministry.

In my separate interviews with ministry physician-administrators, several had spoken disparagingly of health promoter training programs, including the one run by the ministry. But given international development experts' approval of primary health approaches, ministry negotiators rarely offered a public challenge to the concept of community-based health care or of training lay health providers. Their official stance was probably influenced by the fact that USAID, the ministry's largest funder, had been instrumental in setting up El Salvador's national CHP promoter program.[1]

Contesting Ministry Claims of a Monopoly on Competence

In early negotiations the two sides were, as one participant put it, "talking two languages." Popular system negotiators pressed for official recognition (and pay) for promoters, while ministry spokespersons talked doctors. In October 1992 a ministry regional administrator brushed off an appeal of this kind, replying, "We brought up this issue this morning in an organizational meeting. We decided it's better to leave the promoter issue to one side. The first thing is to have ministry physicians working in the [former war] zone for a while. It should be left to the communities to consider their needs for promoters." In another session, a ministry representative said official recognition of promoter roles would require an act of the legislature, and noted that in other areas of the country, "we've concentrated on more practical work."

A popular system physician countered, "But legalization of the promoters is key . . . they are the network between the technical personnel and the communities." A ministry representative then changed the subject, but a diocese physician brought it back up, declaring, "We all know [promoters] can resolve 85–90 percent of these communities' health problems. No institution is capable of putting a doctor in each community."[2]

To help remedy the "two language" problem, in November 1992 popular system leaders took ministry negotiators on a tour of the repopulated communities so that they could meet the promoters and visit popular system clinics. I was invited to go along. The government physicians and nurses were visibly impressed. Each time they entered a popular clinic, the regional director would

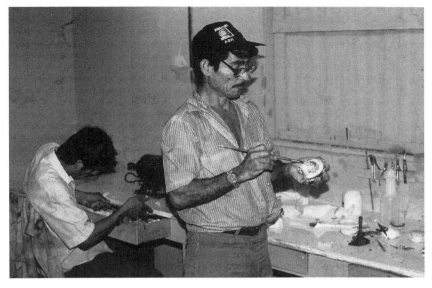

Dental promoter with a mold in lab of the San José Las Flores dental clinic. Besides cleanings, fillings, and extractions, the dental promoters also built partial and total plates for campesinos with missing teeth, including those with facial wounds from the war. The Ministry of Health, in contrast, only offered dental extractions in rural areas. Photograph by Sandy Smith-Nonini.

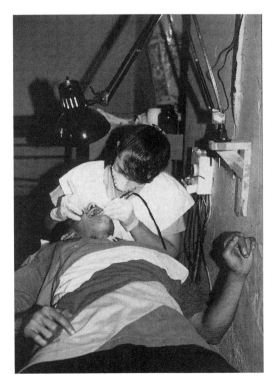

Dental promoter working on teeth of a villager, San José Las Flores. The clinic relied on a generator to power the drill; the water sprayer was powered by gravity, drawing on water stored in barrels mounted in the rafters. Photograph by Sandy Smith-Nonini.

turn to Leo, an ex-FMLN physician, to explain things, but Leo would simply introduce them to the promoter in charge. The biggest hit on the tour was the San José Las Flores dental clinic. The ministry regional director's jaw dropped as he gazed at a pair of peasant promoters wearing face masks, calmly drilling teeth, a service that the ministry doesn't offer in rural areas. He exclaimed, "We have to support this."

First world care in El Salvador

A ministry dentist had come along in response to a request from technicians in the dental lab. They wanted her advice on adapting the bridges and plates that they routinely made to fit peasant patients with facial war wounds. But the dentist said, "I don't know how I can help you. You're doing things here that I don't even know how to do." She gaped at their Bunsen burners, handcranked centrifuges, and plaster casts, then promised to read up on techniques and get back to them.

Under-trained doctors

After this remarkable encounter, ministry negotiators rarely resorted to humanitarian appeals or claims of a monopoly of knowledge for healing. Rather than dispute the merits of lay health workers or question the competence of the popular system promoters, government spokespersons simply tabled the issue. But it became clear that legalization and pay of lay promoters as well as local control of health decision making would remain outside the agenda. The dialectic of the debate became set as the popular health representatives continually pressed on these issues while the ministry resisted and pushed instead for permission to reintroduce ministry physicians to the former war zone. The stalemate was extremely frustrating both for the Chalatenango health workers and for the international development observers. At the end of one 1993 meeting, a normally staid but clearly frustrated PAHO representative stunned the ministry representative by declaring: "I've traveled a lot of places and I've never seen this level of irresponsibility in a ministry. I've been in this process a year and what have we achieved? We haven't sent in doctors. We haven't sent in nurses. We haven't sent in medicines. We haven't trained promoters. We haven't done anything. That's my opinion, even if I lose my job."

The discussion eventually turned toward the ministry's preferred agenda of the criteria for government physicians to enter the zone. This ability to frame the universe of possibilities is a critical element of situated or institutional power. As Foucault's term "medical policing" suggests, issues of scientific efficacy need not be central to state intervention in health (1980). The state's prerogative rests also on the institutionalization of medical expert knowledge and an ethic of social development. In the case of public health in El Salvador, however, this "technology of populations" had become untethered from the real bodies and body politic of rural life.

For the next few months, ministry negotiators continued to insist that itinerant physicians in mobile caravans were all the government could provide in the former war zone, an offering that the popular system spurned as propaganda.

In the course of rejecting the mobile caravans, the popular negotiators challenged the ministry to provide permanent physicians based in the repopulated villages. This impasse led the health committee in the repopulated village of Arcatao to draw up a list of standards for physicians who work with the popular system. Directed specifically at the ministry, the new rules stipulated that physicians would live in the community, that they would allow promoters to serve as gatekeepers (that is, only treating patients referred by promoters), that a physician practicing locally would be subject to community decisions, and that he or she would visit remote hamlets for consults, teach promoters using understandable language, and help plan and cooperate with a community health plan that had both preventive and curative components. (Church and ex-FMLN physicians in the popular system had already become accustomed to working with promoters according to these rules.) While the popular system's negotiators did not wish to discuss physicians because this would mean adopting the ministry's frame of reference, they felt compelled to take the proposal of the Arcatao health committee seriously, since this village had been a standard setter for community participation.

Uneasy Compromise: The Chalatenango Health Accord

In early 1993 the ministry modified its stance and offered permanent physicians, specifying that access to medicines and other government aid in the former war zone would be tied to the presence of a government physician in each municipality. The popular system committee, conscious of the long-term need for physicians in the former war zones (and under some pressure from FMLN leadership to reach an accord[3]), signed an agreement with the ministry that April that committed the ministry to placing physicians and medical supplies in eight repopulated villages. Many popular health organizers, however, were unhappy with the agreement because the language on how physicians would collaborate with promoters was vague, implying that the ministry personnel in each village would respect both ministry practice norms and popular health norms, which seemed a contradiction in terms. Conversely, a negotiator for the popular system told me that as long as ministry physicians were assigned to well-organized communities, he felt confident to leave it to local leaders to judge how well the physician abided by local popular health norms.

The accord was signed by the ministry regional director and the popular health negotiations committee in a public ceremony in San José Las Flores. The bishop of the Chalatenango Diocese spoke at the gathering, underscoring the Church's approval of the agreement. After the signing, a ministry employee raised a few local eyebrows when he walked over and hung a sign on the local clinic that read "Ministry of Health." The promoters were appalled at the arrogance but held their tongues.

Fight to distrust gov't plans

Two months passed and the promised physicians and medicines failed to materialize. Meanwhile, the ministry regional director declined to attend three consecutively scheduled negotiation sessions. Ministry employees sent in his place claimed they had no decision-making power. I gained an interview with the regional director and asked about the delay. He initially told me that several social service physicians he had assigned to the former war zone had resigned their postings because the towns were too remote or out of fear, not wanting to be the sole government representative in a rebel area. But he also acknowledged that the ministry central office had not allocated adequate funds to staff the positions.

Frustrated at the delays and stalled negotiations, the popular health committee took out a newspaper ad in the capital denouncing the ministry's failure to comply with the accord. In San José Las Flores, where the agreement with the ministry had been signed, promoters had their own joke on the ministry. On top of the new "Ministry of Health" sign on the front wall of their clinic, they hung there a second hand-lettered sign that read: "This sign is the Ministry of Health's only investment in this community." Reports of the San José Las Flores sign and the newspaper ad angered ministry officials, who said it was "a show of bad faith" on the part of popular health workers.

Under-staffed

The first ministry medical team arrived in Arcatao in July 1993, and others gradually arrived in five other repopulated villages, although supplies of medicines were further delayed, and only two of the six promised sanitation inspectors showed up. Curiously, the ministry sent an oversupply of nurses to three villages, leading some in the popular system to believe this was a strategy to make the lay promoters superfluous.

Ministry Physicians Enter the Repopulated Villages

Subsequent local-level "negotiations" in Arcatao provide a glimpse of the structural (and, indirectly, political) barriers within a health ministry that prevent health workers from developing flexible programs that can adjust to local-level needs. The new ministry physician, Herberto, fresh out of medical school, was sympathetic to the goals of popular health, but he expressed conflicted feelings about his position. On his first visit to Arcatao he told me: "I feel as if my hands are tied and I'm being pulled in two directions at once." In a meeting that day between the new ministry team and the promoter team, Herberto worried aloud about how he would comply with ministry paperwork requirements on each patient if the promoters continued to see patients. "Teach us the paperwork," suggested a promoter.

Health care is not affordable by design

"But what about the charges for consults?" Herberto asked. "We're supposed to ask for five colones [US$0.62] per consult. And the system Arcatao residents have approved is five colones per month per family. [The ministry] is just going to pull me out if I go along with the popular standards and reassign me to a really remote spot as punishment."

The promoters asked the physician and nurse to give them classes on biology and medical techniques, but the ministry personnel said they weren't authorized to teach. The ministry nurse said she would be required to take over the pharmacy from the promoters as soon as ministry medicines arrived. I ran into Herberto a week later as he was leaving the ministry's regional headquarters. He was frustrated because he had just been rebuffed when he sought guidance from his supervisor on how to accommodate popular health practices without violating ministry standards. He told me, "I honestly think the purpose of the ministry in sending me to Arcatao is for propaganda reasons. The government wants to announce in the newspapers that it now runs the clinic in the rebel town of Arcatao. I don't think the ministry sees any future role for popular health promoters."

[margin note: Self Doubt]

This last sentiment was confirmed in an interview with a ministry administrator. "Within a year, he predicted to me confidently, "you will not be able to tell a clinic in a repopulated village from any other ministry clinic." His prediction of the demise of the popular system proved premature, but in the longer run the ministry's influence did indeed weaken the popular system greatly.

What productive collaboration did come about between the two sides occurred at the local level and took place out of sight of ministry administrators. Ministry personnel and the promoters in Arcatao eventually settled into a working relationship. With the support of Leo, an ex-FMLN doctor, the promoters convinced both Herberto (and his successor) to share responsibility for consults with promoters, and they secured the physician's commitment to hike to outlying hamlets twice a month to see rural residents. The ministry nurse insisted that the promoters stop rotating duties and specialize in different areas, which they did. And, after many local discussions, she finally agreed to share control of the pharmacy.

[margin note: Specialization works or sharing duties]

There were some improvements: In addition to a regular physician presence and medicines (relieving some of the financial burden on the diocese), vaccinations became a daily affair in the clinic, with better recordkeeping and improved well-child care.

In the months that followed, Herberto became convinced that the popular system approach had much to recommend it. He decided to resist propaganda efforts of the ministry directed at the town, including the banners, loudspeakers, and TV coverage the ministry arranged for a government-sponsored vaccination drive that the church and local health workers argued was unnecessary because it was in an area they had already covered. He also joined villagers in resisting pressure from the ministry headquarters to paint the clinic in the national colors and hang a flag and portrait of the ARENA president.

As in Arcatao, the promoters in San José Las Flores achieved a tense but productive working relationship with their social service physician. Although not as cooperative as Herberto, the physician complied with many popular system "norms." Inez, a promoter in Las Flores, told me, "The doctor doesn't like to hike for vaccinations. We have to pressure him. But we're not receiving any salary and he is, so we insist he go too. But he complains, 'You all do it, I can't manage, and so on.' "

Sidelining the Popular Health Promoters

Although assertive popular promoters in these two well-organized villages managed to develop working relationships with ministry personnel, in four other repopulated villages less-assertive promoters had been sidelined when I visited in the fall of 1995. They no longer participated in medical consultations or planning and had been relegated to chores like mopping floors and hiking on vaccination drives. The promoters complained about the tendency of the supposedly full-time physicians to only come to town one to two days a week and said that many physicians refused to hike to hamlets to give consults, forcing sick people there to walk or be carried for one to three hours to see a doctor.[4]

In Las Vueltas, for example, Lidia, a ministry physician, took over prenatal care from the two promoters who had specialized in midwifery. Up until then the promoters had held a single prenatal day each month when pregnant women from the countryside came to the clinic for check-ups, vitamins, socializing, and educational talks. Since prenatal care had little precedent in Chalatenango, this approach had worked well to accustom women to preventive care and educate them about the need for iron-rich foods and a varied diet.[5] Lidia elected instead to handle prenatal care individually, whenever women came for clinic visits, a strategy that the promoters worried about since women in more remote areas tended not to undertake the long trip to the clinic except when they were sick. Lidia also told the promoter midwives to stop handling local births, saying she would oversee them.

But as the months passed, Lidia stopped handling births at night, she was not willing to leave the clinic to walk to laboring women's homes when it was raining or if they lived outside of the immediate village, and she was not in town at all on weekends. For a while, the physician, who slept in the clinic, stopped even answering the door when villagers came with health problems at night, but after people complained to the town council, a meeting was held and the physician agreed to resume taking care of emergencies at night.

Unable to rely on Lidia, pregnant women again turned to the promoter midwives to handle their births, but the promoters felt handicapped in taking on the responsibility because Lidia controlled the women's prenatal care and their records. Mariana, one of the midwives, complained to me, "This puts us in a bad position. Something bad is going to happen with a birth and then people will blame us."

In daily work at the clinic, Lidia assigned the promoters routine support duties but took on all the planning and diagnostic duties herself. During a morning of consults that I attended in Las Vueltas, she rarely spoke to the attending promoter. One of the promoters who had gained the physician's favor had been granted a position as her special assistant—with divisive results as the other three promoters became more and more angry and alienated but felt powerless to do anything short of gossip and complain in popular health meetings.

In mid-1993, in lieu of accrediting and paying popular promoters, the ministry had invited repopulated villages to choose a few promoters to attend the three-month course of the ministry's CHP promoter program. The ministry offered to waive the normal requirement for a ninth-grade education for trainees (because few in the former war zone had achieved that grade level). This invitation was debated at length by promoters in local and regional meetings. One concern was that the ministry was only interested in training a handful of individuals, and many felt this would create two levels of expertise and authority—with a few promoters identifying as employees of the ministry rather than as primarily responsible to their community. Also, these few would receive government salaries equivalent to $150 per month while the majority scraped by with minimal stipends equivalent to $18–$40 per month. They felt this would be divisive.

In addition, popular system workers were aware that ministry CHP promoters had a reputation in rural areas as being unable to solve people's health problems. The duties of ministry promoters were to vaccinate, promote latrines and hygiene, and do well-child checks, but the only medicines they were allowed to handle were vitamins, malaria pills, aspirin, and one antiparasitic drug. In contrast, popular promoters had a wider range of responsibilities and were trained to use about thirty-five medicines including antibiotics and antispasmodics. The popular system negotiators agreed that a handful of highly paid promoters working for the ministry in a reduced capacity was not the best solution to the region's health problems, and they declined the ministry's offer.

Soon rumors were flying that ministry personnel had shown up in several villages recruiting potential CHP trainees. Popular system negotiators felt deceived. Confronted about this in a meeting, a ministry employee acknowledged that he was under orders to find trainees even if he had to bypass existing popular promoters and recruit people with no health background. Contrary to its own guidelines, the ministry recruited CHP trainees in at least two cases from outside the villages they were to work in. Residents of one village signed a petition protesting ministry plans to send a CHP promoter with no knowledge of the community to work there, claiming that they had been well served for the last two years by two popular promoters who were natives.

Finally, in mid-1994, as a means of obtaining some level of salary support for promoters, the popular negotiators agreed to recruit twenty-two promoters from repopulated villages for the ministry CHP course. Upon graduation, however, only eleven of those finishing the program were offered paying jobs by the ministry. As is customary with the government CHP program, they were expected to work the first month for free "to show good faith."[6] Their initial duties were to do a household epidemiological survey. In a surprise move, however, two months later the ministry laid off all the popular promoters it had hired, citing cutbacks in USAID funds (a step in the shifting of the CHP program to ministry control, which had been long expected). Resecuring these jobs became the top item on the popular health agenda in 1995. By this time, however, promoters throughout the popular system were unhappy and grumbling about the collaboration with the ministry. They felt marginalized by the ministry, which had never recognized their health work or offered them even minimal salaries. Adding to the demoralization, a small NGO fund that paid small stipends to promoters in repopulated villages was due to run out in December 1995, shortly after I left the field.

Some popular system negotiators remained hopeful because new reforms being considered by the ministry held prospects for future contracting with NGOs and giving more decision-making power to regional health offices. But in the fall when negotiations resumed, representatives from the ministry's regional office still claimed they had no power to act. One ministry administrator claimed to sympathize with the goals of popular health, even agreeing that many popular promoters were "more capable than new nursing graduates." He called the selective firing of popular promoters a "dirty trick" but then, citing budgetary constraints, said there was little he could do.

Containing the Popular Health Movement

Like other branches of the Salvadoran government, administrators of the Ministry of Health talked of new beginnings following the cease-fire. The regional director readily conceded that the civil war grew out of deep socioeconomic disparities and acknowledged that public health indices had not improved over thirty years using traditional models of service delivery. But under testing in negotiations, the ministry's actual "political will" to consider alternative approaches appeared weak as government negotiators repeatedly broke off talks.

A remarkable aspect of the negotiations was how easily the two sides agreed in theory, at the October 1992 negotiation session, on the need for a more locally responsive model of health delivery with strong preventive and public education components. And yet, despite cheerleading from PAHO and the UNDP about the great opportunity the popular system presented, the course of events over the next year suggests that the ministry saw the popular system as more of a threat than an opportunity.

The PAHO "integrated local health" model that the ministry had recently endorsed (but had not yet put into practice) was viewed with suspicion by many health workers who feared that local control under the model would become a

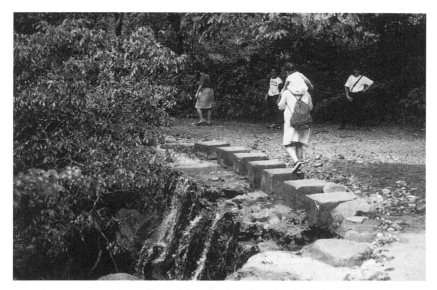

A health promoter with medical kit in a backpack and baby on her shoulders, hiking to a remote cantón. Providing care for residents in remote areas was a priority for the popular system, but this caused controversy when Ministry of Health physicians took over municipal clinics in the former war zone in 1994. The physicians did not want to hike to remote hamlets, but popular system leaders put pressure on them to do so. Photograph by Sandy Smith-Nonini.

Fear of private enterprise health care

prelude to privatization and further shirking of government responsibility for rural health. As Godfrey Woelk pointed out, fostering the rhetoric of community participation often serves ruling elites by helping create the illusion of democracy and enable resources (for reform) to be expended on development projects favorable to them and other dominant vocal groups (1992, 420).

Popular health proponents were suspicious of the ARENA government's rhetoric about health reforms, and some believed there was little point in negotiating. But the majority felt that the possibility of collaborating with the ministry had to be tested. In addition, there could be no stronger public relations ploy for the FMLN than to do a better job at providing health services than the government. But as early as the first negotiation session, it became clear that the ministry had not been willing to consider regularization of lay promoters or local control of health decision making. While the popular health representatives continually pressed for inclusion of these issues, the ministry resisted and pressed instead for an accord that would allow ministry physicians to reenter the former war zone. Rather than dispute the merits of lay health workers (which would not have been politic in the presence of international development experts who observed the talks) or question the competence of the popular promoters, ministry spokespersons simply tabled the issue.

The ministry's decision to send mobile medical caravans into the former war zone early in 1992 reflected in part the government's modus operandi for rural health in formerly conflicted areas where it had closed clinics during the war. It also reflected a perhaps willful ignorance of the competency of the popular health system and the unity of the repopulated villages. The medical caravans were better received on the outskirts of former rebel territory, in less organized and more heterogeneous towns, than by the returned refugees who shared a history of poverty and experiences of poverty and repression. For the villages, rejection of traditionally valued resources such as medicines and physicians' services required organization. Just as the new concepts of health as a social good were discussed in village assemblies, the assemblies were also the sites in which the boycotts of state medical offerings were organized.

Medical aid from the state in this case failed to accrue the necessary symbolic capital to shore up dependency. As Pierre Bourdieu wrote, possession of wealth only translates into long-term political power when it is converted into "symbolic capital" (1977, 195). That is, the arbitrary nature of the connection between the gift and countergift must be misrecognized and the relationship cast instead as a natural one. Otherwise the veil of generosity is telescoped into a socially scrutinized calculated exchange so that no debt or power differential accrues. As A. E. Komter (2005) noted, efforts of the powerful party in a relationship to impose a moral obligation can poison social ties. After all, revolution is about scrutiny of the social contract, or, in the case of a historically repressive state such as El Salvador, the assertion that there ought to be one.

For many Chalatecos, the prospects of the Ministry of Health returning to the former war zone raised the specter of government surveillance. Many expressed to me their preference for health workers "*de confianza*" (who could be trusted). Promoters shared this sense of loyalty. One popular promoter who was assigned to do household surveys during her brief stint as a ministry CHP (prior to the firings) told me she had felt a bit like a spy and pointed out that the information she had gathered had not stayed in the local clinic where it would be useful in health planning but had been taken away to ministry headquarters with no follow-up.

Her words recalled those of Jaime Briehl writing about government-run PHC programs that served a "medical policing" role: "The medical bureaucratic apparatus, when penetrating into the poor urban districts or rural village, is tantamount to an invisible surveillance network that penetrates the daily lives and families . . . [and serves to] assert the present and hierarchical role of state representation among poor populations [and] to feed back to the state's information system relevant social data by formal and informal channels" (1979, 232).

The ministry's change of heart in 1993, when administrators offered to provide permanent physicians, actually reflected a new policy throughout rural areas affected by the war. Bolstered by postwar foreign aid for reconstruction and a long overdue increase in its budget, the ministry increased the number of social service physicians based in Chalatenango by more than a third in the three years after the cease-fire. Many long-term observers feared, however, that this attention to rural areas would be short-lived. Indeed, within a year most of these "permanent" physicians were adopting the long-standing ministry practices of limiting their time in the rural post to two days per week.

The ministry's insistence on physicians as the central component of rural health recalls Sandra Morgen's conclusions from a study of feminist health centers in the United States (1990). When the grassroots health centers sought federal funds, they found support for direct service provision but none for advocacy or community outreach. "[The process] tended to underwrite the very kinds of social relations feminist health activists sought to change—hierarchical, one-on-one, provider-client relationships" (Morgen 1990, 172). Likewise, Salvadoran popular system leaders had long maintained that the state should have financial responsibility for health services. So they challenged the ministry to send permanent doctors to the repopulations, never believing the ministry would comply. But they were trumped when the ministry agreed. And the popular negotiators found themselves trapped in this frame of reference—forced to negotiate over the details of physician-centered services rather than their preferred agenda of support for a network of lay promoters and community participation in health.

The patronage-orientation and politicized nature of the Salvadoran medical bureaucracy required that medical professionals practice within rigid norms. In such a culture, complaints were unwelcome, and each level blamed the next level of bureaucracy, or "la politica," for problems. This forced personnel to adopt a kind of "structured ignorance"—the term that Taussig (1978) used to describe structurally inhibited ideation. As Herberto discovered, bureaucratic restraints such as rigid practice guidelines and excessive paperwork diminished the possibilities of collaboration between ministry physicians and promoters or local health committees. Arthur Rubel (1990) documented similar dilemmas that constrained Mexican social service physicians from addressing preventive health issues in rural Mexico. However, when Herberto was rebuffed by his supervisor for seeking guidance on how to collaborate with the popular system, he became convinced that the problem was more ideological than structural.

The efforts of USAID to promote the CHP program within the ministry since 1990 at first seemed to signal a shift toward community health as a priority within the ministry. But after January 1995, when USAID shifted responsibility for the program to the ministry, the CHP program was put on the back burner while the ministry shifted resources to hiring more physicians and improving physician salaries. This appeared to be a reversion to prewar priorities, which long-term observers blamed on the ministry's extremely centralized hierarchy, a reality that USAID-sponsored reforms have failed to change (Fiedler 1987; and Hanania de Varela 1990).

In public evaluations of the ministry's CHP program in 1995, it emerged that high-level administrators in the ministry viewed CHP promoters as ineffective, an assessment that was shared by a community health development specialist I interviewed who had studied the program. But unlike ministry physicians, he blamed the problems on inadequate training and support rather than lack of promoter capability. Such restrictions on PHC promoter roles have been observed in many countries. As David Werner observed, instead of being agents for political change, lay health workers trained by health ministries in many Third World nations tended toward another mold:

> For all their international funding . . . and glossy bilingual brochures portraying community participation . . . there was usually a minimum of effective community involvement and a maximum of dependency-creating hand-outs, paternalism, and initiative-destroying norms. . . . A different breed of village health worker is being molded; one who is taught a pathetically limited range of skills, who is trained not to think but to follow a list of very specific instructions or "norms" . . . who is subject to restrictive supervision and rigidly defined limitations. (1981, 47)

Authoritative Knowledge and Bureaucratic Power

A popular system official assured me in 1992 that if ministry physicians in the repopulations did not toe the line with respect to popular system norms, the communities would throw them out. I was not so sure. I had begun to worry about this during the tour the popular system gave ministry officials in November 1992. In the Arcatao clinic that day, two rather overbearing ministry nurses had converged on poor Francisca, the promoter coordinator. I was shocked to see this highly competent, ordinarily assertive peasant woman withdraw into a shell. She was so intimidated by the "professionals" and their barrage of pointed questions that she blushed and trembled, answering in halting sentences. I wondered how villagers would continue to have faith in their promoters when they saw them intimidated so easily by the experts. My concerns, unfortunately, were warranted.

In 1992 many residents of these villages openly opposed letting the Ministry of Health into the zone. One told me, "It's fine for the ministry doctor to come, but he won't get away with kicking out the promoters." But by 1995 peasants had gotten used to having a local physician. In less well-organized towns like Las Vueltas, many peasants would only visit the clinic when they knew the doctor was in, not bothering to consult with promoters except in an emergency. Although at least two villages protested to the ministry about individual physicians' behavior, most people I talked to valued having a physician based there and saw this access as an achievement of their struggle. These sentiments led promoters to fear they would not have their communities' support in a confrontation with the ministry about the problems.

The mood of promoters at a June planning meeting in Arcatao was despondent. One after the other they voiced complaints about the ministry and the fact that nothing had been achieved in two years of negotiation. The recent firings of the promoters hired by the ministry had added insult to injury. In addition, applications for legal status for the new union of health promoters (formed in 1994) faced delay after delay in government offices.

ISABEL: We should go on strike, not let the [ministry] doctors into the clinics.

MAURICIO: I don't like the idea that the repopulations are leaving health up to the ministry. We don't want to commit the same errors as in the east where the ERP [the FMLN faction in Morazán] practically gave its clinics to the Ministry of Health. Now [health] promoter work hardly exists there.

FRANCISCA: What are we going to do to defend what we've struggled for?

ISABEL: The problem is a lack of financing; I'm afraid the community will say, well the doctor is here and the medicines, so what else do we need? That's why the ministry sent nurses. We never asked for nurses.

FRANCISCA: So what do we do? The population says thank you very much for saving us from dying of cholera during the war, but now the state has taken over and you're not needed.

A ministry nurse in the zone who had impressed me with his keen political sense was also convinced that prospects for community-based health had worsened. He told me, "The mistake of the negotiations was to accept physicians here. The ministry knew NGO donations would drop off in the postwar period, and that's why they tried so hard to put in doctors. They figured people would get used to them little by little and they would lend influence to the government. They have wanted to throw out the promoters from the beginning."

Given the popular system's long-term position that the government had a responsibility in health, perhaps it is not so surprising that sick peasants should seek out the most expert treatment they can get, a tendency that was reinforced by the Salvadoran peasant's historical almost magical faith in medical authority—a form of dependency that the popular health system had only begun to subvert. This is also likely related to a general decline in solidarity that accompanied peace and the return of the (individualizing) market economy to the former war zone.

Dialectics of Medical Orthodoxy and Heterodoxy

Notions of medical progress are based on the premise of a "community of practice" through which practitioners weigh claims and arrive at a consensus on standards (Jordan 1993). In Chalatenango, despite the presence of international observers from PAHO and a clear interest in issues such as efficacy on the part of negotiators for the popular system, there was no "neutral" scientific community to weigh competing claims. Rather, claims of interest in the public welfare or of essential expertise became reduced to a power exercise—and the state was the only entity in a position to guarantee long-term health services.

In a society such as El Salvador, where state coercion rather than a social contract has been the more commonly experienced governing relationship, patronage has often been the mechanism for relating to the state. The Ministry of Health was structured along these lines, and physician expertise was embedded in institutional patronage hierarchies. Unlike the U.S. model of professional dominance in which physicians are autonomous, self-regulating professionals (Friedson 1974), in El Salvador (and much of Latin America) organization of medical professionals has been weak and the influence of medical expertise has long been mediated by the state and allied elites. The alliance with professional healers enhances state influence, which is often exercised as a form of "situated social power" (Wartenberg 1990). The relative unimportance of information about actual effects on the public's health in this struggle underscores Thomas Wartenberg's (1990) claim that "there is no necessary connection between the expert knowledge possessed by the empowered agent and the structure of the power relationship itself. [Expertise becomes] indistinguishable from the authority [that accrues] as a result of being situated as an empowered agent" (154).

Conflation of bureaucracy with biomedical professional authority in Latin American Ministries of Health has often achieved for state physicians what Bourdieu called "institutional legitimacy"—releasing them from having to endlessly reconfirm their claims to expertise (1977, 63). At the macro level in Chalatenango, this meant that access to medicines and funds became directly tied to the repopulated communities' acceptance of physicians. At the local level, a priori institutional legitimacy allowed Lidia, for example, to retain status as the preferred health care provider in spite of her growing reputation as neglectful of health needs outside of clinic hours. Association with the ministry (which sought to maintain a monopoly on both claims of efficacy and control of health in El Salvador) allowed Lidia to cut back her hours and turn away emergency patients.

Conversely, the prestige adhering to provision of biomedical services achieved a form of badly needed legitimacy for the Salvadoran state. Bureaucracy alone, unlike professional authority, is often regarded negatively by citizens. Eliot Friedson (1974) observed that whereas citizens may consider bureaucracies arbitrary because their workings are subject to appeal and modification, professional practices are viewed as having objectivity because of their reliance on expertise and scientific truth. As a result, they are not routinely subject to higher review or change by virtue of outside appeal (157). Hence, influence gained by the state by association with healing generates little resistance (Wartenberg 1990). But an important caveat is that such influence is only cheap (for example, compared to coercion) if it can be maintained without large expenditures for development.

The popular health system challenged the ministry's legitimacy by training lay workers who gained a reputation as effective, thus claiming the symbolic mantle of healing authority for a radical social movement. Then, during the negotiations over a health accord, popular system advocates openly challenged the ministry in front of international observers to live up to its own promises by diverting more state funds to development so that officially stated goals for public health could be met. If the two systems had coexisted in a shared system of knowledge with a common ideology of scientific criteria, the popular system would have prevailed.

But it did not prevail. As Friedson made clear, "there is no pure knowledge—there is only knowledge in the service of a practice" (1974, 159). In the case of the biomedical system, the simultaneous social and political consequences of knowledge production have often been the production and reproduction of elite structures and hierarchical systems that frustrate efforts at democratic participation.

Taking the democratic scientific community as an ideal, the desired end result of alternative approaches to healing such as midwifery or primary health care would be the nourishment of "new communities of practice" in which the physician and other specialists become "expert consultants, guides thru the maze of specialized information, rather than functioning as privileged decision-makers" (Jordan 1993, 167).

Such pedagogical goals cannot be teased apart from their political consequences. An integrated system of authoritative knowledge, while benefiting from top-down knowledge, must base itself in the grassroots (Jambai and MacCormack 1996). As Frankenberg noted, the association of radical politics with public health "highlights the state of the individual somatic body affected by events in the recent personal past." When epidemiological notions of future risk coincide with present discontents, such a combination may legitimize radical claims of causation, creating an "explosive" situation (1993, 235).

The Chalatenango negotiation process demonstrated well that the locus of conflict between a grassroots PHC project and the capitalist state may have more to do with local control of health and the community-based nature of popular health promoters than with the existence of lay workers per se. The Salvadoran Ministry of Health, like other health ministries in developing countries, was willing and ready (at least as long as USAID funds held out) to train lay health providers and to foist unimportant and underfunded preventive health tasks on them, but it was not willing to restructure programs in rural areas around the need for comprehensive approaches to health or to share health decision-making authority with local providers or organized community structures (Matomora 1989; and Sauerborn, Nougtara, and Diesfeld 1989).

Despite the ministry's reassertion of dominance, the Chalatenango popular health experiment demonstrates that comprehensive PHC and community participation is not an illusion. Although faced with resource constraints and a hostile national government, the popular health system made remarkable progress in less than a decade. This account has focused on the repopulated villages because those communities were most active in negotiations with the government. But outside of the repopulated area, by 1995 popular promoters were already serving more than eighty rural communities throughout the province, which lacked access to health services.

Ironic though it may be, the war actually helped create the conditions for such a project. Scott notes that dissident subcultures are more likely to form under conditions of "isolation, homogeneity of conditions, and mutual culture—often one with a strong 'us vs. them' social imagery" (1990, 135). It is also reasonable to view the negotiation process, in Giroux's words, as "both a site and a type of engagement" in the ongoing political struggle for social reform (1988). For the popular promoters, it was a participatory process: The progress of negotiations were regularly reviewed at promoter assemblies and community health meetings, where promoters gave feedback to negotiators. Those willing to volunteer for organizational and political tasks were welcomed by the overworked participants. Thus, the process itself, while disappointing in its concrete results, fostered solidarity among those participants. It constituted what Scott (1990) described as a "public declaration of the hidden transcript."

Also, through this process the ministry was forced to publicly acknowledge the competence and experience of the popular promoters—a few hundred unsophisticated, relatively uneducated peasant men and women—and take them seriously. The negotiations also likely reinforced promoters' self-respect and a sense of the importance of their work to their communities. In the absence of a polarizing influence like a war, and with little or no financial rewards for their work, a sense of common struggle may be a vital ingredient to holding a popular health system of this sort together. Scott wrote: "Solidarity among subordinates, if it is achieved at all, is thus achieved paradoxically, only by means of a degree of conflict. Certain forms of social strife, far from constituting evidence of disunity and weakness, may well be the signs of an active and aggressive social surveillance that preserves unity" (1990, 131).

This sense of commonweal, however, became more difficult to maintain in the neoliberal 1990s, when peasants faced a rural cost of living that was higher than before the war, and rural dwellers felt the lure of the city where a former health promoter might acquire educational credentials for a paying job as a nurse (a goal some promoters saw as a possible future).

This ethnography of the postwar negotiations over health in Chalatenango helps shed light on mechanisms by which authoritative medical knowledge can obscure the exercise of political power. In El Salvador, long-standing elite control over social services had created a reality in which the "political will" of the ruling ARENA party was all too clear. Often poorly run government programs were shored up by the very international funders that later feigned surprise and cried "lack of political will" when programs failed. The popular system's achievements were a bottom-up technology of populations, which meshed innovative community-building ideologies of a grassroots rebellion with transnational forms of social capital and material aid. Social change in El Salvador, when it has occurred, has only rarely come from government-administered development aid. It has come from the ground up, and it has always been fought for.

Grass roots has been low charge facilitators in El Salvador, not because the gort deems it so.

9

Disinvesting in Health

Multilateral Lending and the Clientelist State

We are not enemies of the NGOs, but we are friends of order.

–Dr. Eduardo Interiano, minister of health, 1995

The problematic peace process negotiations between the Ministry of Health and community health leaders in Chalatenango were not surprising given the strained political relations between the right-wing ARENA government and its former enemy, the FMLN, whose leaders remained popular in this former rebel stronghold. To gain a wider perspective, in fall 1995 I examined postwar changes in less controversial parts of the country, focusing on the two largest community health programs in El Salvador: the community health promoter (CHP) program in the Ministry of Health and the Maternal Health and Child Survival Project (known by its acronym, PROSAMI), which was a consortium of NGOs specializing in community-based health. Both programs relied on lay workers and both were initiated by and received funding from USAID, although the ministry was in the process of taking over support for the CHP promoter program, and its future was uncertain.

The timing was apt since in 1995 the ministry, under tutelage of World Bank and USAID advisors, was considering how to reform the health system. Structural reforms were seen as critical if El Salvador was to be eligible for a multimillion-dollar health development loan package. Health ministries throughout the Global South were being encouraged by the World Bank to enter into contracts with NGOs for health service delivery to poor populations. The PROSAMI network of NGOs was considered by many to be a prime candidate for such a contract because the program had been designed to fill a clear need and to compliment ministry programs. However, the prospect of contracting with NGOs was controversial for a government that had until recently regarded NGOs that served the poor as politically suspect.

To gain insights on the politics of community health and proposed reforms, I interviewed observers of the process, including staff in the ministry, consultants, and staff in development agencies who participated in health reform negotiations, as well as critics of the process, many of whom were linked to nonprofit health NGOs. Given the potential for bias, I adopted the practice common to investigative reporters of confirming factual assertions with multiple sources. I followed the reform process for three months and conducted followup interviews by phone from the United States.

This chapter begins with a brief history of the crisis in funding inside the Ministry of Health that resulted from poorly planned development projects, followed by war-related budget cuts, which led to dependency on USAID. I then describe the ministry's half-hearted foray into community-based health through its own promoter program beginning in 1989, the new neoliberal conditionalities in international health lending that favored decentralization, and the controversial turn to NGOs. This combination produced the ironic situation encountered by the PROSAMI network, which, despite a reputation for effectiveness at low cost, ended up losing funding due to the ministry's distrust of grassroots organizing. Although administrators in the Ministry of Health had concerns about working with NGOs, the ministry needed development loans and played along with the reform game in public while quietly making their own plans, which had little to do with the agendas of lenders or community health advocates. I conclude by discussing implications for community health work in the neoliberal era.

Govt funds with a catch

USAID and the Ministry of Health

It was ironic that USAID began embracing community-based health at such a late date in El Salvador. During the 1980s the USAID mission had tailored its programs to strengthen the Salvadoran government at any cost—including making up a massive funding shortfall in the Ministry of Health, which resulted from wartime budget cuts and a questionable Inter-American Development Bank (IDB) building project that planned to add more than one hundred (mostly rural) health facilities between 1975 and 1985 but that included no support for recurrent costs (Fiedler 1987, 1988). To staff the new clinics, the ministry shifted funding to personnel at the expense of other needs such as maintenance, supplies, and pharmaceuticals. By the late 1980s USAID was picking up the tab for many of these costs, including up to three-quarters of all pharmaceutical purchases. The USAID intervention kept the ministry functioning but relieved pressure on administrators to institute needed reforms (Fiedler, Gomez, and Bertrand 1993).

To make up for the shortfalls, staff salaries were also cut, especially those for the part-time physicians the ministry now relied on to make weekly visits to rural clinics (Fiedler 1988). This led many physicians to cut back the time they devoted to ministry work (relative to more lucrative private practices in urban settings). As a result, rural clinics gained a negative reputation with poor Salvadorans due to irregular physician coverage and shortages of medicines and supplies.[1]

Cut salaries, receive fewer amenities

According to a USAID health sector review, between 1987 and 1992 significant declines occurred in many ministry preventive services, including percentages of pregnant women registered in prenatal care; well child coverage; enrollment of malnourished mothers and children in feeding programs; and immunization coverage for DPT, measles, and polio (Fiedler, Gomez, and Bertrand 1993). Even after the war, although in theory the ministry covered health needs for 85 percent of Salvadorans, a USAID household survey revealed that only 40 percent of citizens said they went to public health clinics when they got sick (ADS 1994).

Affordable healthcare but many do not take advantage

After the 1992 cease-fire, USAID mission officers began frantically backpedaling in an effort to distance themselves from the "Frankenstein" that U.S. wartime economic aid had helped create. In interviews they emphasized USAID efforts to upgrade the ministry's cost accounting and optimistically predicted that the ministry would be able to take over 100 percent of drug purchases and funding of the CHP project as USAID funds were phased out in 1995—goals that outside evaluators called unrealistic.

The ministry's CHP program, which dates to 1989, was designed and initially funded by USAID with the goal of bringing primary health care to remote villages that lacked access to services. By 1995 there were 1,432 ministry promoters working in rural areas and charged with making house visits, especially in rural cantóns, promoting latrines, advising families on hygiene and well-child care, checking on vaccination coverage, and referring pregnant women for prenatal care. As discussed in chapter 8, although ministry promoters were also to offer first aid, an in-house evaluation of the program in 1995 showed that they had few supplies for this other than analgesics, nor were they able to evaluate infants. Plans to equip them with thermometers, baby scales, and blood pressure cuffs never came to fruition. Likewise, because so many rural families lacked funds to build latrines and the ministry had no supplementary funds for this purpose, the promoters were hampered in latrine promotion as well.[2]

Lack of sanitation

In interviews with me, government physicians openly opposed the policy of training lay promoters, and they stated this openly in the 1995 roundtables of health ministry employees set up to evaluate the program. The doctors maintained that the twelve-week CHP training course was inadequate to prepare promoters to respond to patients' curative needs (a conclusion also reached by outside evaluators).[3] Insiders in the ministry reported that physicians also resented the promoters' relatively high salaries (equal to more than a third of the salary of physicians in their social service year at that time).

Higher-level physician-administrators had expressed skepticism about the program since its creation, and one result was a stripped-down program design that restricted promoter training and duties to a far greater extent than programs for promoters in NGO-operated community health initiatives. Because the promoters were not able to respond to common curative care demands, many community health advocates predicted they would find it difficult to gain status and trust in villages. As noted in chapter 8, a 1995 USAID proposal that promoters' duties be broadened to include emergency use of sulfa drugs or antibiotics for serious respiratory infections was vetoed at top levels of the ministry before the evaluation got under way.[4]

The CHP promoter program also received a negative review by outside experts (Lewis, Eskeland, and Traa-Valerezo 2004), and members of a multilateral donor mission that traveled to rural areas to evaluate the ministry promoters described the program to me as "almost dysfunctional," noting that personnel in rural health clinics could not even tell the mission how many promoters worked in the area or where they were based. When villagers living in towns where ministry promoters were based were interviewed by the mission, many could not describe what promoters did. When asked who they had consulted the last time they were ill, most reported seeking care from private or NGO clinics.

People, trusted American method of medicine

In late 1994, when USAID turned over to the ministry full responsibility for promoter salaries, the program entered a crisis for lack of political support at high levels of the administration.[5] Despite USAID enthusiasm for the program, Health Minister Eduardo Interiano insisted that promoters lacked the skills needed to deliver health care properly. When I left the field in November 1995, plans were under way to quietly lay off most promoter supervisors and shift funds toward physician salaries.[6] Although the program continued to function after 1995, it did not grow, and promoters received little continuing education.

Neoliberal Health Reform and the Turn to NGOs

This was also a time of ferment in other ways for the Ministry of Health, which was negotiating with the World Bank and the IDB about a loan to finance health sector reforms. Critics from both ends of the political spectrum agreed that the incessant flow of U.S. economic aid during the war, combined with former President Duarte's policies of growing the civil sector, had worsened bureaucratic corruption and inefficiency. So while the end of the war held promise of greater social spending, government officials were under pressure from major foreign donors to downsize and rationalize public sector expenditures (Boyce 1995; del Castillo 2001; and Pastor and Conroy 1995).

Plans under discussion for reforming health included a new system for fee collection from public patients, privatizing some ancillary hospital services, contracting with NGOs for community health, and *departmentalización*—the local term for decentralizing decision making in the ministry's notoriously rigid and politicized central office. Many of these new prescriptions had been formalized in the World Bank's 1993 development report, *Investing in Health*, which called on countries to prioritize health interventions that had proven cost-effective, and expressly linked decentralization with use of outside contractors, including

NGOs and private entities, with the goal of increasing efficiency. The Bank justi-fied the new approach, citing preliminary data comparing NGO and public sector productivity from Africa (World Bank 1993, 163–164). Applying the butcher-knife logic of the business elite, the changing focus of foreign aid was explained in a *Wall Street Journal* article titled "Developing Countries Pass Off Tedious Job of Assisting the Poor":

> During the Cold War foreign aid was used as a weapon in the East–West struggle. Huge amounts were spent to win political loyalty, with little regard for whether it helped the poor or lined the pockets of leaders. Now, with the Soviet threat dissipated, the U.S. and many other donor nations have neither the inclination, nor the resources to be lavish with foreign aid. Thus, more governments are tapping into NGOs, paying what amounts to block grants in the hope they can deliver services more effi-ciently. (Greenberger 1995)

[handwritten: NATO has no interest in Latin America post-Cold War]

The article noted that the Clinton administration, feeling pressure from the foreign aid–slashing GOP-led Congress, planned to deliver 40 percent of foreign aid through NGOs in 1996. The turn to NGOs had begun during the 1980s, a decade during which multilateral development funds going to voluntary agen-cies had risen tenfold (Hellinger 1987). The World Bank, which had become the largest external funder of developing countries' health sectors, first linked such health finance policies to conditionality for loans in 1987 (Walt 1994). This shift in Bank policy carried both dangers and opportunities for organizations doing grassroots health work. In Latin America, few advocates for primary health care disputed the need to decentralize inefficient, urban-based, and curative care–oriented health ministries in poor countries. But health rights advocates saw the push to decentralize while privatizing as posing a serious danger to equity—especially if governments delegated responsibility for health services to private entities without the necessary funding, technical support, regulatory oversight, or mechanisms for local accountability.

The case of health in El Salvador provides an example of the complex poli-tics involved when bilateral and multilateral donors pressure a conservative ministry to restructure itself internally to improve efficiency while giving up control over some services to nonstate providers. Issues of control were espe-cially sensitive within the ministry after the cease-fire because, as noted, USAID's recent largess had come with many strings attached during the civil war. For Salvadoran administrators, although the funding was welcome, the intervention in sovereignty was greatly resented.

[handwritten: Like hate loss of sovereignty]

USAID also served as the conduit for most of the $250 million in recon-struction aid pledged by the United States after the 1992 cease-fire, $55 million of which was slated to be dispersed through NGOs (GAO 1992). Likewise, the World Bank had already made El Salvador a structural adjustment policy (SAP) loan of $100.3 million in 1992 (a small portion of which was earmarked for social services). But donor agencies had not made postwar reconstruction aid conditional on internal reforms to strengthen equity. Nor had Salvadoran government leaders been willing to cut military spending—which remained at twice as high a proportion of GDP as in the prewar period—or to levy higher income taxes (historically very low in El Salvador) to help finance reforms agreed to in peace talks with the FMLN. Instead the ARENA-controlled government chose to rely entirely on foreign donors, primarily the United States, to pay for reforms.

The resulting shortfall in foreign aid, combined with right-wing political opposition in El Salvador, slowed crucial peace programs such as land transfers, training of the civilian police force, and justice system reforms (Boyce 1995). In general, reform of social services was secondary to other peace plan goals. And since ministry officials could see their budget was unlikely to increase greatly while external funders were leaving (or cutting back support), it was logical that potentially expensive health promoter programs—previously nurtured by USAID and lacking a strong constituency inside the physician-dominated ministry—were first on the chopping block.

War and Proliferation of NGOs in Central America

In much of Central America, the irony is that international and domestic NGOs had already been substituting for states in providing critical basic (often constitutionally guaranteed) services to poor populations. NGO activity in the region grew in direct relation to the regional conflicts. By 1992 there were at least three hundred development NGOs in Nicaragua, seven hundred in Guatemala, and around seven hundred in El Salvador (Sollis 1996).[7] The picture is complicated by the diverse political and religious groups involved in development. While a plethora of international NGOs such as Oxfam, American Friends Service Committee, and Catholic Action supported liberation theology–style initiatives on behalf of grassroots organizations, USAID and the region's military governments responded by encouraging a wave of conservative evangelical NGOs to begin or expand programs. Some right-wing NGOs in El Salvador and Guatemala worked closely with national army civic-military actions, which offered one-day food giveaways and medical consultations in rural areas where antigovernment rebels were active. Thus policies of diverting public funds into NGO activities could cut either way on the political spectrum.

Nevertheless, during the 1980s NGO-supported grassroots activism succeeded in drawing unprecedented levels of international attention and resources to rural populations in the region that had suffered from economic exploitation and military repression. In El Salvador alone, a 1995 Ministry of Health survey found 171 health-related NGOs operating. If we consider only primary health-oriented programs in which lay workers received significant training, and the programs were

village-based and could count on referral systems to resolve residents' more serious health problems, studies suggest that more than two thousand such NGO-
supported community health workers were serving more than half a million
Salvadorans in underserved rural communities (IPM 1995).

In El Salvador, the dollar value of NGO interventions sometimes rivaled
that of progovernment development projects. For example, the Diaconía, a
Salvadoran ecumenical organization that funded NGO programs of humanitarian assistance for displaced peasants, received a total of $65 million in foreign
donations between 1982 and 1992, a level of funding that approached the
$75 million USAID spent in the same period on its displaced person's program.[8]
Unfortunately, not long after the Central American peace processes got under
way in the early 1990s—creating opportunities for postwar reconstruction—
many major donors began redirecting their attention and funds to other global
hot spots like Bosnia and Eastern Europe, forcing national NGOs in the region to
seek out new sources of support.

A persistent uncertainty in the post–Cold War period was the degree to which
NGOs in El Salvador could remain effective advocates for the poor, given the
onslaught of globalizing neoliberal policies and pressures to align with powerful
donors or governments to obtain funding. Ironically, in the case of health, the efficiency and high patient acceptance of many NGO operations was directly tied to
their local grassroots orientation, and health advocates feared this effectiveness
would be compromised by rapid expansion. Leaders of the popular health system
in Chalatenango worried that the local participation in health they had nurtured in
communities would suffer if the organization suddenly shifted from a combined
advocacy–service role to provision of the vertically administered selected services
favored by most large donors. Furthermore, few NGOs working in the country had
the institutional infrastructure for managing basic health services on a large scale,
as would be needed for Ministry of Health contracts.

The World Bank, the Ministry, and the NGO Network

A physician who had directed a regional office of the ministry (and whom I had
known since 1992) shocked me shortly after I arrived in June 1995 with his
upbeat predictions of more autonomy at the regional level and future ministry
collaboration with health NGOs. "This is quite a change of heart for the ministry," I remarked. "Yes," he replied with a wink, "two years ago it would have
been a sin to talk about these things." But in the months to come, as I followed
events, it became clear that "talking" was about as far as things would go.

The changes he was predicted dated to a set of prescriptions published in
1994 by an international health advisory commission that USAID created after the
war. The group's assessment of the Salvadoran health sector, known as the ANSAL
report ("Análisis del Sector Salud de El Salvador"), identified many inefficiencies

in the Ministry of Health, including high costs, low productivity, poor management, inappropriate technology, and deficiencies in planning and budgeting (ANSAL 1994). However, unlike the critiques coming from the FMLN and the popular health sector, the ANSAL proposals for reforms sidestepped issues of broadening services to the one-third of the population in extreme poverty. The report, based on a USAID epidemiological study of the country, downplayed the role of poverty and inequality as contributors to ill health (Ayalde 1994).

In 1995 the recommendations of the ANSAL report became the guidelines used by a World Bank–initiated health reform group. This group, appointed by the ARENA president, Armando Calderón Sol, but outside of the health ministry, undertook its deliberations in secret, keeping a broad spectrum of interested health workers and policy analysts in the dark for most of a year about what reforms were being proposed. In the end, the group, led by an architect and a pediatric neurologist—neither of which had any experience in public health (Homedes et al. 2000)—concurred with the ANSAL findings and designed a set of reforms based around decentralizing and privatizing some administrative units as well as health service delivery for uninsured patients while transforming the ministry from responsibility for public health for the poor to a role as a "coordinator" of services provided by outside contractors (see also Selva-Sutter 2000).

The Ministry of Health dutifully played along with these international advisors, setting up a reform office and issuing white papers during 1995. The carrot in this relationship, from the point of view of the ministry, was a proposed joint loan package from the World Bank and the IDB that some estimated would amount to $40 million. The reforms were presented as a way to achieve such lofty goals as extending services to the 37 percent of the population estimated to lack any health coverage and creating a safety net insurance system for the poor. Details on how this would be done remained hazy.

Health advocates for the poor were wary of the ministry's decentralization talk, fearing it might provide a rationale for the government to further shirk responsibility for public health. On the other hand, many community-based workers were hopeful that the promises would mean more autonomy and efficiency in regional health offices, and ministry financing for NGOs. Like the government, many NGOs had seen their foreign donations shrink in the postwar period while the actual level of need in the countryside remained acute. The cost of living for peasants had risen dramatically, even compared to the difficult prewar years, while per capita income fell. Many promised peace process reforms, such as transfers of land, were delayed due to shortfalls of funds and political opposition.[9]

Hopes of collaboration with the ministry were especially high for the PROSAMI program that linked thirty-five local NGOs into a network, which USAID had funded since 1989. The NGOs had trained 1,500 lay promoters in an innovative Maternal and Child Health (MCH) program aimed at remote rural communities. By 1995 the community-based promoters served an estimated 10 percent of the country's population. The primary health orientation of PROSAMI promoters was very similar to that of the Chalatenango popular promoters, except that PROSAMI promoters had more limited prescribing and curative duties (although they did handle antibiotics in cases of severe respiratory infection). While they were based in historically underserved cantónes, most PROSAMI promoters did relatively little community organizing, although a number of administrators of PROSAMI NGOs believed that this aspect of their work should be expanded.

Preliminary evidence from an evaluation by international health consultants showed decreasing infant death rates from diarrhea and acute respiratory disease in areas served by the PROSAMI network compared with areas served only by the ministry. The reviewers also gave the NGO network high marks for efficiency in providing a wide array of educational and preventive MCH interventions with a high degree of community acceptance (Thornton, Boddy, and Brooks 1994). Many observers credited the NGO network's success to the fact that the program circumvented the government's rigid health bureaucracy and patronage system.

With USAID funds for PROSAMI promoters slated to run out in early 1996, advocates for rural health waited impatiently for favorable news from the ministry about future collaboration. But insiders reported that Dr. Interiano, the health minister, disagreed with development experts from USAID and PAHO on the viability of community-based health models and challenged the findings of the PROSAMI evaluation (which, although carried out by outside consultants, carried the onus of having been paid for by USAID). Instead he favored policies of hiring more physicians for regional hospitals and increasing physicians' salaries (which had declined in purchasing power during the war years). This stance frustrated advocates for community health. One international consultant predicted to me that the hidden support costs for each new physician brought into the system would effectively double that professional's base salary—a sum adequate to support six promoters. "If the ministry really had cost-benefit at heart," she said, "it would be much more cost-effective to hire promoters."

Dr. Interiano, who had gained a reputation even within ARENA for his ultraconservative views, made no secret of his distrust of NGOs, many of which had long been regarded by El Salvador's government as "leftist." A *Wall Street Journal* article quoted Interiano as saying, "We are not enemies of the NGOs, but we are friends of order." The ominous term (*orden*) was well known in El Salvador as right-wing code for authoritarian policies. An insider to the health reform negotiations told me, "The minister thinks all NGOs are guerrillas, but most of the PROSAMI network NGOs' politics are more like those of Jimmy Carter."

A health planner close to these discussions in the ministry explained that high administrators were "afraid to deal with NGOs because their funders are leaving, and NGOs will begin to pressure the ministry for full support." There were, in his opinion, no serious plans to contract with NGOs. Shaking his head, he predicted, "Most of this NGO work will disappear." Members of multilateral donor missions interviewed later confirmed that the minister remained firmly opposed to contracting with the PROSAMI NGO network.

One USAID-funded development expert who advised the ministry laughed at my naiveté when I kept asking when the reform office would publish its long-delayed, much-talked-about reorganization scheme. Officials in the ministry's reform office had just told me they were expecting a $40 million loan from the World Bank and IDB that would pay for upgrading regional health centers to small hospitals, with placement of several medical specialists at each site. Expansion of hospital capacity is, from a public health standpoint, a question-able prioritization of funds, given El Salvador's large underserved rural popula-tion and recent history of expanding hospital infrastructure.[10] But putting that question aside, I wondered aloud, "Doesn't the ministry have to put these reforms into effect to get that loan?" The development consultant replied, "The reform office is to please the banks, but they're never going to follow through. The banks just emphasize reforms to maintain their international image."

Around that time, the government budget for 1996 became public. Instead of the much-heralded downsizing, the national budget actually grew by several thousand jobs, a fact that generated a flurry of derisive newspaper articles. The health ministry also grew, as it should have, given President Calderón Sol's pledge to dedicate more funds to social services. This new influx of funds, how-ever, did not translate into better health care for the 37 percent of predomi-nantly rural citizens whom ministry services failed to reach. In fact, in Chalatenango, historically one of the most underfunded provinces, the regional health director claimed that his budget had been cut, forcing him to freeze hir-ing and lay off a dentist and several sanitation inspectors.

Likewise, departmentalización, the reform intended to give more auton-omy to ministry administrators in regional offices, was proving to be, as one observer put it, "a map on paper." Representatives of the Chalatenango popular health system had been assured that after the reforms the regional director would be empowered to hire popular health promoters to work with ministry clinics. In a formal negotiation session, however, the director claimed that departmentalización meant little. "The reality is that administratively we're totally dependent on the minister's decisions. There is no money. Who knows when there will be?" he said, throwing up his hands in a meeting with frustrated popular health negotiators.

To their credit, World Bank and IDB officials took the advice of their health teams and balked on the planned loan once the minister's attitudes about reform became clear. An observer at the November 1995 talks between the ministry and representatives of the two banks later reflected on the meeting, "They wanted hospitals. [The minister] said 'I want four hospitals in time for the next elections.' And he wanted them in areas where the ARENA party was weakest! Imagine telling that to a joint bank mission! . . . He really showed his colors. The minister is not interested in reform."

The observer claimed that the banks considered government collaboration with NGOs to be "part and parcel of our program," but he lamented that the ministry never seriously evaluated NGO health promoter activities or considered how coordination with NGOs might maximize coverage in rural areas. Shortly after the joint mission left the country, the head of the ministry's reform office quit in disgust and afterward spoke out about politicization within the ministry. Members of the joint bank mission, however, told me that higher-level administrators in the World Bank and IDB were not pleased with denial of the loan and immediately began planning another mission to El Salvador to, as one said, "try [to] make something work."[11]

In summary, after a year of debates over health reform in postwar El Salvador from 1995 to 1996, the national budget grew, but historically underserved rural regions like Chalatenango saw budget cuts. Decentralization of ministry decision making turned out to be a "paper reform" with little reality in practice. And instead of collaborating with an existing NGO network such as PROSAMI, which was based on promoters whose effectiveness and low cost had been demonstrated, the ministry rejected contracting with NGOs for political reasons. At the same time, it began downsizing its own community health promoter program while shifting funds to doctor salaries and a questionable new plan for a more medicalized approach to rural care.

Community Health NGOs in the Neoliberal Period

In the 1990s, an ongoing debate among Salvadoran health activists centered on what kind of strategies small NGOs with social justice agendas should pursue. During the last half of the war in particular, hundreds of professionals and community-level health workers had registered their disgust with discredited public services by forming NGOs, through which they sought political support, human rights protections, and funds from foreign donors. The goal of replacing the government through revolution failed, although the rebellion did succeed in dismantling the military's repressive apparatus. Now, with the war over, it was clear that a second phase of struggle would be needed to achieve key social reforms. Community health advocates, frustrated with the highly centralized and clientelist health ministry, held out hope that some aspects of neoliberal reforms such as decentralization and contracting with NGOs could work in favor of their struggle to expand coverage for the poor and build networks for community participation.

Unfortunately, high-level administrators in the ministry were also aware of these possibilities. Interiano's opposition to reforms recalls Kurt Weyland's study of failed health reform in Brazil (1995) in which he concluded that clientelist politicians opposed health reforms for fear that if decentralized services succeeded in improving health of the poor, this would weaken peoples' dependence on patrons and undermine dominant politicians' electoral position. Peter Sollis viewed this intransigence as a regional pattern: "The dilemma for urban elites who monopolize political and economic power is that organized beneficiary participation creates conditions for greater grassroots democracy and broader local autonomy at the same time as it facilitates smaller, cheaper and more cost-effective government. A consensual solution to this contradiction is the problem of governance in Central America today" (1996).

For the Catholic Church and European NGOs aligned with the popular movement in Chalatenango, the strategy chosen in the early postwar period was one of officially confronting the ministry at the local level. As shown in chapter 8, this played to the strength of the locally based health system, allowing popular system leaders to reinforce solidarity at the community level through continuing "a kind of war" with the government while showing off their model of community health to observers from the United Nations and PAHO. But then outside donors cut funding to the community-based NGOs, and FMLN physicians involved in the negotiations began to feel pressure to compromise with the government, which they believed would strengthen eligibility for external funding from international development institutions.

Neither the Catholic Diocese health office nor FMLN-affiliated health NGOs working in Chalatenango trusted USAID overtures. They had boycotted invitations to join the PROSAMI network because of its USAID connection, despite the attraction of steady funding. Some other FMLN-aligned health NGOs did join the USAID-funded PROSAMI network, as did groups affiliated with more social democratic factions.[12] These groups reaped the benefits of several years of financial support, allowing training for their promoters and extending their outreach into new communities that lacked health coverage. The tradeoff (for USAID support) was a requirement that promoters in the network adopt a more service-oriented approach, with less emphasis on community development or health problems outside of maternal and child health. Many NGO promoters and their supervisors also found it a burden to manage the USAID paperwork. But the primary downside for most was the looming cut-off in funds. (After I left the field, PROSAMI funding was extended two more years, then permanently discontinued in December 1998.) Unlike the Chalatenango popular system in which promoters began as volunteers and had never been able to count on more than nominal stipends, PROSAMI network NGO administrators feared that their more recently recruited promoters thought of their work as "a job" and would discontinue health work when funds ran out.

To the credit of some PROSAMI leaders, representatives of member NGOs began meeting together in 1995 to form a health coalition—a strategy to facilitate economies of scale for purchasing and to strengthen their chances of obtaining funding abroad. Dr. Hector Silva, a future mayor of San Salvador, played a key role in this effort. They also met with their health counterparts in the Catholic Church. Nevertheless, as I went back and forth between Chalatenango and San Salvador, I was constantly struck by the lack of communication between programs—a tendency that grew out of overwork, understaffing, rivalry over constituencies and resources, and the persistent distrust of other organizations that the civil war engendered.

No one talked to each other

By then it had become clear to health activists that gaining more resources at the community level would depend on overcoming regional and organizational fragmentation and building a broad-based coalition that could confront both the ARENA regime and the international finance banks. In the postwar period, health advocates realized that primary health care needed to be carried out at the national level to have equitable planning and resource allocation.

As El Salvador's case shows, under neoliberal development, the goal of decentralization served ARENA's political agendas by providing a rationale for the health ministry to abandon burdensome functions through privatization and/or funding cuts. A similar process took place during Chilean and Guatemalan health reforms (Vergara 1997; and Maupin 2008). Likewise, in Colombia, geographic decentralization of sanitation services was used to defuse political protest and reinforce the power of local authorities and private landowners.[13] These examples point up the potential for loss of accountability when individual community health NGOs contract with the state to provide services. A contracting relationship carries the additional risk of diverting a grassroots NGO from a social justice orientation to one of direct service delivery.[14]

Reliance on the Big Man

Although some scholars of globalization have predicted the decline of the state as a power base (relative to increasingly unfettered transnational corporations), this account supports the view that states will continue to be important strategic power blocs in their own right as well as sources of legitimacy for capitalist projects (see Sunkel 1995). Most social movements channel demands for a more democratic order through states, and NGOs continue to be critical actors in this struggle precisely because of their potential to extend strategic alliances borders. Without these alliances, which provide volunteers, resources, and human rights scrutiny, dissident Salvadoran peasants would have found it much more difficult to build model health systems that challenged government models of service delivery.

Thesis that globalization will not diminish sovereignty

The viability of the state as an equitable service provider and the importance of incorporating health struggles into multisectoral struggle are well illustrated by Kerala, the impressive Indian state in which health expenditures per capita grew to thirty-five times the national norm, with exemplary morbidity and mortality indices following suit (Franke and Chasin 1994). But no single health initiative or campaign could take credit for Kerala's enviable statistics, which reflected decades of land reform, relatively high minimum wages, high female literacy, a popular health education movement, and a declining birth rate. Ratcliffe (1978) argued that the causes of social development in cases like Kerala must be thought of as "synergistic"—in this case involving a forty-year tradition of social activism and mass organization that has forced even conservative state administrations to adopt strong social programs. And, contrary to the neoliberal paradigm, Kerala's development progress was not dependent on economic growth alone—Kerala remains a relatively poor state within India— but was related to more equitable distribution of existing resources and a history of policies favoring education and land reform.

Both the Kerala model and the Salvadoran popular system are examples of "evolutionary revolution"—a term used by Skalnick (1989) to refer to continuous innovations in political culture and social order in a situation in which leaders are responsive to the changing expectations of the people. In the long run, such advocacy models may prove more fruitful for community health NGOs in the Third World than the "replace the state" service delivery functions envisioned for NGOs by neoliberal experts. As networks, health NGOs can also be effective at advocating for reforms in the policies of major donors (see Walt 1994; Epprecht 1994; and Hellinger 1987). Arguments for donor attention to such concerns is strengthened by a review of twenty-five World Bank projects that found a strong correlation between project success and participation of grassroots organizations (Cernea 1988).

Neoliberal "Reform" as Performance

Many of the reforms that USAID and the World Bank recommended to the Salvadoran Ministry of Health followed from the prescriptions for cost-effective health development outlined in the World Bank's 1993 development report, *Investing in Health*. In a review of that document, Marc Epprecht (1994) pointed out the contradictions posed when public health is bent into a neoliberal mold, such as the report's failure to mention data showing that Africans' health had been damaged by SAP loans, and free trade policies that favored Northern exports of high-priced pharmaceuticals, tobacco, and polluting industries. *Investing in Health* conveniently blamed Africa's declining health indices on corrupt governments, ignoring histories of colonialism, unfavorable trade policies, arms exports, and failed development projects that contributed to famine.[15]

Cost-effectiveness criteria also led the World Bank to promote questionable public health priorities. For example, the Bank advised countries not to spend loan funds on rural water and sanitation infrastructure, the very interventions that community health NGOs in Chalatenango considered to be most important in preventing diarrhea—one of the largest killers of rural children. Citing a history of ineffective water project loans, *Investing in Health* blamed corrupt public ministries for siphoning off funds instead of providing responsive services, then went on to acknowledge that "demand-driven" water initiatives seemed to be more efficient than "supply-side" projects. But rather than use this evidence to argue for more development work at the grassroots level, the report's authors simply concluded that in rural areas "health benefits alone do not generally provide a rationale for public subsidy of water and sanitation" (1993, 93). The report's own statistics failed to support this finding since it found diarrhea, primarily due to poor sanitation and water supplies, to be responsible for 10 percent of the disease burden in developing countries.

This ideology permeated the Salvadoran health reform plan. In a discourse analysis of the 1994 ANSAL report, Luis Aviles (2001) noted that, in contrast to trends in international public health of treating poverty as tightly linked with health, the USAID epidemiological report on El Salvador "presents general statistics that completely ignore health inequalities in the country and their social and historical determinants . . . problems of social class inequalities remained unnamed, unanalyzed, and invisible. . . . The 70-page report has no single table in which health indicators are related to any measure of social class, whether it is education, occupation, income, or poverty level" (2001, 165). The ministry's health care reform office issued draft documents stating clearly that a primary objective of reforms was to formalize the privatization process that was already under way, according to Ernesto Selva-Sutter (2000), who led creation of the country's first public health school at the University of Central America in San Salvador in the 1990s.

Thus, beginning in 1995, El Salvador's health development goals shifted abruptly from a target of basic health and sanitation services for the majority to an emphasis on downsizing Ministry of Health staff and implementing user fees and financial tracking systems. In a conversation that fall with a USAID staffer about El Salvador, I observed that cost-benefit seemed to have replaced epidemiology as the goal of development in USAID and World Bank documents. I asked, "What is the evidence that privatization will improve services in rural areas?" He seemed annoyed that my question had veered outside the ideological framework of neoliberal *Realpolitik* and responded curtly: "Look, first you have to accept the premise that this is all based on: that ministry-delivered health nationwide is not the cheapest and best way to do it." Minutes later I asked if USAID projected future profitability for basic services. He replied, "The idea that health care is profitable anywhere is not true. After all, we subsidize health in the [United] States." No argument there, but I couldn't help wondering, if not the state, and not business, then to whom are impoverished rural peoples of the Third World supposed to look for basic health services? To charities? An answer for the nineteenth century, perhaps, but in the twenty-first century, it's a stretch to call this development.

One might assess the Salvadoran health ministry's intransigence at actually working with community-based NGOs as a failure of neoliberal reform. However, the reforms only "failed" if the stated goals (for example, decentralization and subcontracting rural health to NGOs to obtain more efficient services for the poor) are taken to be the real aims of structural adjustment. Certainly limited redistribution of wealth was a major goal of World Bank policies during the Robert McNamara era, and there was no doubt in my mind that the middle-level staff of major donor agencies who talked to me were sincere in their desires to alleviate poverty. Nevertheless, by the late 1990s it had become apparent to many observers that solving the problems of poverty was not the goal of the "Washington Consensus," as the prevailing view favoring free trade came to be known in the international community.

This is particularly apparent when one tallies the human consequences of structural adjustment policies (SAPs), as the comprehensive shift to privatization and deregulation has become known. A study reviewing a decade of neoliberal SAPs in eight Latin American countries found that in the name of extracting interest payments for northern banks—amounting to a sum several times the size of the Marshall Plan in constant dollars—social expenditures were drastically cut across the board, including reductions in health budgets over ten years that averaged 67 percent of what was spent in health in 1980 (Petras and Vieux 1992); this in an ex-colonial region that in the last thirty years had come to have the worst disparity in income between rich and poor anywhere in the world. Epprecht cited similar erosion of essential services in Africa, including declining life expectancies since 1986 in eleven countries with SAPs (1994). In the end, neither Latin American nor African countries reaped higher national GDPs for all that reform; most countries with SAPs saw GDPs fall (see also Kim et al. 2000; and Fort, Mercer, and Gish 2004).

After all the talk of economic growth as the key to development, one is forced to ask, where is the development in this picture? In practice, structural adjustment in combination with the neoliberal forms of modernization and economic growth it facilitated has often functioned to undermine social welfare for the majority. Neoliberal policies thus perverted the very meaning of development by harnessing tools of intervention in ways that created poverty rather than alleviating it.

Given the major donors' "pressure to lend" and the records of approving loans even for governments with abysmal human rights and development records (see Walt 1994, 157–159; Justice 1986; and Danaher 1994), we can understand why El Salvador's minister of health was not rushing to implement reforms that would hurt his own power base. The rhetoric of reform served ARENA well in giving the new civilian government a badly needed veneer of social responsibility, both for domestic consumption (in El Salvador's new era of electoral politics) and in reassuring foreign donors and investors, many of whom had previously been put off by ARENA's history as the party linked to death squads. But like high-level administrators in many formerly colonized states, Dr. Interiano had patronage hierarchies to protect. For example, in 2007 local news stories reported that several ARENA businessmen, including former president Alfredo Cristiani, had invested in private pharmacies well positioned to benefit from privatization of state health functions. Interiano also oversaw a professional constituency of physicians who saw state-supported promoters as competition. Thus, he had little reason to jeopardize these relationships by contracting with the "wrong kind of NGOs" for community health; instead of taking the more politically feasible option of boosting ministry physicians' salaries and using loans to expand the number of full-time doctors on the ministry staff.

He also was no doubt reassured by USAID's decade-long history of pumping funds into government social services as the pacification arm of U.S. low-intensity war strategy. Such a history made it sound a bit disingenuous when the World Bank official whom I interviewed in 1996 blamed the failure of health reform on "a bad egg" of a minister, rather than on a history of policies that undercut democratic forces seeking to oust "bad eggs" from power.

Hence, the development establishment's turn to NGOs notwithstanding, this tale of health "antireform" adds to a long stream of evidence that decision making by large donor institutions pursuing neoliberal goals has often been less concerned about outcomes of proposed reforms, or even their cost-effectiveness, than with the political stability of Third World governments allied with major donor nations.

While the turn to NGOs for development has opened up opportunities for channeling funds and expertise into grassroots projects, benefits are likely to be short lived if, in the rush for funds, NGO health planners sacrifice community development goals and become mired in the role of charitable "service provider." Just as true social development is always based in participation, in the long term, the leverage an NGO is able to weld in the political arena will always rest on the organization and political participation of its constituents.

10

The White Marches

Healing the Body Politic

O paga, o se muere. [Pay or die.]
—slogan in White Marches

Vice President Dick Cheney's description of El Salvador as a "success story" (see chapter 1) is a revisionist nugget that neatly sums up the two countries' foreign relations in recent years—based on renovation of ARENA from the party of death squads to advocates for a neoliberal business model. Wielding control of the legislature during most of the 1990s, ARENA (allied with small parties on the right) oversaw the doubling of the GDP, proliferation in free trade zones, rampant privatizations of public infrastructure, and, in 2001, the switch from colones to dollars as the national currency. In the run-up to the 2004 Salvadoran presidential elections, two high-ranking Bush administration officials made public statements threatening U.S. retaliation in the form of restrictions on Salvadoran immigration to the United States and punitive foreign investment policies if the FMLN were elected. The threats frightened voters because a quarter of the Salvadoran population lives in the United States, and remittances have become essential to family survival strategies (Rodriguez 2009).

While Latin America, as a region, edged away from the Washington Consensus on free trade policies, El Salvador, under ARENA, remained the Bush administration's darling—the only country in the region to send troops to Iraq and the first to put the Central American Free Trade Agreement (CAFTA) into effect. Official U.S. and Salvadoran reports emphasize this commercialization, describing El Salvador in glowing terms. The *Wall Street Journal* and *Moody's* ranked El Salvador as second only to Chile for having the most "open" economy in Latin America.

The other side of the coin is the country's continued rankings for social development among the four poorest countries in Latin America. While poverty rates declined and health indices improved relative to the war years, overall the poorest half of the population lost ground in purchasing power compared to

1980. The lack of social reforms in the peace agreement contributed to this disparity. Promised land transfers to families of guerrilla combatants, for example, were held up for years; a 13 percent sales tax has substituted for comprehensive tax reform (there is no property tax); and the much touted *maquila* sector has disappointed in terms of job creation and continues to be associated with abusive conditions and repressive antiunion tactics. Homicide rates, now due to crime and gang activity rather than to military violence, are the highest in Latin America; however, as Moody noted, unlike the war deaths, the deaths due to sickness or crime in the postwar period have less value for public consumption and are mourned in the private sphere (2005).

As of 2007, the same wealthy families—now with diversified holdings that balance agricultural interests with a range of other business investments—retained political power. The middle class expanded as former exiles repatriated their savings to buy houses and open businesses near the capital. But economic growth remains concentrated in urban enclaves where developers and commercial investors have been best positioned to benefit from neoliberal reforms. During a six-week research visit in mid-2007, high prices for food and medicine were inescapable themes in conversations with urban cab drivers and poor rural families, who tend to cite the 2001 shift to the dollar as the moment inflation increased. While the minimum wage increased slightly, it only reached half the level needed to keep the average family out of poverty. The situation has inspired a new wave of migration to United States by workers whose families have come to rely on their cash remittances to make ends meet. As of 2005, remittances accounted for 17 percent of the GDP.

As the opposition has repositioned itself in the political arena, the increasingly desperate situation of poor families and a steady drumbeat of scandals linking ARENA officials to corruption and profiteering began to threaten the right-wing coalition. The FMLN, which suffered a debilitating split in its ranks right after the war and a slow transition to political party status, made gains during the late 1990s, winning the mayorship of the capital and a growing power in the Legislative Assembly. The 2003 elections gave the FMLN a majority (eighty) of the country's municipalities and enough legislative seats to pass laws by forming coalitions with smaller parties. Interestingly, two recent leftist mayors of San Salvador, Hector Silva (1997–2003) and Violeta Menjívar (2006–2009), were former physicians with a history of support for community-based health work, whose public agendas emphasized improving access to health care in barrios of the capital.

By the late 1990s, public health had become the unlikely bailiwick for a wide range of struggles over privatization. From 1999 to 2003, radicalized health workers led a series of strikes and street demonstrations—the largest and most fractious social mobilizations since the war years—focused on stopping privatization of the social security health system. The most impressive show of force took place between September 2002 and June 2003, when a prolonged health strike shut down most hospitals and clinics nationwide, and periodic roadblocks interfered with business and tourism. A series of White Marches (Marchas Blancas) against privatization brought hundreds of thousands into the streets month after month dressed in white as a show of solidarity with hospital workers. Police raids on hospitals, threats and arrests of health workers, and hunger strikes became headline news. The level of political polarization reminded many of the civil war years.

Eventually the progressive health coalition won several of its demands. ARENA President Francisco Flores backed down from his privatization agenda in 2003, and negotiators for the popular sector also got rare concessions from the World Bank, removing privatization conditions from loan agreements. But both sides took political losses from the prolonged showdown, which put thousands of patients with chronic problems at risk and paralyzed national affairs. As of 2007, government promises of collaboration on health reforms remained unfulfilled, and ghosts of privatization continued to haunt the agenda; however, the ARENA party, under incoming President Antonio Saca, perhaps haunted by its own specters of mass protests, adopted a much more restrained tone on health reforms.

The first round of debates over World Bank–sponsored health reform in the mid-1990s is recounted in chapter 9, with special attention to rural health needs. Organized health workers, both professionals and community-based providers, were vital actors in that struggle. But whereas in 1995 debates over health reform were the domain of a few specialists and had little popular appeal on the national agenda, in this chapter we see organized health workers emerge as national leaders of coalitions working for social change, upstaging even the FMLN leadership—which adroitly forged a collaboration to take advantage of and lend mobilizing strength to the health unions that led these protests. Although health policy is often complex, issues of access to care and constitutional guarantees of health rights became the rallying cry for the movement.

For the most part, the mainstream U.S. media, which retreated from coverage of Latin America after Bush's "War on Terror" took center stage, ignored the White Marches and health and transport strikes that shut down entire sectors of the economy multiple times in 1999–2000 and 2002–2003. Other than Paul Almeida's 2006 historical sociology on the country's waves of protests since 1925, which includes a chapter on antiglobalization struggles, these mobilizations have likewise received little attention from academics. Nevertheless, ramifications of the uprisings for ARENA, for the World Bank's neoliberal health agenda, and for the opposition party have been pivotal. In this chapter I draw on a range of sources, including forty-six interviews conducted in 2000, 2002, and 2007 with march participants, movement leaders, health officials, and political/health analysts to reconstruct events and analyze how concerns about access to health came to stand in for a wide range of policies seen as impacting social life in negative ways since the end of the civil war.[1]

In thinking about these mobilizations, it is important to acknowledge the historical legacy and practical knowledge that many health activists gained from the Latin American Social Medicine movement, which in the 1990s produced a variety of analyses and critiques of neoliberal health reforms in the region (Tajer 2003). But as Joan Nelson points out, health has seldom been an arena for mass mobilization in Latin America during the neoliberal period (2004). The arcane nature of policy debates about privatization, the dominance of professional interests in medicine, and the uncertain political gains for politicians who take stands on the issue usually preclude mass participation. A goal of this chapter is to examine what circumstances in El Salvador cast healing as the central metaphor in debates about the role of the state and public patrimony in a period dominated by demands of transnational institutions and finance markets that have gained unprecedented control over the policies of states.

Privatization and Radicalized Doctors

Neoliberal privatization efforts in El Salvador date to the election of the ARENA party in 1989. The banking system, which had been nationalized under Duarte, was the first to be sold to private investors, and it is not incidental that former ARENA president Alfredo Cristiani now owns Banco Cuscatlán, one of the country's largest banks. Postwar loan agreements with the World Bank and the International Monetary Fund committed the country to pursue privatization in other sectors, and since then telephone services, electricity distribution, pensions, a distribution service for subsidized goods, and an institute that made affordable housing loans have all been sold off. Ports and the international airport were partially privatized. Unionized workers and the FMLN opposed the sales of government infrastructure, but the fact that many of these sectors had been corruptly managed and inefficient as government entities helped to mute public criticism.

Privatization lived up to some promises but failed in other areas. For example, new private providers improved access to phones in urban markets, but service to some rural areas was suspended because it was deemed unprofitable (Prokosch 1997), and rates charged to customers soared after the deals were closed. By 2002, the cost of telephone service had doubled and electric rates had risen fivefold over levels in the late 1980s (Schuld 2003). The new corporate owners also laid off large sectors of the predominately unionized workforces. In a five-year period, the number of telephone workers was cut from 7,000 to 3,200 (Equipo Maiz 2005). Nor did the privatizations realize the efficiencies that proponents had predicted would occur as a result of increased competition to provide the services. Because the national electric utility was sold, mergers and buyouts reconsolidated most holdings under control of the American-based AES Corporation (Equipo Maiz 2005). A study by the Center for Constitutional Studies for Human Rights, a Salvadoran NGO, concluded that rather than spur competition, privatization led in several cases to public services becoming private monopolies (Creedon and Ney 2003).

By 1994–1995 the ideology of privatization became incorporated into health reform proposals in the form of the ANSAL report (see chapter 9), which explicitly acknowledged that the Ministry of Health lacked adequate funding to provide primary services to rural residents who lacked access to care, and advocated for a complete restructuring of the system, including privatization of public hospitals (including services and administration), contracting out of primary health services to organizations managed at the municipal level, which could be either private or nonprofit, and transferring of the Health and Social Security Institute (ISSS) from the Ministry of Labor to the Ministry of Health (ANSAL 1994, 15–22). While privatization may result in the loss of sovereignty from a government standpoint, many analysts have noted that in the case of government health plans, this move is seen as an ideal scenario for profit generation from the viewpoint of a corporate insurer or health maintenance organization because the state becomes responsible to channel tax proceeds directly to the company that contracts to provide services, minimizing the costs of collecting premiums from individuals. This likely explains the considerable interest on the part of multinational health insurers in expanding into the Latin American market (Waitzkin and Iriart 2001).

The Salvadoran Ministry of Health's concerns about opposition from organized health workers led to an official discourse that substituted a variety of less offensive terms for "privatization" or "contracting." In interviews with me and in public statements, officials in charge of implementing ministry reforms insisted that "privatization" was not an accurate description of their goals because nonprofit NGOs as well as businesses would be eligible to "gestionar" (manage) health services. When asked questions about proposals that seemed to call for "contracting out" services, ministry spokespersons said "contracts" were the wrong term. The preferred language, they said, was "concesiones" (grants). This doublespeak was maddening to the growing coalition of health workers who sought reforms that would improve services for the poor. The ministry's euphemisms for privatization became a joke among activists, but the muddled language was hopelessly confusing for anyone relying on media coverage of the issue.

As noted in chapter 9, the initial World Bank loan for health under consideration in 1995 was scaled back when the bank team balked at ARENA's agenda of diverting funds to hospitals in key electoral districts where the party had weak support rather than focusing on public health needs. Around this time, a number of ministry and social security system physicians had been meeting secretly to develop strategies to counter what they saw as a further dismantling of a system that was already in crisis for lack of state support. In 1998 a slate of these progressive physicians was elected to lead the Colégio Médico (the national medical association), which previously had a reputation as an elite social club. For the next five years the Colégio Médico became a bully pulpit for critique of ARENA's health policies. The colégio doctors issued a Citizen's Proposal (Propuesta Ciudadana) for Health, which applied a socially conscious epidemiology in interpreting national indices for public health. Unlike the ANSAL report, the Citizen's Proposal soundly condemned the lack of national commitment to resolving health problems of the poor (Colégio Médico 1999; and Aviles 2001).

In 1998 the Inter-American Development Bank (IDB) again proposed a health loan conditional on the ministry contracting out service delivery, and the following year proposals emerged for privatizing ancillary services at two hospitals in the ISSS network. As in the past, the multilateral banks failed to seek feedback from health workers or citizens (Homedes et al. 2000). The social security health system is seen as an attractive target for privatization, and has long been at the center of health activism and proposals for health reform. This is true for the same reason cited by New York gangster Willie Sutton when asked why he robbed banks: in the Salvadoran health system, the ISSS is where the money is. Less than 5 percent of Salvadorans have private health insurance, and in the early 2000s, the ISSS provided health services to another 17 percent of the population—mostly government and private employees in urban areas—yet it had a budget five times the size of the health ministry. This fact alone is galling to most health advocates because the ministry is charged with serving the remaining three-quarters of the population, including the half of the population that the United Nations Development Program estimated was scraping by on less than $2 per day. The ISSS system receives funds from employers and the government for one million people covered by the plan, but there are enduring problems in the system. For example, insured workers in the maquila industry complain that their employers impose a months-long waiting period before new workers can obtain coverage, and that even when that period is up, some companies delay issuing workers their social security cards. Maquila workers also complain of supervisors who deny time off for workers who become ill, or who have sick children, to visit a clinic.[2]

A militant social security workers' union, known by its Spanish initials, STISSS, has also long denounced the poor law enforcement that allows some companies to avoid paying their full share of health benefits to the social security system. The union also charges the ISSS administration with corruption. Upper-level ISSS administrative posts are reputed to be plum appointments for bureaucrats with close ties to pharmaceutical and medical supply houses owned by elite families, and their high salaries are disproportionate to those of ISSS staff physicians and other professionals.[3] Also, STISSS has had a longstanding dispute with the government over a debt of $280 million that the state owed the ISSS after borrowing from the social security reserve fund in the 1980s. Social security workers and patients encounter these budget shortfalls in the form of understaffed clinics, crowded facilities, and often daylong waits for patients seeking clinic appointments.

The 1999–2000 Health Workers' Strike

When the ARENA plan to privatize ISSS hospital ancillary services became public in mid-1999, STISSS held a series of short protests actions, and social security administrators retaliated by firing several union leaders. This retaliation triggered the first long-term health strike that fall. The focus on privatization sharpened when the government announced plans to reopen two closed hospitals as ISSS facilities under "new administration," which would give concessions to private health providers to bid on various procedures, including hysterectomies, surgeries for varicose veins and hernias, and some ambulatory care.

The STISSS mobilization was strengthened later that fall by an alliance with a newly formed union of social security system physicians known as SIMETRISS. Concerned about the privatization talk, 1,200 out of the 1,500 total social security physicians had unionized in 1997, forming the first union of professional workers in the country. Leaderships of both unions acknowledged in interviews that they initially distrusted each other. STISSS, made up of nonphysician health workers, had a three-decade history of militant struggle, and some of its members feared that the more privileged physicians' union included members who stood to gain from privatization. For their part, many physicians were wary of STISSS's confrontational tactics, such as reliance on strikes and marches. But their alliance grew out of a sense that health worker jobs and, indeed, the future of the union movement were at stake. The Colégio Médico also joined forces with SIMETRISSS and STISSS.

The two main demands of the strike that began in November 1999 were no privatization, and improvement in the doctors' perennially low salaries, which at the time were only 1,400 colones (US$243) per month for seeing patients two hours a day. The strike resulted in closure of all ISSS ambulatory services and elective surgeries for four months. During this time striking health workers provided basic care for in-patients, but the only new patients accepted were emergency cases. The ISSS administration responded by firing 221 employees accused of supporting the strike. So a central demand of the strikers in the months that followed was recovering the jobs of these workers, most of whom belonged to STISSS. The government held firm, however, and this issue of lost jobs haunted the union, hurting support for the leadership among workers.

In June 2000 interviews with workers at an ISSS clinic in the northern barrio of Zacamil, the financial hardships to families caused by the firings were a central topic. Even those who kept their jobs claimed that the ISSS discounted paychecks of employees suspected of sympathizing with STISSS. One couple, both health workers, adopted a strategy of the husband supporting the strike while the wife continued to work, so that at most they would only lose one salary. Fear of a lost job was even cited by a union steward who said, "If I had supported the strike, I'd be in the same boat as those who were fired."

It was an attempt to end this strike in the weeks before the March 2000 presidential elections that led to the incident described in the prologue, when riot police used rubber bullets, tear gas, and water cannons to disperse strikers blocking the streets outside the emergency room at the Medical-Surgical Hospital. At least two teargas grenades exploded inside the hospital, injuring several dozen people. The news media reported that two patients died of heart attacks during the attack, but it remained unclear whether the deaths were due to the attack or unrelated health problems.

Negotiations began a few days later, and government authorities signed an agreement in late March promising not to privatize services at the two hospitals (however, within five months, ARENA reneged on the accord, opening bidding to privatize ancillary services—security, laundry, cleaning, and food services—at the same hospitals). The settlement did not restore the 221 fired workers' jobs, and although a labor court later found the firings illegal, the government refused to rehire them. Thus ended the first round of health mobilizations.

Dolarización, Disasters, Drought, and Dengue (2001–2002)

Political mobilization was put on hold during 2001 as "survival" took precedence. For the majority of poor and near-poor citizens, the bad news began in January with the advent of *dolarización*—the switch from colones to dollars (which also involved a slight devaluation due to the exchange rates used for the conversion). Although heralded by the Bush administration and ARENA as a boon for attracting foreign capital, the switch to the dollar was immediately blamed by poor consumers for increased inflation affecting common items such as beans, produce, and over-the-counter medicines. (As late as 2007, urban residents I spoke with still expressed anger over the conversion, which they saw as a turning point, after which prices rose overnight.)

Salvadorans also endured a string of natural and economic disasters in 2001, including two earthquakes in January and February that killed 1,246 and injured 8,000, leaving hundreds of thousands homeless.[4] One earthquake caused a landslide that obliterated part of a middle-class suburb in Santa Tecla, just a few miles from the capital, generating a public debate about the role of deforestation tied to a development project that critics charged had made the hillside unstable. Then a persistent drought, also worsened by deforestation, led to loss of 60 percent of the corn and beans crops, and spurred the government to import food from Mexico. These events generated much public debate about the role of profiteering and lax regulation in exacerbating natural disasters and droughts.[5] Also, in the aftermath of the World Trade Center disaster that September in the United States, tourism and international trade took a hit, creating a recession that lasted for many months in El Salvador and other countries of the region.

During the summer of 2002, a dengue epidemic became headline news, prompting another flurry of debate on public health. San Salvador's popular mayor, Dr. Silva, who had initiated a string of reforms in municipal sanitation and urban community health, called on Cuban doctors, who had extensive experience with dengue, to advise the Salvadoran health ministry on how to deal with the epidemic. Right-wing politicians and administrators were aghast at the suggestion that Cuba might have more expertise on the disease than El Salvador.

Negotiations over CAFTA gained momentum in 2002. The Bush administration counted on Salvadoran governmental support in lobbying for the pact throughout the region. Debates over CAFTA provoked splits within the FMLN, which eventually came out in support of the pact as a party, alienating many of its supporters. It was in this context that the Salvadoran private business association, known by its Spanish initials ANEP, met to discuss privatization of the social security health system, opening what became "round two" of the national health mobilizations.

The White Marches (September 2002–June 2003)

By late summer 2002, President Flores announced that he would push for a law to set up a private voucher system for social security health services and pensions. Some provisions of the plan, such as a $50 million concession to private insurers to pay for start-up costs and another $10 million for a media campaign to sell private insurance to the public, were immediately denounced by organized health workers (Schuld 2003). In September, doctors at the ISSS Oncology Hospital walked out, and shortly afterward they were joined by doctors at the medical, surgical, and specialty hospitals. The approximately seven hundred doctors on strike announced that they would not accept new patients or do ambulatory care, and they would limit their work to attending emergencies and basic maintenance care for hospital patients.

In October, a standoff between doctors and police at the Oncology Hospital erupted into violence when police attempted a raid on the hospital. Then President Flores announced that the military hospital would offer services to patients closed out of ISSS clinics. For their part, the strikers announced a series of health fairs "to bring health to the people." In mid October more than two dozen striking doctors affiliated with the Colégio Médico received death threats. The same week, in the Legislative Assembly, opposition leaders countered the voucher plan with a bill backed by the Colégio Médico that stated the government would guarantee health and social security services, and ruled privatization

Privatization of health:

unconstitutional. The bill reaffirmed a right of citizens to health services already stated (if nominally) in the national constitution. By this time, the health worker unions had built alliances with many other sectors on the left, including umbrella organizations representing alliances of smaller organized groups (Almeida 2006). Unions representing truck and bus drivers, market vendors, and municipal workers also loaned their support. The first White March, in which protesters dressed in white to show solidarity with striking health workers, was called for October 16 in support of this legislative bill, dubbed Decree 1024. The event brought fifty thousand doctors, nurses, and citizens into the streets chanting slogans such as "Privatization: Pay or Die" and "Health is not for sale. It's a right." Strike supporters set up fourteen blockades on highways, bridges, and border crossings, bringing road traffic to a standstill around the country. The next day—to the surprise of many—FMLN lawmakers managed to forge a political coalition, including smaller parties, in defense of health care as a state guarantee. The Legislative Assembly passed the antiprivatization decree, which provoked wide celebrations on the left.

One participant in the marches who spoke with me remembered the fall marches as provoking feelings of "effervescence." She said, "People had grown distrustful of politics after the war. But there was a real feeling that this was winnable. The marches were peaceful, and they had clear demands. And people trusted the movement's [physician] leadership in part because it was *not* led by a political party."

One advantage that organized health workers had over the government was knowledge that ARENA sought to boost the country's international image through hosting the Central American and Caribbean Olympic Games, slated to take place November 8, 2002, on the newly renovated campus of the national university. A week after passage of Decree 1024, the University of El Salvador, long a center of dissident activity, suspended classes so students and faculty could attend a second Marcha Blanca, which journalists reported as drawing fifty thousand to eighty thousand people. Many private medical clinics also suspended activities for twenty-four hours, and the Legislative Assembly was paralyzed when fifty leftist deputies walked out as a group to join the march, provoking a flurry of media attention and laying to rest any questions about the FMLN's position on the issue.

A mid-level ISSS administrator who supported the strike spoke nostalgically about the solidarity: "Our White March stretched for sixteen blocks, from Hospital Rosales to the Casa Presidencial, everyone dressed in white! We had representatives from every health center in every department of the country!"

Police set up rural roadblocks to stop buses of marchers from other regions en route to the capital. When buses were stopped, anyone dressed in white was detained, in actions eerily reminiscent of military tactics used during the civil war. The key issue in the second march was the president's threat to veto Decree 1024, so the slogan on banners and on strikers' lips was "No al veto presidencial."

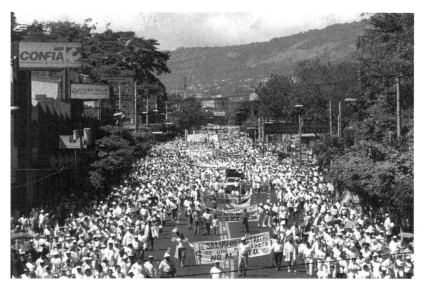

In the largest street demonstrations since the end of the war, tens of thousands turned out for a series of White Marches held between September 2002 and March 2003 to protest government plans to privatize portions of the social security health system. Marchers dressed in white to show solidarity with striking health workers. Photograph courtesy of Edgar Romero.

In the face of widespread opposition, a week later Flores withdrew his privatization bill.

The third White March was designed to coincide with opening ceremonies for the Olympic Games. Police blocked the streets to prevent marchers from approaching the stadium full of dignitaries. On November 14, Decree 1024 was again voted on in the assembly, and this time it passed with a veto-proof two-thirds majority, obligating the president to sign it into law. The vote prompted a night of celebrations by the opposition, but it also heralded a spate of violent actions by paramilitaries against opposition leaders, including shooting into the front of a leader's house, raids on another's home, and threats. Overall, Amnesty International documented thirty threats against members of the health unions, including many from a new death squad that called itself Comando Extermino.

This began a period of heated confrontations that lasted into 2003 as the president stepped up pressure on the unionized doctors to settle. On November 27, police staged a raid on strikers during a peaceful protest at the Maternity Hospital, which resulted in thirty-five people injured from rubber bullets and more than one hundred infants inside the hospital exposed to tear gas. The angered protesters marched to the Legislative Assembly, broke the gate, and occupied the building, gleefully burning a framed photo of Roberto D'Aubuisson, a deceased former ARENA politician (and infamous death squad leader).

In December, during a fourth White March, police again set up roadblocks to keep buses away from the capital. Two weeks later the U.S. government announced a donation of $1.7 million in supplies and equipment for the National Police, in spite of recent violence by police against strikers. The legislative tables then turned against the opposition on December 19 when the PCN, a small party traditionally allied with the military, withdrew its support for Decree 1024 and assisted ARENA in overturning the new law against privatizing government health services. After the vote, over a dozen union leaders were arrested. President Flores also stepped up his media campaign to discredit striking physicians by threatening to fire strikers who did not go back to work. He offered bonuses of US$1,500 to any doctor who quit the strike. The physicians had already achieved higher salaries as a result of the first health strike that ended in 2000, and some of them took him up on the offer, but around 550 remained on strike (Creedon and Ney 2003). In late December and early January police conducted a series of raids on ISSS clinics and hospitals occupied by strikers.

A fifth White March was held in February, and later that month a University of Central America public opinion poll showed that two-thirds of Salvadorans opposed the president's handling of the strike. A sixth White March the next month took place only three days ahead of municipal and legislative elections in which ARENA lost ground to the FMLN in the legislature and municipal mayoral contests. Later that spring, media accounts commented on widespread public fatigue over the stalemate. Several strike leaders offered to return to work, even though no formal settlement had been reached, but now Flores maintained that they had been fired. Hunger strikes ensued over the firings, and the Legislative Assembly passed a decree reinstating the doctors' jobs.

Winning the Strike, Losing the Presidency

The strike finally ended in June with a signed agreement between the president and the strike leaders. In addition, Dr. Guillermo Mata, president of the Colégio Médico, achieved a commitment from officials of the World Bank in Washington, D.C., to remove privatization conditions from a forthcoming health sector loan (Wolfwood 2003).

Public health observers and political analysts generally agree that the scale of the 2002–2003 White Marches dwarfed any previous mobilizations since the end of the war, establishing radicalized health workers as the new leaders of the militant left in the country. This is one of the few cases in which mass mobilizations have set back a privatization agenda backed by both the ruling party and multilateral lending banks. In an interview, Ricardo Monge, secretary general of the STISSS union, described the marches as sending "a message to all of Latin America, to show that it is possible to fight neoliberalism."

But both political parties and the radical health alliance paid political costs for the long strike. By the previous December it had become clear that the wider public was weary of the long lines and delays in medical appointments that the strike caused for ambulatory patients, especially those with chronic problems. Also, hostile rhetoric in headlines, traffic stoppages, and violent confrontations in front of hospitals led to denunciations of the polarization that plagued national affairs. San Salvador's popular physician mayor, Hector Silva, who many regarded as the most likely next FMLN presidential candidate, was among those calling on all parties to negotiate in late 2002, but his effort backfired. In a meeting with the president about mediation, Flores reportedly encouraged Silva to step into the breach and lead a mediation effort. Since any successful mediator of the long strike would emerge a national hero, this may have appealed to Silva as a move that could boost his presidential ambitions. But Flores slyly insisted that Silva would have to step down from his position as mayor to play this role. Flores was essentially setting a trap for Silva, and he caught him.

Silva, who had been seen by the U.S. Embassy as a more acceptable leftist presidential hopeful than FMLN hardliners, agreed to this role. But his overtures were rejected by leaders of the health coalition, who had not been consulted in advance and distrusted Silva's motives in reaching out to Flores. FMLN leaders broke with Silva openly in a breach that some predicted would end his political career. As one long-time observer put it to me, "In this country, you have to consult with other leaders on the left [before reaching out to their opponents] and Silva should have known that."

ARENA also paid a price for its intransigence in the 2003 municipal and legislative elections. For the first time in history, the FMLN received more votes than ARENA. Many analysts blamed the right-wing party's poor showing on Flores's rigidity in handling the strike. This led to reassessments of strategy within ARENA. The party's winning presidential candidate in the 2005 elections, Antonio Saca, won plaudits from all sides for his more moderate tone in public discourse, compared with the hard-nosed positions President Flores was known for.

The breach with Silva hurt the FMLN in the 2005 elections. The party ended up backing Shafik Handal, an ex-guerrilla commander from the war years and head of the FPL (the FMLN's largest faction), for the presidency. Since Handal was known as a hardliner, this played into the hands of ARENA propagandists, who predicted a Handal victory would upset the Bush administration and lead to U.S. legislation hostile to Salvadoran immigrants to the United States, many of whom enjoyed Temporary Protected Status. Dr. Guillermo Mata, who had achieved a public profile speaking for the Colégio Médico during the strikes, was chosen to run as Handal's vice presidential candidate. This also proved controversial because the party did not consult with health movement leaders about the decision, and the choice of Dr. Mata provoked a backlash among conservative members of the Colégio Médico, who later won control of the med-ical organization back from the leftist contingent.

Setting aside political ramifications of the events, there were undoubtedly many public health ramifications from the disruptions in regular services of clinics and hospitals. During the strike the two conservative newspapers in the capital, *La Prensa Gráfica* and *El Diário de Hoy*, carried stories of desperate patients shut out from hospitals who waited long hours for care at private clin-ics or makeshift health fairs. I have found no data from which to estimate the impact of the strike on public health. (Conversely, it is also difficult to estimate the health consequences of routinely rationing care according to ability to pay, which occurs in a privatized medical system that lacks adequate access for unin-sured and poor patients.)

White Marches and the Body Politic

In interviews with participants and observers of the health mobilizations I sought to reconstruct events (for there was no comprehensive coverage of the strike by reputable media sources) and I sought insights into key questions rele-vant to the themes driving this book: (a) What conditions led to the radicaliza-tion of physicians and facilitated their leadership of this movement? (b) Why did the public turn out in such large numbers, filling the streets month after month over as arcane an issue as privatization of health services? (c) What do the mobi-lizations say about the state of El Salvador's body politic, and prospects for the future? Are there lessons here for a wider social science of the neoliberal era?

The Radicalization of Salvadoran Physicians

As accounts in this book attest, health workers of various stripes have been at the forefront of struggles for social justice in El Salvador for many years. Dr. Miguel Saenz Varela, a physician and ex-legislator for the FMLN who com-mented on the health strikes, has himself lived such a life, tracing his medical activism to 1965, when he and other medical students took part in a health strike that paralyzed the country's health system for ten days to gain govern-ment improvements in hospital care. Colonel Rivera, the country's military president in the mid-1960s, agreed to the demands rapidly, noted Saenz, who commented, "That military man had more political vision than [President] Francisco Flores!"

Although STISSS has a long history of dissident struggle against conserva-tive governments, the union had never previously been able to forge a broad coalition with other health workers and the public as occurred in 2002. Most observers of the strike concurred that it was the physicians' leadership that ral-lied such wide public support. Several physicians I spoke with echoed Venício Cabrera, medical advisor to SIMETRISSS, who said, "Because of the work they do, doctors are more vulnerable to suffering of the people, so doctors come to have common interests with their patients." It is an argument reminiscent of Rudolf Virchow who wrote that physicians were the "natural advocates of the poor" (1985, 4). In a country like El Salvador, where poverty is abundant yet upper classes cloister themselves in urban enclaves, certainly doctors are among the few professionals who encounter human suffering on a daily basis. Julie Feinsilver (1993) noted a similar radicalization effect in Cuba when revolutionary guerrillas from middle-class backgrounds first encountered rural poverty—an experience that helped build a consensus in the new government for postrevolutionary health reform.

One might counter that working with the sick has hardly produced class solidarity between physicians and poor patients in industrialized countries, where professional dominance is the more common relationship (Friedson 1974). But Saenz went further in his analysis, arguing that doctors themselves have been proletarianized in El Salvador, and have come to share many of the insecurities of the marginalized classes. He was referring to a situation that developed after the University of El Salvador (UES) was occupied by the military from 1980 to 1984 (the second such occupation in a decade). I was part of a small U.S. medical delegation that in 1985 investigated effects of that militarization on the UES School of Medicine, and so gained some insights into what took place. After closing the UES, the government lent support to new ventures to start small private medical schools, and by middecade the small country of El Salvador had five medical schools turning out graduates. Meanwhile, influenced by leftist administrators and the urgent need created by the war, the UES Medical School, which reopened in 1984, adopted an open admissions policy, greatly enlarging its entering classes and offering aid to poor students to enroll.

The result was a significant increase in trained physicians and increased competition both for government-controlled residency slots and for the limited number of salaried positions. Today there are roughly seven thousand physicians practicing in the country, or roughly twice the number in the mid-1980s. Unfortunately, both the new medical schools and the UES have been criticized for their low quality of instruction, especially during the war years, and competition between the public and private medical schools over limited hospital residency slots has meant delays in training. So more physicians has not translated neatly into rising quality of care.[6]

On top of these problems, low salaries of public sector physicians, especially in the Ministry of Health, led many to cut their public service hours and rely more heavily on a second income flow from private clinics or NGOs. As a result, many physicians are underemployed, and some have gone into other lines of work. Remarking on the change in medical culture, Saenz noted, "In the 1960s all physicians had automobiles. Now they ride buses and live in Zacamil [a working class barrio]!" An administrator in the ISSS spoke of the White

Marches as especially meaningful for physicians who had been relegated to driving taxis or working in labs because the mobilizations helped them to "recover their dignity as doctors."

Why Did So Many People Participate in the White Marches?

The first health strike (1999–2000) brought issues of health reform to public attention, but the mobilizations during that period were much smaller than in 2002–2003. One popular health educator I spoke with, who was a leader in the White Marches, had become convinced that the large public response in 2002 was linked to the traumatic series of public disasters that began with the earthquakes and dolarización in January 2001 and lasted until the dengue epidemic of summer 2002. "It was a period of huge crises and it affected the whole country," she said.

Certainly, as Americans learned after 9/11, one outcome from a widely publicized disaster can be a strong sense of public unity, as human suffering on a large scale and humanitarian responses to suffering are catapulted to the center of the body politic. It is in those moments that the public turns to the state as the broker of last resort. The switch from the colón to the dollar during the same period as poor people encountered postearthquake inflation in food and housing further drew public attention to ARENA's policies. Although the Legislative Assembly voted to freeze prices for basic goods right after the disaster, the price freeze was reversed by President Flores, who called it *inconveniente* (improper). After the Santa Tecla landslide, much public controversy centered on the role that politically connected commercial developers had played in destabilizing the hillside that collapsed burying dozens of suburban houses. Then the drought and the post-9/11 recession pointed up the country's vulnerability to a food crisis. When a government fails to respond to suffering or, worse, seems to have contributed to the disaster thorough corrupt policies—reminiscent of the Duarte government's failures after the 1986 earthquake and the Bush administration's incompetence after the Hurricane Katrina floods—one result may be wide-scale disillusionment with national leaders.

Another development seems to have been a growing public understanding of the consequences of privatizing public services. By 2002, after huge hikes in utility rates for phones and electricity and an ongoing discussion about privatizing water and health services, a large sector of the public had gained personal experiences with this new concept. In 2002 I sat in on a health rights conference in San Salvador that featured several speakers describing privatization struggles in other sectors. Later, a social security hospital nurse I interviewed spoke knowledgeably about many high-paying administrative jobs that she said had been suddenly created in the newly privatized telephone and electrical companies. "Profits will leave the country and they will leave us here bankrupt like Argentina," she predicted. Paul Almeida (2008) concluded that public dissatisfaction over higher utility rates had helped the medical unions gain multisectoral support. Public opinion surveys on privatization of utilities conducted by the Catholic University of Central America showed a shift from 60 percent opposition to privatization in the late 1990s to 80 percent opposed during the period of the White Marches (Wolfwood 2003).

Had the marches been organized by the FMLN alone, most observers doubt that the party could have built such a wide coalition opposing privatization. Many remarked that, despite the hardships caused by the strike, the public seemed to respect the credibility of the physicians of the Colégio Médico and SIMETRISSS. As one observer commented, "People have a lot of faith in doctors. Like education, health is ideological—to the people, health is important because it is connected with their personal life, so it's more simple and straightforward."

Dr. Saenz concurred with this view: "Health is something you feel everyday. Although the services here are sadly inadequate, given our political and economic situation, health is seen as a public good. People don't distinguish between public health and medical services, and that doesn't matter. What is important [to the public] is that they are good services, because people know health is related to development." He went on to cite statistics of twelve thousand child deaths a year from respiratory illnesses and thirteen thousand from diarrhea and gastrointestinal problems, and noted that tuberculosis, which had been well controlled, was making a comeback.

Dr. José Santamaría, the current president of the Colégio Médico who was regarded as a political moderate, put it this way: "Health is neither left or right. It is a matter of cultural patrimony; a fundamental right. That's why so many came out to the marches."

By the second White March, the striking health workers had gained a formal alliance with the FMLN, but they had specifically requested that party members dress in white and avoid traditional revolutionary symbols. Several observers I spoke with saw the FMLN's agreement to these conditions and respect for the health worker leadership as critical because of widespread public frustration over the polarization between the political parties. But the FMLN's so called *poder convocatorio* (ability to call people into the streets) was likely a critical factor in allying the physicians with transport unions, who could close the roads, and in boosting the size of marches and sustaining public support month after month. Almeida (2006) noted that this mobilization capacity was aided by the proliferation of "organizations of organizations" in El Salvador in which an umbrella group can rapidly call members from several smaller unions into the streets when a march is announced. The lack of such broad multisectoral support in a previous failed struggle by the telephone workers union (against privatization of the phone service in the mid-1990s) was a key weakness that the health union leadership sought to overcome (Almeida 2008). A former member of the health coalition observed that this would not have been possible if the public had not trusted the credibility of the physicians. "We're no longer in a civil war. Nowadays, when the party calls people out, people choose whether they want to comply or not. And when people don't trust the [opposition] leaders they stay home."

In addition, beyond issues of the physicians' credibility with the public was an important objective reality of the health strike that many believed also helped to force President Flores to the negotiating table: the simple fact that the government did not have the means to fire and replace the striking doctors.

Significance of the White Marches

Although parries and feints over privatization have continued to bedevil debates over health reform in El Salvador, many health workers regard the period of mobilization as a symbolic victory that greatly reduced ARENA's political capital. "If not for the marches in 2002, everything in health would have been privatized!" said Carmen, a former Chalatenango sanitária and former president of the health promoters union, who was attending medical school at the time of the events.

Many observers of the political scene who were not directly involved in the marches commented on how privatization of health has come to stand in for a wide variety of sins blamed on the ARENA government. A spokesperson in the U.S. Embassy noted that "privatization has become an emotional issue here, sort of like gun control or family planning in our country." While his words seemed intended to emphasize the irrationalities of the movement, his observation held important insights about the ways that health rights have come to represent a fundamental patrimony in El Salvador—a kind of line in the national sand beyond which ARENA (and the World Bank) have been warned not to cross.

The Salvadoran White Marches have similarities with the doctors' mobilizations in Chile in the early 1970s that played a role in the overthrow of a military government and elevation of Salvador Allende, a physician and social democratic leader, to the presidency (Anderson, Smith, and Sidel 2004). More recently, in 1990 a Nepali doctors' movement drew on social justice concerns combined with the symbolism of science and modernization to help instigate the mobilization that overthrew that country's Hindu monarchy (Adams 1998). In all of these cases, the medical workers' leadership grew out of their credibility both as professionals who wielded prestige and expertise and as bearers of medicine's moral symbolism as a defender of life and hope—a form of power that purports to be above politics (in the sense of manipulative power brokerage) and yet, as Adams observes, is inherently political in that the physician leaders often end up in positions of political influence. In San Salvador, the 2005 election of Dr. Violeta Menjívar, previously a guerrilla physician based in FMLN-controlled Arcatao, to replace Silva as mayor continued this trend.

Likewise, the doctors in these struggles have embodied a vision of modernity widely associated with democratic ideals. There is, of course, a potential contradiction when claims of moral standing linked to scientific expertise become linked to movements for democracy. As noted in chapter 5, medicine's symbolism can also be used to further undemocratic political regimes. The reprehensible cases of Nazi medical experiments in Germany, South Africa's apartheid medical system, and the doctors assisting in torture chambers in Pinochet's Chile come to mind (see Zwi 1987). More recently, the irony of this symbolism was noted in the case of U.S. senator Bill Frist, whose credibility as a surgeon helped him rise to the position of Senate majority leader in spite of a history of ruthless politics and his family's partial ownership of a for-profit HMO charged with orchestrating massive fraud against Medicare (Grann 2003). In contrast to these cases, the Salvadoran, Nepalese, and pro-Allende Chilean doctors' movements have contained strong elements of class consciousness and have defended access to basic services for the poor as an inherent aspect of the body politic.

The struggle over health reform in El Salvador ebbed after 2003, but access to health services and medicines remained a topic of heated public debates. When I arrived in the capital in June 2007, the country was abuzz with recent scandals. Investigative reporters had documented the minister of health's channeling public patients needing nuclear magnetic resonance scans into his private practice. Accusations flew about $400 million in missing international donations that had been slated for reconstruction of hospitals damaged in the 2001 earthquakes.

A new national university study showed Salvadoran inflation in medicine prices to be the highest in Central America, and both urban hospital workers and the staffs of rural clinics complained in interviews that the Ministry of Health and the social security health system were creating artificial shortages of medicines to justify the need for privatization. Meanwhile, recent rises in prices for medical appointments and common drugs were being felt even among the middle class. A private medical consult now ran around $25–30—out of reach for poor families—and a prescription for antiparasitics or antibiotics filled at a private pharmacy could easily double that cost.

Although health reform negotiations with the ministry had stalled, popular health organizers were meeting and building support for a bill to set national standards and quality control for pharmaceuticals. These were sensitive topics because a number of wealthy families that supported ARENA also owned pharmacies that supplied government clinics. Under the new CAFTA agreement, the country was obligated to abide by new rules protecting patents of imported medicine. Unlike Costa Rica, which specified exclusionary situations in which these rules would not apply (for example, an epidemiological emergency), El Salvador had not negotiated any exceptions. This concerned health advocates because the country lacks pharmaceutical manufacturing facilities. Discussing with me the new bill for quality control, Dr. Santamaría, who represented the

Colégio Médico in the coalition, declared firmly, "We need, as a state, to declare some areas to be outside the market!"

The coalition that led the White Marches had lost much of its cohesion. The new leadership of the Colégio Médico sought to maintain a reputation as politically neutral and had expressed openness to the ISSS and Ministry of Health developing "concessions" with NGOs. SIMETRISSS had also lost its radical edge and much credibility since a new law was passed allowing social security doctors to see public patients in their private clinics yet receive capitation fees from ISSS as if they had been seen in a social security clinic.

Trying to resurrect the popular strategies of 2002–2003, the FMLN called a White March for a Saturday in mid-June. Although some derided the effort as a party project that lacked the backing of the health coalition, to the surprise of many, the march filled ten or twelve city blocks. The crowd blocked the street in front of Rosales Hospital for much of the morning. One factor that likely boosted turnout was SIGESAL (Sindicato General de Empleados de Salud), a newly emergent health workers' union based inside the public health ministry, which had recently expanded its membership to hospitals around the country. In September 2007, eight SIGESAL leaders were arrested and charged with disorderly conduct because of prior participation in a July protest. The arrests relied on a revised penal code allowing ten-year sentences for political crimes (a variation on antiterror measures adopted since 2001 that are similar to legal codes used during the war).

Clearly, struggle was continuing, and health symbolism continued to serve as a standard for democracy and political morality that held more resonance than older symbols of revolution. The movement had shifted subtly from a partisan conflict over which party controlled the state to the responsibilities of the state to the body politic, not unlike the peasant "globalization from below" in Costa Rica described by Edelman (1999).

The White Marches and privatization debates helped to put clothes on the slippery agenda of neoliberal reforms (and their corporate sector backers), and they undermined support for ARENA, bringing together a new coalition of political actors who, while aligned with the FMLN, are not dominated by the old-guard left. The visibility of the mobilizations has helped to bring the realm of postwar individualized or private suffering and death back into the public sphere. The potency of the movement to date suggests that a successful counterpolitics to economic globalization must center on debate over the role of the state in building a humane future—a true body politic—in which governance is held to a popular standard that links the welfare of the population more closely to the ideal of the nation.

Epilogue

Toward a Moral Politics

Chalatenango, June 2007

When I got off the bus in San José Las Flores, it was clear something was going on. The square was empty, but amplifiers waited next to chairs and tables under a canopy. A man set off bottle rockets near the church, where a crowd spilled out of the open doors. Inside, sunlight filtered through open windows; dozens of paper streamers danced in the breeze over the heads of villagers packed into pews. I marveled at the beauty of the reconstructed building that had been a ruin at the end of my field research, its roof fallen in from neglect and war damage.

June 20th. Of course! I had forgotten the date. It was the twenty-first anniversary of the town's repopulation. There lined up against the side wall were the health promoters. Cristina's eyes met mine and I ducked and ran over to join them in a flurry of whispered greetings and hugs. She and Inez were preparing for a procession, which was now an occasion for educating young children about the town's revolutionary legacy. Groups who took part in the town's lucha walked down the aisle in turn—guerrilla fighters, farmers, child care workers, popular educators, and, of course, the health workers. Holding hoes, stethoscopes, and schoolbooks, the costumed group joined the priest and nun around the flower-filled altar while the congregation applauded and sang. The promoters had wrapped gauze around the head and arm of a young boy who limped along beside Inez, pretending to be wounded.

In many ways Las Flores was clearly thriving, with new houses and paved streets. The soccer field was now a proper stadium, and a remote university campus now permitted students to study closer to home. A long-delayed sewer system was being built by European NGOs, and most village collectives were now self-supporting, including a restaurant, tailor shop, two stores, a chicken coop, and a communal bank that ran a rotating loan fund. Most families farmed private plots, but fifty families remained active in the cattle cooperative.

However, in conversations with Cristina and her husband, Rigo, economic disappointments loomed large. The land redistribution promised in the peace accord had initially left many families saddled with loan payments they could not afford. Popular resentment led the ARENA-led government to forgive the loans in 1998; even so, Cristina's family had received a plot so far from town that it made no sense to farm it. Rigo pulled me aside to ask advice about his prospects for migrating to the United States for work, a strategy now common throughout the country, especially in rural areas like Chalatenango, where a quarter of families depend on remittances from abroad (Kandel 2002). Cristina explained that while they were lucky to have jobs, their minimal salaries—$200 a month—barely covered the inflated prices for food and necessities for the family, which includes their six-year-old son and her elderly parents. She held up a $5 chunk of cheese to make her point: "Five colones bought a larger piece than this ten years ago! And everything in the canasta básica [minimum household needs basket] has gone up!"

At the local Ministry of Health clinic, Cristina—reputed to be among the most competent popular system promoters—is no longer allowed to treat patients today, but works as an *ordenanza* (health aide), vaccinating children, cleaning floors, and running errands for the nurse. Although the 1993 accord that popular system leaders signed with the ministry specified a permanent physician, the young social service doctor continues to work only part time in Las Flores, often leaving a nurse in charge who is not allowed to prescribe or handle most medications.

I caught the next bus to Guarjila, where the only remaining "popular" clinic continued to function, still located in the building built in 1991 with funds that Dr. Ana Manganaro had raised during the war years from Catholic parishioners in St. Louis, Missouri. Since Guarjila had not been a large settlement prior to the war, it had never been incorporated as a municipality and was bypassed by the Ministry of Health in its drive to reestablish control over rural clinics. In the interstices, "popular" health continued to thrive, and the Guarjila team still worked closely with the Catholic Diocese's technical team, now run entirely by Salvadorans, which also supported health promoters in dozens of rural cantóns. The clinic, recently featured in a short film on primary health made by the University of El Salvador, had gained a reputation as far away as Honduras as a place where a poor family would not be turned away.

Today the clinic is vividly painted with a likeness of Dr. Ana, who died tragically of cancer in mid-1993. Michaela, a former FMLN doctor, took over Ana's post until 2005 when she was lured away to newly revolutionary Venezuela where the Ministry of Health under President Hugo Chávez was expanding community health services. The person I had come to see was Guillermo, a former popular system health trainer I had known since 1992 who had struggled to complete medical school in the capital and now worked as Guarjila's permanent physician. For me, it was very special to see this tall, handsome son of a campesino family practicing medicine in rural Chalatenango where he was raised. As a young man during my fieldwork, he had been a favorite of the diocese's technical team for his love of learning and dedication to rural service. The child of a large poor family in a remote town, Guillermo still recalled his shaking knees when he was presented to the local priest for catechist training at age thirteen. One of the students in his first adult reading class was his own father. In 1992 he became the first health promoter instructor in the diocese's basic health course, but by then his health work had already led to clashes with conservative landowners in his town who had spread vicious rumors attacking his integrity. When he first dreamed of medical school, it seemed impossible, and probably would have been had not Michaela and other international volunteers raised funds abroad to help pay his university fees.

I arrived in time to sit in on a workshop in the courtyard that the promoters conducted on how to avoid intestinal parasites. About a dozen local women were in attendance. The promoters' latest project is promoting trash collection; Guillermo estimated that about 80 percent of the four hundred households in town were participating to date. Most houses were larger now, with concrete floors and enclosed by fences to keep animals outside (finally putting in effect the goals of the campaign that promoters had begun in 1995, discussed in chapter 7).

Over dinner, Guillermo noted that Guarjila families were struggling economically; about 16 percent of households had sent members abroad to work. The repopulated villages continue to wrestle with the hot potato of whether families receiving remittances should pay into a fund to assist widows and families who cannot raise the thousands of dollars charged by the smuggling companies. The financial risks of a migration are also substantial. The family of Margarita, a local promoter, had accrued a debt of $6,000 after her husband migrated to the United States only to be imprisoned and deported before he had earned enough to pay off the coyote.

The burden of a busy medical practice combined with constant proposal writing to keep international donations flowing was taking its toll on Guillermo. Padre Jon Cortina, a local Jesuit priest who had spearheaded many local development projects, had died of a stroke in 2005, and since then Guillermo had done his best to fill the gap. But he was now working seven-day weeks and had little time to spend with his adolescent son or his wife, who worked in the capital. He said NGO support for the clinic had been dwindling, and he worried how much longer he could keep things going.

I thought back to the struggles with the Ministry of Health in the 1990s to preserve the popular health model that had succeeded so well in demonstrating how a truly community-based health service might function. Much had changed for the better in these resettlement villages, but too much still depended on transnational efforts, with one or another humanitarian NGO or European agency filling in for a government that had long disregarded the welfare of most of its citizens.

Constructing the Body Politic

The goal of this research has been to elucidate the relationship between humanitarian beliefs and practices and political power. Although I had documented many cases of health work targeted in warfare prior to my research, the notion of the "body politic" held little resonance in studies of culture in the 1990s, so I began my work thinking of such a social materiality as a cultural ghost, a vague projection on a screen. How, exactly, I wanted to know, could humanitarian work pose a threat to established orders? After all, as Farmer noted, access to health is the "least contested" human right (2003, 19). Thus, my ethnographic focus on contestation about rural health work allowed a line of inquiry into notions of moral order at the most basic level in a deeply divided society.

Part One of this book traced the forms of symbolic, structural, and overt violence that have shaped Salvadoran culture, with special attention to the very material role that modern agricultural development—specifically the expansion of export crops and beef cattle production—played in creating new rural poverty, and the role that both liberation theology and repressive force played in the formation of solidarities in opposition to military rule. Part Two followed the development of guerrilla medicine and origins of "popular" health practices that helped shape new social identities and practices around bodies and a reconstituted body politic. Chapter 4 documented the ways that El Salvador's militaristic state, backed by U.S. military aid and advisors, systematically violated international law protecting health work, and discussed the role of humanitarian narratives in challenging the legitimacy of militarism. Chapter 5 examined how the transnational militarism of low-intensity conflict uses medicine and humanitarian goals as a weapon to objectify bodies and reinforce state power.

Part Three examined in more detail a model for an alternative body politic through the case of popular health practices in communities that were resettled by refugees in rebel-held territory beginning in 1987. My ethnography compared the popular system's concept of community participation with government-run rural health programs that "mass-produced" lay health workers, and explored the lessons for international health development offered by the popular health model. In Part Four we saw many of the tensions of the war continue into the peace process as the popular system found itself gradually marginalized by the state. Then, as neoliberal programs came to dominate multilateral lending, the study documents how promising rural health programs were abandoned so that the ARENA government could reinforce its clientelist base. Finally, in chapter 10 the theme returns to solidarities as advocacy for health reform becomes the face of national resistance during the massive White Marches against privatization in 2002–2003. Just as human rights advocacy articulated a resistance based on humanitarian narratives during the war, the White Marches demonstrated the potential power of solidarity around basic needs and the assertion of moral order as counterpoint to the politics of exclusion. As a national movement, these mobilizations, which reflected real networks of human cooperation and resistance, injected new life into the phantom of the body politic.

Diversity and difference are easy to find. Solidarity requires a wide-angle lens to see. Only after returning again and again to the resettled villages of Chalatenango did I appreciate the power in the density and level of organization that made up the popular health system, and the increasing sophistication in their debates and collective practices, strengthened by transnational alliances. In the last half of the 1980s, a period of stalemated military struggle, such moral counterhegemonic challenges to state authority was as important as militarism in the balance of power.

"By fostering new forms of organization and bypassing official institutions," wrote Arturo Escobar, grassroots organizations threaten to undermine hierarchies of both the developmentalist state and dominant international structures of dependency (1992). It was for these reasons that health work in the FMLN-controlled zones became such a high-level target (second only to a command post). The cultural capital and moral authority attached to healing lent legitimacy to new counterhegemonic forms of authority in this setting. But symbols became material in the form of the new practices and understandings that the popular system promoted, and in the leadership that health promoters represented in these communities, all of which offered a reproach to the poorly run Ministry of Health after the war.

The development process allows the state (and World Bank) to incorporate elements of counterhegemony such as "community health" programs, local control over health, and collaboration with NGOs as "legitimating devices," which, while closing some avenues, also open up new spaces for struggle. Of course, as Sayer (1994, 376) has noted, such moves by the state (and transnational) elites both empower and constrain new forms of struggle, particularly as the shifting fields and visibilities of globalization open up new grounds for contestation. The greatest challenge facing Central American urban elites, according to Peter Sollis (1996), is the fact that the neoliberal push for greater decentralization and NGO participation creates conditions for greater grassroots democracy and broader local autonomy at the same time as it facilitates smaller, cheaper, and more cost-effective government. (190). (The shift to the left in the last decade in many Latin American countries is testimony to popular disillusionment with the still dominant framework of neoliberal globalization.)

The concept of the body politic can serve as a useful tool for thinking about hegemonic power. While there is a history dating to Aristotle of references to the "body politic" as analogous to the political organization of society, it would be a mistake to dismiss the concept as metaphorical. I draw heavily on practices and material aspects of populations in this study precisely to ground the analysis in the reality of bodies and earth. It is an irony that the merit in conceiving of society as "somatic" lies in rediscovering a framework and methodology for study of human agency (Turner 1996).

Following Bryan S. Turner, the focus on the body is not intended to highlight individualized agency to the exclusion of solidarities (1992), and therein lies an important difference between this concept and that of Foucault's biopower, which he envisioned as capillary in its nature and strangely lacking in subjecthood. Biopower, in Foucault's analysis (2003), carries a sense of top-down imposition of diffuse (institutional or state) power acting on docile bodies with their assent or collusion (Hogle 2002). I think of the body politic, conversely, as bottom-up in its constitution and corresponding to Scheper-Hughes's rhetorical question (1994, 232) "What kind of society does the body wish, need, dream?" Unlike Foucault's industrializing European state, I argue that in a society with a legacy of poverty and state coercion in which capitalist development has been a cruel disappointment (or, worse, a destructive force), this question has been dangerous to talk about because it is fraught with moral power and pregnant with collective agency.

The principal work done by the body politic is to transcend dualistic thinking, reasserting the materiality of the social. It also serves as a corrective for a recent historical bias toward analyzing difference as the primary method for understanding culture. The framework for a nondualistic analysis requires a dialectical perspective, which emphasizes the relational and fungible aspects of power as well as the role of practice and experience in construction of the social. The focus on experience and recovery of the material aspects of discourse requires consideration of coercion and structural violence as formative in cultural hegemonies. Likewise, this focus pushes us toward holistic notions of health and well-being, and an acknowledgment that humans share a common set of biological and psychic needs and live in interdependent relationships with other humans and as participants in a wider ecological order.

I end this book at a moment of rapid change with great potential for progressive reform. In late 2008 we witnessed massive failures of unregulated capitalist markets in the United States and public repudiation of Bush administration policies as the electorate rallied to support Barrack Obama for the presidency. Then in March 2009 the FNLN-allied reformist candidate, Mauricio Funes, won a close presidential race in El Salvador, ending twenty years of ARENA rule. The moment calls for new thinking about the politics of possibility.

Like all theories, the concept of the body politic has political implications. In that spirit, I wish to join Bryan S. Turner (1992), who saw his theorizing on the body not only as an attack on a "Cartesian utilitarian paradigm of social relations" but also as "an attempt to establish a basis of political action" (257). He spoke of the need to assert the existence of a shared ontology around the human experience of pain and suffering. Such a framework, he argued, offers hope for replacing natural law with new moral agendas. "The current debate about globalization points toward the idea of a shared set of problems, and in some circumstances, shared cultures. . . . I want to retain the foundationalist view of that frailty of the human body in order to have a politics, on the one hand, of ecology, and, on the other hand, of human rights" (Turner 1992, 254, 256).

The pretence that social science is outside of politics holds no water in Central America. This was made clear to me on my first visit to El Salvador in 1985, when, after touring the firebombed social science building and the destroyed medical school at the national university, we sat down with the U.S. ambassador who told us that the government was trying to get the medical school "to focus on the medical sciences rather than the social sciences." Only a few years later, in 1989, Martín-Baró and his fellow Jesuit scholars—social scientists all—were murdered for continuing to insist that the social sciences belong in the public sphere. That is a powerful legacy for scholars in the North who enjoy far more privileges and are far less likely to pay such high prices for acts of courage. Of all citizens, social scientists are well positioned to see these linkages and to recognize that forms of economic tyranny, including the so-called free market of neoliberal discourse, depend on rocket launchers as well as business degrees, and on state and transnational forms of coercion as well as hegemony and consensus.

NOTES

PROLOGUE

1. The full title of the Ministry of Health is Ministerio de Salud Pública y Asistencia Social.

CHAPTER 1   MANUFACTURING ILL-BEING

1. Citing the Salvadoran Ministry of Planning 1986 Proyecto: ELS/78/P04. "Politicas de poblacion: estimaciones y proyecciones de poblacion 1950–2025." San Salvador.
2. El Salvador had fertility rates of 6.3 in 1970, dropping to 4.1 by 1991. This is the average number of children born to a woman during her lifetime, according to the World Bank (1993).
3. Pion-Berlin (1991) notes that Kjellin's belief in the organic metaphor was not shared by Friedrich Ratzel, the founder of geopolitics. Kjellin's ideas, however, became adopted by Gen. Augusto Pinochet, of Chile, who promoted them in Latin America. See Pinochet's book *Geopolitica* (Santiago, Chile: Gabriela Mistral, 1968).
4. Durham (1979) also found no evidence to support the theory that Salvadorans' high fertility resulted from peasants continuing to have large families after advances in health care had reduced the number of deaths among young children. His study of two generations of Salvadoran peasants in the Tenancingo area showed that as child mortality inched down in the decades since the 1930s, peasant families had fewer children, maintaining the same family size with fewer births.

CHAPTER 2   REPRESSION'S REPERCUSSIONS

1. Analysis of the bombing was done at the University of Central America (UCA), in San Salvador, in 1985. See Edwards and Siebentritt 1991, 18.
2. Guarjila's original church had been destroyed by aerial bombardment.
3. This category includes deaths from hardships related to violence, such as babies who died of dehydration while the family was fleeing the army.
4. The number of killed or wounded who were guerrillas is probably underreported.
5. This roundup of civilians took place in Guazapa during the army's 1986 Operation Phoenix. It debuted a new policy to forcibly remove civilians from conflicted areas rather than kill them.
6. Spanish acronym for the United Nations High Commission on Refugees, which ran small camps along the Honduran border to aid fleeing Salvadorans.

7. Radio Venceremos (Spanish for "we will win") was operated by the ERP faction of the FMLN out of Morazán. The FPL later set up Radio Farabundo Martí, which broadcast clandestinely from Chalatenango.

8. In the late 1980s a trick reporters used to get around an army roadblock was to drive through at 5 A.M., before the soldiers had crawled out of bed.

9. After the 1987–1992 repopulation of northeast Chalatenango, the structures of the PPLs were resurrected. The term directiva was used to refer to village's town councils.

CHAPTER 3   INSURGENT HEALTH

1. Many were interviewed on multiple occasions; about a third were taped. Most were conducted between 1992 and 1995, although a few date to the war years, and a few (mostly follow-up) interviews were done in 2007. When I began fieldwork many who had worked in rebel-controlled areas were circumspect about their roles during the war, but with each subsequent visit I found people more willing, even eager, to discuss this period, which most recalled with both angst and nostalgia.

2. "Sanitarios" was the term commonly used for both guerrilla paramedics and civilian lay health workers up until the large-scale repopulation of communities in 1987. Health promoters (*promotores de salud*) became the common term in the repopulated communities.

3. Because many foreign physicians who worked with the FMLN remained in the country after the cease-fire and tended to be locally known and identifiable by country of origin, I changed both the names and the countries of origin for the doctors quoted. However, my pseudonyms for countries reflect their continents of origin—e.g., Michaela, who I identify as Danish, was a European.

4. Frieden went on to play a key role in identifying the economic and political roots of New York City's tuberculosis epidemic in the 1990s. He later served as the city's commissioner of health and was nominated recently to head the CDC.

5. Among topics we discussed were medical ethics. I asked about triage of badly wounded patients. Sanitarios, Leo said, were trained to transport patients that the medical staff was equipped to help. So if they had to decide between two patients, a patient with an abdominal wound would take precedent over one with a head wound because FMLN surgeons regarded neurosurgery as too difficult for field hospital conditions. Ex-FMLN health workers I spoke with said that they did not have a policy of, or a practice of, mercy killing, even with badly wounded individuals.

6. Margarita, who arrived in the camp after these problems were resolved, said she eventually learned a lot when the MSF physicians gave her work in the camp's medical laboratory.

7. The study was done by Giora Keinan, of Tel Aviv University, based on a survey of 174 Israelis (see Carey 2007).

8. For example, see McGuire (1988) on the role of order and power in healing (235–236) and for a list of key references from the medical anthropology literature (317).

CHAPTER 4   LOW-INTENSITY CONFLICT AND
THE WAR AGAINST HEALTH

1. The task forces were organized through the National Central American Health Rights Network, a coalition of committees of U.S. health workers in forty cities that sent

medical aid to the region and did public education about the civilian toll from U.S. military intervention. Our report on the University of El Salvador, "Education under Fire," was circulated with a slide show narrated by Ed Asner. My 1987 report on contra attacks targeting Nicaraguan clinics, published in *American Medical News*, was part of a series that won the Peter Lisagor Award, in the Society of Professional Journalists' Chicago chapter.

2. Interestingly, Herman's comparative survey of the 1984 Nicaraguan elections that Washington had dubbed a "farce" turned up a different alignment, with 80 percent of direct quotes in articles taken from U.S. officials and the Nicaraguan opposition, which together constituted 60 percent of all sources (Herman 1984).

3. To aid the bombing campaign, U.S. military aid was raised to $260 million in 1984 (equal to total U.S. aid for the previous four years). The air war intensified from 1984 to 1986 as the Salvadoran Air Force made use of new intelligence from U.S. surveillance flights at night, and new fleets of sixty Huey helicopters, thirteen A-37 fighter planes, and five rapid-fire AC-47 planes. Flights by Huey helicopters and A-37 strike planes increased by 220 hours per month between July 1983 and February 1984 (Montgomery 1995; and Stanley 1996).

4. Clements (1984) reported that multiple witnesses saw a cigar-shaped object dropped from an A-37 bomber, which burst into a rolling fireball, emitting black smoke. The contents stuck to an adobe wall and kept burning. He photographed the burned vegetation and aluminum container, which had a filling port and contact detonator. For Salvadoran soldiers commenting on the army's routine use of incendiary weapons, see Hedges 1984.

5. Testimony taken by a Medical Aid for El Salvador delegation that visited El Salvador September 10–22, 1984, to investigate bombings of civilians.

6. This was a response to a U.S. State Department query from Washington about human rights reports of civilian casualties from bombs.

7. The army press office routinely photographed people killed in army attacks in this manner.

8. *Informe de los Derechos de Salud*, August–September 1989, Chalatenango Catholic Diocese. I interviewed one of the captured promoters in November 1995.

9. During my visit to the controlled zone in July 1989 residents reported (a) army abductions of eight people, including a dental promoter, who were tortured and asked about health work; (b) army detentions of three health workers during a vaccination campaign; and (c) three cases of soldiers who broke into clinics and robbed supplies.

10. For example, Tommie Sue Montgomery cites a 1980 meeting in which the U.S. *chargé d'affaires* James Cheek pushed Salvadoran Christian Democratic officials to reform the country's penal code to allow the military to retain prisoners for an indefinite period of time.

11. These modifications in death squad and security force activities during the mid-1980s were noted by human rights specialists in interviews with the author, San Salvador, 1987.

12. An adaptation of the military term "total war" used to refer to a nuclear confrontation. See Wagelstein 1985, 42.

13. Also see two unsigned articles in the *Washington Post*, "Gunships for El Salvador Protested," September 8; and "U.S. Rejects AC47 Gunships for El Salvador," September 11.

14. But see Suarez-Orozco's (1992) critique of Taussig's writings on terror for paying little attention to contemporary Latin America's dirty wars (225–229).

15. However, the subsequent Iraq War and the failure of the United Nations to intervene effectively in the Darfur massacres in Sudan point up the role political interests play in shaping application of international law and the need to continually refine human rights policies.

16. Human rights observers I spoke with noted that a government that adopts genocidal tactics against dissident leaders eventually runs out of people to kill, making it easier for officials to adopt moderate policies to accommodate international criticism.

CHAPTER 5   PACIFICATION

1. See Manwaring and Prisk (1988, 226) on the importance of securing these provinces (especially Usulután) because of their economic importance. The plan was never extended into Usulután, as was originally planned.

2. The USAID health initiative being addressed was a proposed project that was estimated to cost US$24 million.

3. Ministry rural clinics were poorly supplied and staffed during the first half of the 1980s as the health budget was cut by half in a four-year period. However, a long-term study of the health system by John Fiedler and colleagues concluded that the roots of the ministry's recurrent cost crisis date to a poorly designed Inter-American Development Bank loan for rural health infrastructure in the 1970s (1993, 28). (See also chapter 9.)

4. See Second U.S. Public Health Commission Report 1983; by 1993, when funding came through to resupply and restaff facilities that had been closed during the war, the number of clinics and health posts affected numbered 122 located in 115 municipalities (APSISA 1994).

5. Interviews with UNICEF staff in San Salvador and New York.

6. I changed names of the local health workers to pseudonyms in excerpting this segment from Ana's diary.

CHAPTER 6   THE ANATOMY OF "POPULAR HEALTH" IN THE REPOPULATED VILLAGES

1. Diarrhea gradually declined as a major cause of child morbidity each year after the town was repopulated, according to my study of clinic records from 1987 to 1992 (see figures 1 and 2 in chapter 7).

2. Additional problems in a formal epidemiological survey involve finding an appropriate control population. There was little independently obtained epidemiological data on effectiveness of health services in rural El Salvador; figures used by international organizations were extrapolated from small samples. Other problems were poor recordkeeping in both popular and government systems and incompatible records.

3. I attended village health assemblies, vaccination campaigns, training classes, health planning meetings, and negotiation sessions between the ministry and popular health representatives. I conducted more than 120 interviews with different participants in the popular system and their patients, including twenty-five lay promoters, thirteen former FMLN physicians, six church-affiliated physicians, and a variety of

other technical team members. I conducted a written survey of forty-one health promoters administered orally at meetings. In the Ministry of Health, I interviewed twelve physicians (including six administrators), seven nurses, three technicians, and four health promoters, and I attended evaluation sessions of the government health promoter program. I interviewed specialists in health at USAID, PAHO, the UNDP, at universities, and with development or relief NGOs.

4. To be without a government-issued cédula during the war was treated by authorities as evidence of guerrilla activity. Thousands displaced by violence lost their cédulas. Despite government promises that new ones would be issued, this process was very slow.

5. Nurses and midlevel ministry employees seldom agreed to an interview with me without having it okayed by a supervisor. Likewise doctors in their social service year were nervous about offending supervisors. But Consuelo had been in her position for many years. Also, the regional health director for Chalatenango approved my request to observe a clinic and specifically recommended this clinic.

6. This was a straightforward disease to treat since it was self-limiting as long as the patients were kept from becoming dehydrated due to the constant watery diarrhea.

7. In 1993, after a negotiated agreement between the popular system and the ministry, government physicians returned to many villages and took over many tertiary care responsibilities formerly managed at the Guarjila clinic (see chapter 8).

8. In 1995, after the return of the Ministry of Health to the zone, a new health clinic was built in San José Las Flores.

9. Since the Church anticipated a drop-off in foreign donations after the war (and since negotiations with the ministry on state funding were stalled), a debate was under way in 1993 on how to transition to a more self-financed system. Villages held health assemblies to discuss this, and most clinics opted to ask for voluntary donations from patients to build clinic funds to supplement purchases of medicines from the Diocese.

10. Some latrines served multiple households. The presence of a latrine did not mean that families used them. Some latrines filled up, and some campesinos rejected them as smelly.

11. The Technical Team adopted this policy because of studies showing that injections led to side effects such as small skin infections in a minority of patients.

CHAPTER 7   THE ELUSIVE GOAL OF
COMMUNITY PARTICIPATION

This chapter is a revised version of Sandy Smith-Nonini, "Primary Health Care and Its Unfulfilled Promise of Community Participation: Lessons from a Salvadoran War Zone," *Human Organization* 56, no. 3 (1997): 364–374. The author received the Peter K. New Prize from the Society for Applied Anthropology for this paper.

1. Especially Spanish editions of *Where There is No Doctor* (Werner 1981) and *Helping Health Workers Learn* (Werner and Bower 1982).

2. In contrast to promoters in resettlement villages, popular promoters in other parts of Chalatenango were volunteers. The Catholic diocese stressed volunteer work and resisted proposals to pay stipends to new promoters entering training outside the former war zone, a stance that created some tensions between promoters in the two areas.

3. Consultants hired by USAID organized a few village assemblies and focus groups of physicians and nurses to evaluate the CHP promoter profile in 1995. I attended two sessions and interviewed staff involved in the review process.

4. Twenty-two popular promoters took the ministry's three-month CHP course in the capital, but in contrast to its usual practice of hiring promoters trained, the ministry only offered jobs to eleven and fired them three months later in late 1994, citing funding shortfalls. (See chapter 9.)

5. Often one promoter at each clinic specialized in natural medicines and made supplies of cough syrup, skin cream, or liquid vitamins for the clinic dispensary. The Lutheran church in El Salvador had identified about twenty herbal remedies that the popular system promoted through workshops and herb garden projects. Not all clinics were well equipped to make natural medicines, and sometimes supplies ran low because promoters lacked time to make them.

6. The number of clinic visits doubled in the same period, from roughly 150 per month in 1987 to 300 per month in 1992. The epidemic of conjunctivitis was probably self-limiting, and since numbers of cases of conjunctivitis and malaria were very low, it is uncertain whether these declines in incidence reflected improved preventive health measures.

7. Written recordkeeping was a difficult task for many promoters, and while records of use of medicines had to be kept in order to be resupplied, promoters were more lax about records of community education activities.

8. See Wellin (1955) for discussion of how Peruvian women responded to advice of health officials about boiling water. Some residents in town centers did not boil water because they believed that the promoters adding chlorine to the central water tank was sufficient; however, the health team advised residents to boil water anyway. None of my informants mentioned humoral beliefs that boiled or "cooked" water becomes "hot" and therefore not good to drink, as some Peruvian women did in Wellin's study, although one insisted that boiling changed the taste.

9. A study by Nichter (1986) of a PHC center "as a social system" is an exception, as is Morgan's (1989) work on state-supported community participation in Costa Rica.

CHAPTER 8   POPULAR HEALTH AND THE STATE

This chapter is based in part on Sandy Smith-Nonini, "'Popular' Health and the State: Dialectics of the Peace Process in El Salvador," *Social Science and Medicine* 44, no. 5 (1997): 635–645.

1. El Salvador's CHP program differed significantly from the popular health system in Chalatenango in that promoters had far less responsibility and support, few curative duties, and were not allowed to organize locally to build community participation. The program was being cut back in late 1995, less than a year after USAID turned responsibility for funding the program over to the ministry. (See chapter 9.)

2. The role of the Catholic Church in the peace process health negotiations was ambiguous. The Catholic diocese, which had by far the largest financial investment in training and supplies for the popular health system, described its role as an observer rather than a partner in the negotiations. Although members of the Catholic technical team were active in early stages of the negotiations, they became less active as promoters were recruited to fill these roles.

3. Not all factions of the FMLN were as committed to community-based development as the FPL. In Morazán Province, where the second-largest FMLN faction, the ERP, was the dominant political group, negotiations between the Ministry of Health and local health promoters went extremely rapidly since the local health system was not well organized. Chalateco health workers saw the Morazán situation as a disaster because ministry physicians simply moved into the popular clinics and took them over. However, when nearly a year had passed since the cease-fire without a negotiated accord on health in Chalatenango, the ex-FMLN physicians and sanitarios (involved in the negotiations) began to gain a reputation within the FPL as "hardliners." This contributed to a hasty accord in 1993 that many in the popular system later came to regret.

4. Ministry of Health social service physicians rotated in and out of their rural postings each January, creating problems for the repopulation communities. The ministry did not brief new physicians on the regional health accord, so local efforts to coordinate the two health systems were forced to start over from scratch each year.

5. Anemia is a frequent problem in this undernourished population. Some older women and those in more remote areas still adhered to folk beliefs about "hot" and "cold" foods, which prohibit pregnant women from eating a wide variety of foods, including fish, beef, acidic fruits, fresh vegetables, and in some cases even staples like beans. The folk diet limits lactating women even more drastically—some consuming only chocolate, dry cheese, and tortillas in the forty days after birth.

6. Popular promoter graduates of the CHP course resented this requirement because ministry travel stipends had not sufficiently covered their costs for transport, meals, and supplies while studying in the capital. Several had borrowed money or sold things they owned to complete the course.

CHAPTER 9   DISINVESTING IN HEALTH

Portions of this chapter are based on Sandy Smith-Nonini, "The Smoke and Mirrors of Health Reform in El Salvador: Community Health NGOs and the Not-So-Neoliberal State," in *Dying for Growth: Global Inequality and the Health of the Poor*, eds. Jim Yong Kim, Joyce V. Millen, Alec Irwin, and John Gershman, 359–381. Monroe, MN: Common Courage Press, 2000.

1. From 1977 to 1985 the share of the health budget directed to personnel costs increased from 56 percent of the ministry's Centralized Agencies operating budget to 92 percent. This caused a concurrent fall in the budget for pharmaceuticals and supplies from 44 to 8 percent (Fiedler 1987).

2. Based on in-house evaluations of the program that I attended; on interviews with staff, promoters, and USAID consultants; and on an evaluation of the program by Lewis, Eskeland, and Traa-Valerezo (1999). (See also Lewis, Eskeland, and Traa-Valerezo 2004).

3. Based on a focus group meeting in a community served by ministry promoters, a focus group of ministry health professionals that evaluated the program, interviews with staff of consulting firms hired by USAID for the evaluation, and interviews with a World Bank official who oversaw a team evaluating ministry promoters. In the final report, Maureen Lewis and colleagues (2004) argued that Salvadorans' preference for private facilities over the services of ministry health promoters reflected a general failure in the concept of community health, while I would argue that it reflects the

extremely poor version of community health that the ministery created. Mass-produced health promoters trained in a capital city are often poorly prepared and only nominally "community-based" (see Walt, Perera, and Heggenhougen 1989).

4. From interviews with ministry employees and foreign aid consultants, all of whom asked that their identities not be revealed. Over the course of two months, I made multiple requests for an interview with Dr. Eduardo Interiano, the minister of health. His secretary said he was too busy for an interview and referred me to the reform office.

5. Compared with the 1980s, USAID enjoyed declining influence with the government in the post-cease-fire period because the agency was rapidly downsizing its funding. A degree of resistance to USAID was also a matter of national pride.

6. Based on interviews with staff involved in the ministry's community health planning office and information provided by the ministry's reform office and its finance division.

7. In many cases, local NGOs grew out of self-help movements that developed their own advocacy organizations. Many found allies among Northern Hemisphere development foundations that sought alternatives to partnering with corrupt governments.

8. Ibid., 191.

9. The Salvadoran Ministry of Planning estimated in 1988 that two-thirds of Salvadorans lived in poverty, and one-third lived in "extreme" poverty. Average per capita income fell by 25 percent during the war. Although the GDP began to grow again after 1990, little wealth trickled down, and the poor were disproportionately affected by new value-added taxes on basic goods. The San Salvador–based Center for Defense of the Consumer calculated that the cost of the canasta básica for a family of five increased by 11 percent from July 1994 to July 1995.

10. An international consulting team strongly advised against regional hospital expansion in a 1993 study of the health system, noting that occupancy rates for hospital beds had been very low, especially in regional health centers (Fiedler, Gomez, and Bertrand 1993). (A member of the World Bank mission team later told me no exact loan amount was arrived at, nor were uses of the funds for hospitals approved.)

11. In 1996 President Calderón Sol reportedly began pressuring the health minister (an old colleague who played a key role in his presidential campaign) to reach a compromise with the banks, and as a result Interiano resumed consideration of the banks' reform agenda.

12. For example, one PROSAMI NGO, *Fundación Maquillishuat*, was directed by Dr. Hector Silva, who was elected major of the capital with FMLN support in 2000.

13. On the role of the state in equitable primary health care, see Collins and Green (1994). For examples of states using decentralization to cut back health services, see Collins (1989). See Walt (1994) for discussion of the forms decentralized health care can take.

14. For a contrasting case study, see the description of a successful rural health network in Cambodia, where two large international health NGOs successfully bypassed a corrupt health ministry and have done a better job of delivering services in rural areas (Dugger 2006).

15. For other critiques of the post-1993 World Bank's position on privatization of health, see Abel and Lloyd-Sherlock (2000); Kaufman and Nelson (2004); Kim et al. (2000); and Rao (1999).

CHAPTER 10   THE WHITE MARCHES

1. Susan Greenblatt, an American translator and former health educator based in San Salvador, provided research assistance for this study. In 2000 she conducted and transcribed ten interviews, including one focus group session. She also collected news clips and documents on the health mobilizations and assisted me to arrange interviews during visits in 2002 and 2007. I conducted thirty-six interviews and attended a local conference on health privatization.

2. Based on interviews by the author (1989) and on reports by the New York-based National Labor Committee (1995) and the Salvadoran Human Rights Commission (1995).

3. For example, in 2001 the top 108 ISSS administrators earned salaries, benefits, and bonuses that averaged around 280,000 colones (US$48,753), with top compensation packages reaching US$122,000, compared with salaries for staff physicians (providing consults two hours per day) of only 16,800 colones ($2,921 annually), according to charts published by the Secretaría de Prensa y Propaganda STISSS, Boletín No. 2, February 2002.

4 Based on figures from the National Emergency Committee (Bueno 2001).

5. El Salvador, with the densest population in Central America, had lost more native forest and had the highest level of erosion in the region by the mid-1980s, according to the International Institute for Environment and Development (proofs of report on Central America, provided by Dr. H. Jeffrey Leonard, Director of IIED International Programs).

6. Criticisms of the private schools focused on their small size and lack of resources as well as their for-profit status. The deficits cited for the UES, in contrast, were tied to a lack of equipment and resources—the campus was stripped of valuable items during the military occupation, and the government frequently shortchanged the university's budget after it reopened. The UES is also famously rife with political favoritism, biased toward professors well connected on the left, which at times has hurt quality, according to former medical students and faculty (see Grenier 1999).

REFERENCES

Abel, Christopher, and Peter Lloyd-Sherlock. 2000. "Health Policy in Latin America: Themes, Trends and Challenges," In *Healthcare Reform and Poverty in Latin America*, ed. Peter Lloyd-Sherlock, 1–20. London: Institute of Latin American Studies.

Adams, Vincanne. 1998. *Doctors for Democracy: Health Professionals in the Nepal Revolution.* New York: Cambridge University Press.

ADS. 1994. "National Family Health Survey FESAL-93," produced by the Salvadoran Demographic Association ADS with cooperation of the Ministry of Public Health & Social Assistance and the U.S. Agency of International Development.

Agamben, Giorgio. 1998. *Homo Sacer: Sovereign Power and Bare Life.* Palo Alto, CA: Stanford University Press.

———. 2000. "Means Without Ends: Notes on Politics." In *Theory out of Bounds,* ed. Sandra Buckley, M. Hardt, and B. Massumi, 20–31. Minneapolis: University of Minnesota Press.

Agier, Michel and Françoise Bouchet-Saulnier. 2004. "Humanitarian Spaces: Spaces of Exception." In *In the Shadow of 'Just Wars': Violence, Politics, and Humanitarian Action*, ed. Fabrice Weissman, 297–313. Ithaca, NY: Cornell University Press.

Allport, G. W. 1950. *The Individual and His Religion: A Psychological Interpretation.* New York: Macmillan.

Allport, Gordon, J. Gillespie, and J. Young. 1948. "The Religion of the Post-war College Student." *Journal of Psychology* 25:3–33.

Allwood Paredes, Juan. 1969. *Los Recursos de la Salud Publico in Centro America.* San Salvador: Organization of American States.

Almeida, Paul. 2006. "Social Movement Unionism, Social Movement Partyism, and Policy Outcomes: Health Care Privatization in El Salvador." In *Latin American Social Movements: Globalization, Democratization and Transnational Networks*, eds. Hank Johnston and Paul Almeida, 57–73. New York: Rowman & Littlefield.

———. 2008. "The Sequencing of Success: Organizational Templates and Neoliberal Policy Outcomes." *Mobilization: The International Quarterly* 13 (2): 165–187.

Americas Watch. 1986. *Land Mines in El Salvador and Nicaragua: The Civilian Victims.* New York: The Americas Watch Committee.

Americas Watch and Lawyers Committee for Human Rights. 1984. *Free Fire: A Report on Human Rights in El Salvador.* New York: The Americas Watch Committee.

Anderson, Benedict. 1983. *Imagined Communities: Reflections on the Origin and Spread of Nationalism.* London: Verso.

Anderson, Matthew, Lanny Smith, and Victor W. Sidel. 2004. "What Is Social Medicine?" *Monthly Review* 56 (8): 27–34.

Anderson, Perry. 1983. *In the Tracks of Historical Materialism.* London: Verso.

Anderson, Thomas. 1971. *Matanza: El Salvador's Communist Revolt of 1932*. Lincoln: University of Nebraska Press.

ANSAL. 1994. "Health Sector Reform in El Salvador: Towards Equity and Efficiency." Executive Summary. Health Sector Assessment Project of El Salvador. Funded by U.S. Agency for International Development, the Pan American Health Organization/World Health Organization, the World Bank, and the Inter-American Development Bank. San Salvador: U.S. Agency for International Development.

APSISA. 1991. "Apoyo para Sistemas de Salud—APSISA Project." San Salvador: U.S. Agency for International Development.

———. 1994. "Apoyo para Sistemas de Salud—APSISA Project." San Salvador: U.S. Agency for International Development.

Arendt, Hannah. 1963. *Eichmann in Jerusalem: A Report on the Banality of Evil*. New York: Viking Press.

Arias-Peñate, Salvador. 1988. *Los Subsistemas de Agroexportacion en El Salvador: El Café, el Algodon, y el Azucar*. San Salvador: UCA Editores.

Armstrong, J. D. 1985. "The International Committee of the Red Cross and Political Prisoners." *International Organization* 394:615–642.

Atran, S. 2002. *In Gods We Trust: The Evolutionary Landscape of Religion*. New York: Oxford University Press.

Aviles, Luis. 2001. "Epidemiology as Discourse: The Politics of Development Institutions in the Epidemiological Profile of El Salvador." *Journal of Epidemiology and Community Health* 55:164–171.

Ayalde, J. 1994. "Epidemiological Profile." Final report. ANSAL series. San Salvador: U.S. Agency for International Development.

Baer, Hans. 1996. "Critical Biocultural Approaches in Medical Anthropology: A Dialogue," Special Issue of *Medical Anthropology Quarterly*, n.s. 104.

Baer, Hans A., Merrill Singer, and John Johnson, eds. 1986. "Towards a Critical Medical Anthropology." Special Issue of *Social Science and Medicine* 23 (2).

Baer, Hans A., Merrill Singer, and Ida Susser, 1997. *Medical Anthropology and the World System: A Critical Perspective*. Westport, CT: Bergin & Garvey.

———. 2003. *Medical Anthropology and the World System*. Westport, CT: Praeger.

Barnard, Alan, and James Woodburn. 1991. "Introduction." In *Property, Power and Ideology*, Vol. 2 of *Hunters and Gatherers*, eds. T. Ingold, D. Riches, and J. Woodburn. New York: Berg.

Bender, Deborah, and Kathryn Pitkin. 1987. "Bridging the Gap: The Village Health Worker as the Cornerstone of the Primary Health Care Model." *Social Science and Medicine* 246:515–528.

Bergmans, Lonneke. 1995. "Estudio—El Pensamiento sobre la salud de la comunidad en el municipio Las Vueltas, Chalatenango." Unpublished manuscript in author's possession.

Berman, Peter, Davidson R. Gwatkin, and Susan E. Burger. 1987. "Community-based Health Workers: Head Start or False Start towards Health for All?" *Social Science and Medicine* 25 (5): 443–459.

Best, Steven, and D. Kellner. 1991. *Postmodern Theory: Critical Interrogations*. New York: Guilford Press.

Biddle, Wayne. 1984. "Salvadorans Have Napalm, U.S. Ambassador Confirms." *New York Times*, September 30, p. 10.

Binford, Leigh. 1996. *The El Mozote Massacre: Anthropology and Human Rights*. Tucson: University of Arizona Press.

———. 1999. "Hegemony in the Interior of the Revolution: The ERP in Northern Morazán, El Salvador." *Journal of Latin American Anthropology* 4 (1): 2–45.

———. 2004. "Peasants, Catechists, Revolutionaries: Organic Intellectuals in the Salvadoran Revolution, 1980–1992." In *Landscapes of Struggle: Politics, Society, and Community in El Salvador*, eds. A. Lauria-Santiago and L. Binford, 105–125. Pittsburgh: University of Pittsburgh Press.

Blair, Amy R., and Sara A. Siebert. 1999. "Processes, Not Events: The First Ceasefire Immunization Campaign in El Salvador, 1985." Unpublished manuscript, in author's possession.

Blondel, Jean-Luc. 1987. "Getting Access to the Victims: Role and Activities of the ICRC." *Journal of Peace Research* 243:307–314.

Boehm, Christopher. 1999. *Hierarchy in the Forest: The Evolution of Egalitarian Behavior.* Cambridge, MA: Harvard University Press.

Bonner, Raymond. 1984. *Weakness and Deceit: U.S. Policy and El Salvador.* New York: Times Books.

Booth, John A. 1991. "Socioeconomic and Political Roots of National Revolts in Central America." *Latin American Research Review* 261:33–74.

Bourdieu, Pierre. 1977. *Outline of a Theory of Practice.* New York: Cambridge University Press.

———. 1990. *The Logic of Practice.* Stanford, CA: Stanford University Press.

Bourgois, Philippe I. 1982. "Running for My Life in El Salvador: An American Caught in a Government Attack that Chiefly Killed Civilians." *Washington Post*, February 14, pp. C1.

———. 1991. "The Ethics of Ethnography: Lessons from Fieldwork in Central America." In *Decolonizing Anthropology: Moving Further Toward an Anthropology for Liberation*, ed. Faye Harrison, 110–126. Washington, DC: Association of Black Anthropologists and American Anthropological Association.

———. 2002. *In Search of Respect: Selling Crack in El Barrio.* Cambridge: Cambridge University Press.

Boyce, James. 1995. "External Assistance and the Peace Process in El Salvador." *World Development* 23 (12): 2101–2116.

Bracamonte, Jose Angel M., and David Spencer. 1995. *Strategy and Tactics of the Salvadoran FMLN Guerrillas: Last Battle of the Cold War, Blueprint for Future Conflicts.* Westport, CT: Praeger.

Brauman, Rony. 1993. "When Suffering Makes a Good Story." In *Life, Death and Aid: The Médidins Sans Frontieres Report on World Crisis Intervention*, ed. Francois Jean, 218–227. London and New York: Routledge Press.

Brett, Donna Whitson, and Edward T. Brett. 1988. *Murdered in Central America: The Stories of Eleven U.S. Missionaries.* Maryknoll, NY: Orbis Books.

Briehl, Jaime. 1979. "Community Medicine under Imperialism." *International Journal of Health Services* 9 (1): 5–25.

———. 1995. "Epidemiology's Role in the Creation of a Humane World: Convergences and Divergences among the Schools. Editorial." *Social Science and Medicine* 417:911–914.

Bromley, D. W., D. Feeny, M. A. McKean, P. Peters, J. L. Gilles, R. J. Oakerson, C. F. Runge, and J. T. Thomson, eds. 1992. *Making the Commons Work: Theory, Practice, and Policy.* San Francisco: ICS Press.

Browning, David. 1971. *El Salvador: Landscape and Society.* Oxford: Clarendon Press.

Bueno, Pascha. 2001. "Relief Efforts for El Salvador Earthquakes," *CHRIA News* 18 (1): 1, 5–7.

Bulmer-Thomas, Victor. 1987. *The Political Economy of Central America since 1920.* New York: Cambridge University Press.

Burghardt, Walter J. 1981. "Models of Church, Models of Health Apostolate." In *The Ministry of Healing*, 55–69. St. Louis: The Catholic Health Association of the United States.

Butchart, Alex, Brandon Hamber, Martin Terre Blanche, and Mohamed Seedat. 1998. "From Violent Policies to Policies for Violence Prevention: Violence, Power and Mental Health Policy in 20th Century South Africa." In *Mental Health Policy Issues in South Africa*, ed. D. Foster, M. Freeman, and Y. Pillay, 236–262. Cape Town: Medical Association Multimedia Publications.

Cabarrús, Carlos. R. 1983. *Génesis de una revolución: Análisis del surgimiento y desarrollo de la organización campesina en El Salvador*. México, D.F.: Centro de Investigaciones y Estudios Superiores en Antropología Social.

Cagan, Steve, and Beth Cagan. 1991. *This Promised Land, El Salvador: The Refugee Community of Colomoncagua and Their Return to Morazán*. New Brunswick, NJ: Rutgers University Press.

Capps, Linnea, and Patricia Crane. 1989. "Evaluation of a Programme to Train Village Health Workers in El Salvador." *Health Policy and Planning* 43:239–243.

Carey, Benedict. 2007. "Do You Believe in Magic?" *New York Times*, Science Times section D1–5, January 23.

Carrigan, Ann. 1984. *Salvador Witness: The Life and Calling of Jean Donovan*. New York: Simon and Schuster.

Cernea, Michael. 1988. *NGOs and Local Development*. Washington, DC: World Bank.

CESA. 1977. "Sterilization Abuse: A Task for the Women's Movement." Working Paper of the Chicago Women's Liberation Union. Available online at CWLU Herstory Project, www.cwluherstory.com.

Chatterjee, Pratap. 2004. *Iraq, Inc.: A Profitable Occupation*. New York: Seven Stories Press.

Chen, L. 1989. "Comments On: Thoughts on Good Health and Good Government, by N. Birdsall." *Daedalus* 118 (1): 89.

Chomsky, Noam. 1968. *Language and Mind*. New York: Harcourt Brace & World.

Chopoorian, Teresa, and Eli Messinger. 1983. "U.S. Medical Aid to El Salvador Must Be Condemned." *New York Times*, July 9, p. 9.

Clements, Charles. 1984. *Witness to War: An American Doctor in El Salvador*. New York: Bantam Books.

Cliff, J., and A. Noormahomed. 1988. "Health as a Target: South Africa's Destabilization of Mozambique." *Social Science and Medicine* 287:717–722.

Cody, Edward. 1984. "U.S. Considers AC47 Gunships for El Salvador," *Washington Post*, September 1.

Colégio Médico. 1999. "Propuesta ciudadana por la salud." Colégio Médico de El Salvador. San Salvador: Korrekto, Impreso en Tipografía Offset Laser.

Collins, Charles. 1989. "Decentralization and the Need for Political and Critical Analysis." *Health Policy and Planning* 4:168–171.

Collins, Charles, and Andrew Green. 1994. "Decentralization and Primary Health Care: Some Negative Implications in Developing Countries." *International Journal of Health Services* 243:459–475.

Commission on Medical Neutrality. 1990. *Violations of Medical Neutrality*. Seattle, WA: Commission on Medical Neutrality.

Comaroff, Jean, and John Comaroff. 1991. *Of Revelation and Revolution: Christianity, Colonialism and Consciousness in South Africa*. Vol. 1. Chicago: University of Chicago Press.

Conrad, Peter, and J. W. Schneider. 1992. *Deviance and Medicalization: From Badness to Sickness*. Philadelphia: Temple University Press.

Conroy, Michael, Douglas Murray, and Peter Rosset. 1996. *A Cautionary Tale: Failed U.S. Development Policy in Central America*. Boulder, CO: Lynne Rienner Publishers.

Creedon, Kelly, and Chris Ney. 2003. "Marching for Health Care in El Salvador." *The Non-Violent Activist*, May/June: 8–9.

Csordas, Thomas J. 1994. *Embodiment and Experience: The Existential Ground of Culture and Self*. Cambridge: Cambridge University Press.

Cueto, Marcos. 1994. "Visions of Science and Development: The Rockefeller Foundation's Latin American Surveys of the 1920s." In *Missionaries of Science: The Rockefeller Foundation and Latin America*, ed. Marcos Cueto. Bloomington: Indiana University Press.

Dalton, Roque. 1983. *Poemas Clandestinos—Clandestine Poems*, trans. Jack Hirshman and Eric Weaver. San Francisco: Solidarity Publications.

———. 1988. *Las Historias Prohibidas del Pulgarcito*. 9th ed. San Salvador: UCA Editores.

Danaher, Kevin, ed. 1994. *Fifty Years Is Enough: The Case against the World Bank*. Boston: South End Press.

Danby, Colin. 1984. "U.S. Military Health Program Criticized." *Honduran Update*, September 3.

De la Cadena, Marisol. 2000. *Indigenous Mestizos: The Politics of Race and Culture in Cuzco, Peru, 1919–1991*. Durham, NC: Duke University Press.

De Quadros, Ciro, and Daniel Epstein. 2002. "Health as a Bridge for Peace: PAHO's Experience." *Lancet* 360 (9350) Supplement, December 21.

Del Castillo, Graciano. 2001. "Post-Conflict Reconstruction and the Challenge to International Organizations: The Case of El Salvador." *World Development* 29 (12): 1967–1985.

Democracy Now. 2004. "President Aristide says 'I Was Kidnapped'" *Democracy Now* online edition, http://www.democracynow.org/2004/3/1/exclusive_breaking_news_br_president _aristide. March 1.

Desjarlais, Robert K., and Arthur Kleinman. 1994. "Violence and Demoralization in the New World Disorder." *Anthropology Today* 10 (5): 9–12.

DeWalt, Billie. 1994. "The Agrarian Basis of Conflict in Central America." In *Applying Anthropology: An Introductory Reader*, eds. Aaron Podolefsky and Peter J. Brown, 3rd ed., 183–188. Mountain View, CA: Mayfield Publishing Co.

Donahue, John. 1991. "Planning for Primary Health Care in Nicaragua." In *Health Care Patterns and Planning in Developing Countries.*, ed. R. Akhtar, 55–71. New York: Greenwood Press.

Donnelly, Jack. 1989. *Universal Human Rights in Theory and Practice*. Ithaca, NY: Cornell University Press.

Douglas, M. 1984. *Purity and Danger: An Analysis of Concepts of Pollution and Taboo*. London: ARK Paperbacks. First published 1966 by Praeger.

Dow, James. 1986. "Universal Aspects of Symbolic Healing: A Theoretical Synthesis." *American Anthropologist* 88:56–69.

Doyle, Kate, and Peter S. Duklis. 1990. "The Long Twilight Struggle: Low-Intensity Warfare and the Salvadoran Military." *Journal of International Affairs* 12:431–460.

Dressler, William W. 2001. "Medical Anthropology: Toward a Third Moment in Social Science?" *Medical Anthropology Quarterly* 15 (4): 455–465.

Dubois, Marc. 1991. "The Governance of the Third World: A Foucauldian Perspective of Power Relations in Development." *Alternatives* 16I:1–30.

Dugger, Celia W. 2006. "A Cure that Really Works: Cambodia Tries the Nonprofit Path to Health Care." *New York Times*, January 8, p. 8A.

Durham, William H. 1979. *Scarcity and Survival in Central America: Ecological Origins of the Soccer War*. Stanford, CA: Stanford University Press.

Eckstein, Susan. 2001. *Power and Popular Protest in Latin America*. Berkeley and Los Angeles: University of California Press.

Edelman, Marc. 1999. *Peasants against Globalization: Rural Social Movements in Costa Rica*. Stanford, CA: Stanford University Press.

Edwards, Beatrice, and Gretta Tovar Siebentritt. 1991. *Places of Origin: The Repopulation of Rural El Salvador*. Boulder, CO: Lynne Rienner Publishers.

Epprecht, Marc. 1994. "The World Bank, Health & Africa." *Z Magazine*. November.

Equipo Maiz. 2005. *La Privatizacion o el Nuevo Colonialismo*. Asociacion Equipo Maiz. San Salvador: Algier's Impresores.

Escobar, Arturo. 1992. "Reflections on Development: Grassroots Approaches and Alternative Politics in the Third World." *Futures* 245:411–436.

———. 1995. *Encountering Development: The Making and Unmaking of the Third World*. Princeton, NJ: Princeton University Press.

Escobar, Arturo, and S. E. Alvarez. 1992. *The Making of Social Movements in Latin America: Identity, Strategy, and Democracy*. Boulder, CO: Westview Press.

Espinoza, Eduardo. 2007. *Relatos de la Guerra*. San Salvador: Imprenta y Editorial Universitaria.

Farmer, Paul. 2003. *Pathologies of Power: Health, Human Rights, and the New War on the Poor*. Berkeley and Los Angeles: University of California Press.

———. 2004. "An Anthropology of Structural Violence." *Current Anthropology* 45 (3): 305–326.

Feierman, Steve. 1990. *Peasant Intellectuals: Anthropology and History in Tanzania*. Madison: University of Wisconsin Press.

Fein, Helen. 1979. *Accounting for Genocide*. New York: The Free Press.

Feinsilver, Julie. 1993. *Healing the Masses: Cuban Health Politics at Home and Abroad*. Berkeley and Los Angeles: University of California Press.

Ferguson, James. 1994. *The Anti-Politics Machine*. Minneapolis: University of Minnesota Press.

Ferrell, Theo. 2005. *The Norms of War: Cultural Beliefs and Modern Conflict*. Boulder, CO: Lynne Rienner Publishers.

FESAL. 1988. *Encuesta Nacional de Salud Familiar*. San Salvador: Asociacion Demografica Salvadorena.

Fiedler, John. 1987. "Recurrent Cost and Public Health Care Delivery: The Other War in El Salvador." *Social Science and Medicine* 258:867–874.

———. 1988. "El Salvador's Ministry of Health, 1975–1986: A Provisional Performance Assessment" *Health Policy* 10:177–206.

Fiedler, John, Luis Carlos Gomez, and William Bertrand. 1993. *An Overview of the Health Sector of El Salvador*. San Salvador: Clapp and Mayne, Inc.

Fiedler, John L., R. M. Schmidt, and J. B. Wight. 1998. "Public Hospital Resource Allocations in El Salvador: Accounting for the Case Mix of Patients" *Health Policy and Planning* 13 (3): 296–310.

Finkler, Kaya. 2001. *Physicians at Work, Patients in Pain: Biomedical Practice and Patient Response in Mexico*. Durham, NC: Carolina Academic Press.

Firth, Robert. 1929. *Primitive Economics of the New Zealand Maori*. New York: E. P. Dutton and Company.

Fleury, Sonia. 2001. "Dual, Universal or Plural? Health Care Models and Issues in Latin America: Chile, Brazil and Colombia." In *Health Services in Latin America and Asia*, eds. Carlos Gerardo Molina and José Nuñez del Arco, 3–36. Baltimore: Johns Hopkins University Press for the Inter-American Development Bank.

Fort, Meredith P., Mary Ann Mercer, and Oscar Gish. 2004. *Sickness and Wealth: The Corporate Assault on Global Health*. Cambridge, MA: South End Press.

Foster, George. 1982. "Community Development and Primary Health Care: Their Conceptual Similarities." *Medical Anthropology* 63:183–195.

Foucault, Michel. 1975. *The Birth of the Clinic: An Archaeology of Medical Perception*. New York: Vintage Books.

———. 1979. *Discipline and Punish: The Birth of the Prison*. New York: Vintage Books.

———. 1980. *Power/Knowledge: Selected Interviews and Other Writings, 1972–1977*, comp. Colin Gordon. New York: Pantheon Books.

———. 1988. *The History of Sexuality*. New York: Vintage Books.

———. 2003. *Michel Foucault: Society Must Be Defended: Lectures at the Collège de France, 1975–76*, eds. Mauro Bertani and Alessandro Fontana. New York: Picador.

Franke, Richard, and Barbara Chasin. 1994. *Kerala: Radical Reform as Development in an Indian State*. Oakland, CA: Institute for Food and Development Policy.

Frankenberg, Ronald. 1993. "Anthropology and Epidemiology: Narratives of Prevention." In *Knowledge, Power and Practice: The Anthropology of Medicine in Everyday Life*, eds. Shirley Lindenbaum and Margaret Lock, 219–242. Berkeley and Los Angeles: University of California Press.

Freire, Paulo. 1982. *Pedagogy of the Oppressed*. New York: Continuum.

Frieden, Tom. 1985. "A North American Nurse in El Salvador." *LINKS* 25–26:12–13.

Friedson, Eliot. 1974. *Professional Dominance: The Social Structure of Medical Care*. New York: Atherton Press.

Gadow, Sally. 1980. "Body and Self: A Dialectic." *Journal of Medicine and Philosophy* 53:172–184.

Galvin, John R. 1990. "Uncomfortable Wars: Toward a New Paradigm." In *Uncomfortable Wars: Toward a New Paradigm of Low Intensity Conflict*, ed. Max G. Manwaring, 9–18. Boulder, CO: Westview Press.

García Jiménez, Salvador. 2001. "The Immunization Program in Central America and the Keys to its Success." In *Health Services in Latin America and Asia*, ed. Carlos Gerardo Molina and José Nuñez del Arco, 83–96. Baltimore: Johns Hopkins University Press for the Inter-American Development Bank.

Gazzaniga, Michael S. 2005. *The Ethical Brain*. New York: Dana Press.

Geiger, Jack. 1993. Presentation at the University of North Carolina Medical School on recent medical neutrality investigations of Physicians for Human Rights. March 30.

General Accounting Office (GAO). 1992. *El Salvador: Role of Nongovernment Organizations in Postwar Reconstruction*. Washington, DC: U.S. General Accounting Office. GAO/NSAIAD-93-20BR.

Gilson, Lucy, Gill Walt, Kris Heggenhougen, L. Ouwuor-Omondi, M. Perera, D. Ross, and L. Salazar. 1989. "National Community Health Worker Programs: How Can They Be Strengthened?" *Journal of Public Health Policy* 104:518–531.

Giroux, Henry. 1988. *Teachers as Intellectuals: Towards a Critical Pedagogy of Learning*. Granby, MA: Bergin and Garvey.

Glick, Leonard. 1977. "Medicine as an Ethnographic Category." In *Culture, Disease and Healing: Studies in Medical Anthropology*, ed. David Landy, 58–70. New York: Macmillan.

Golinger, Eva. 2008. *Bush vs. Chavez: Washington's War on Venezuela*. New York: Monthly Review Press.

Gordon, Deborah. 1988. "Tenacious Assumptions in Western Medicine." In *Biomedicine Examined*, eds. Margaret M. Lock and Deborah Gordon, 19–42. Boston: Kluwer Academic.

Gorostiaga, Xabier, and Peter Marchetti. 1988. "The Central American Economy: Conflict and Crisis." In *Crisis in Central America: Regional Dynamics and U.S. Policy in the 1980s*, eds. N. Hamilton, J. A. Frieden, L. Fuller, M. Pastor Jr., 119–135. Boulder, CO: Westview Press.

Gramsci, Antonio. 1971. *Selections from the Prison Notebooks of Antonio Gramsci*. Edited and introduced by Quintin Hoare and Geoffrey Nowell-Smith. New York: International Publishers.

Grann, David. 2003. "The Price of Power" *New York Times Magazine*. May 11, p. 48–55, 68–69.

Gray, Bradford. 1992. "World Blindness and the Medical Profession: Conflicting Medical Cultures and the Ethical Dilemmas of Helping." *The Milbank Quarterly* 70 (3): 536–555.

Green, Linda B. 1989. "Consensus and Coercion: Primary Health Care and the Guatemalan State." *Medical Anthropology Quarterly* 33:246–257.

———. 1994. "Fear as a Way of Life." *Cultural Anthropology* 9 (2): 227–256.

———. 1998. "Lived Lives and Social Suffering: Problems and Concerns in Medical Anthropology." *Medical Anthropology Quarterly* 12 (1): 3–7.

Greenberger, Robert S. 1995. "Developing Countries Pass off Tedious Job of Assisting the Poor." *Wall Street Journal*, June 5.

Greenhouse, Carol J., Elizabeth Mertz, and Kay B. Warren. 2002. *Ethnography in Unstable Places: Everyday Lives in Contexts of Dramatic Political Change*. Durham, NC: Duke University Press.

Grenier, Yvon. 1999. *The Emergence of Insurgency in El Salvador*. Pittsburgh: University of Pittsburgh Press.

Gudeman, Stephen, and Alberto Rivera. 1990. *Conversations in Columbia: The Domestic Economy in Life and Text*. Cambridge: Cambridge University Press.

Habermas, Jürgen. 1989. *The Structural Transformation of the Public Sphere: An Inquiry into a Category of Bourgeois Society*. Cambridge, MA: MIT Press.

Hahn, Robert. 1995. *Sickness and Healing: An Anthropological Perspective*. New Haven, CT: Yale University Press.

Hahn, Robert A., and Arthur Kleinman. 1983. "Belief as Pathogen, Belief as Medicine: 'Voodoo Death' and the 'Placebo Phenomenon' in Anthropological Perspective." *Medical Anthropology Quarterly* 2 (2): 3, 13–19.

Hammond, John L. 1998. *Fighting to Learn: Popular Education and Guerrilla War in El Salvador*. New Brunswick, NJ: Rutgers University Press.

Hanania de Varela, Karla. 1990. *Analisis de la cooperación externa para el Ministerio de Salud Publica y Asistensia Social, 1985–1989*. Documento 15, Fundacion Salvadorena para el Desarrollo Economico y Social FUSADES.

Harrington, A. 1999. *The Placebo Effect: An Interdisciplinary Exploration*. Cambridge, MA: Harvard University Press.

Hatfield, Mark O., James Leach, and George Miller. 1987. "Bankrolling Failure: United States Policy in El Salvador and the Urgent Need for Reform." Report submitted to the Arms Control and Foreign Policy Caucus, U.S. House of Representatives, U.S. Congress 100th, 1st Session, November.

Hedges, Chris. 1984. "Salvador Charged with Dropping Incendiary Bombs." *Christian Science Monitor*, April 27.

———. 2002. *War Is a Force that Gives Us Meaning*. New York: Public Affairs.

Heggenhougen, H. K. 1984 "Will Primary Health Care Efforts Be Allowed to Succeed?" *Social Science and Medicine* 193:217.

———. 1995. "The Epidemiology of Functional Apartheid and Human Rights Abuses. Editorial." *Social Science and Medicine* 403:281–284.

Hellinger, Doug. 1987. "NGOs and the Large Aid Donors: Changing the Terms of Engagement." *World Development* Supplement 15:135–143.

Herman, Edward S. 1984. "The New York Times on the 1984 Salvadoran and Nicaraguan Elections." *Covert Action Information Bulletin* 21:7–13.

Herve-Bradol, Jean. 2004. "Introduction: The Sacrificial International Order and Humanitarian Action." In *In the Shadow of 'Just Wars': Violence, Politics, and Humanitarian Action*, ed. Fabrice Weissman, 1–22. Ithaca, NY: Cornell University Press.

Hirschman, Albert. 1983. "The Principal of the Conservation and Mutation of Social Energy." *Grassroots Development* 7 (2).

Hoffman, Lily. 1989. *The Politics of Knowledge*. Albany: State University of New York Press.

Hogle, L. F. 2002. "Introduction: Jurisdictions of Authority and Expertise in Science and Medicine." *Medical Anthropology* 21 (3/4): 231–246.

Homedes, Núria, A. C. Paz-Narváez, E. Selva-Suter, Olga Solas, and Antonio Ugalde. 2000. "Health Reform: Theory and Practice in El Salvador." In *Healthcare Reform and Poverty in Latin America*, ed. Peter Lloyd-Sherlock, 57–77. London: Institute of Latin American Studies.

Hook, Derek. 1997. "The Politics of Psychotherapy: An Historical Surface of Emergence." Paper presented at the 3rd Annual Qualitative Methods Conference: "Touch Me I'm Sick." Durban, South Africa, September 8 and 9.

Hornborg, Alf, and Carole Crumley. 2007. *The World System and the Earth System: Global Socioenvironmental Change and Sustainability since the Neolithic*. Walnut Creek, CA: Left Coast Press.

Hyde, Lewis. 1983. *The Gift: Imagination and the Erotic Life of Property*. New York: Random House.

ICMN. 1991. *Violations of Medical Neutrality: El Salvador*. Seattle, WA: International Commission on Medical Neutrality.

IDHUCA. 1992. "La salud en tiempos de guerra." *Estudios Centro-Americanos* 513–514: 653–673. Institute of Human Rights of the University of Central America Jose Siman Canas.

IMF. 1999. "Editorial" citing International Monetary Fund Balance of Payments Statistics Yearbook, Part 2, 1999, *Monthly Review* 53 (2).

Inhorn, Marcia C. 1995. "Medical Anthropology and Epidemiology: Divergences or Convergences?" *Social Science and Medicine* 403:285–290.

———. 2008. "Medical Anthropology against War." *Medical Anthropology Quarterly* 22 (4): 416–424.

IPM (Investigaciones de Población y Mercado). 1995. "Revisión y Evaluación de Promotores de Salud Comunitaria: Ministerio de Salud Pública y Asistencia Social y Organizaciones No Gubermentales, Informe Final (borrador)." San Salvador: Investigaciones de Población y Mercado.

Iunes, Roberto F. 2001. "Health Sector Organization/Reorganization in Latin America and the Caribbean." In *Health Services in Latin America and Asia*, eds. Carlos Gerardo Molina and José Nuñez del Arco, 203–222. Baltimore: Johns Hopkins University Press for the Inter-American Development Bank.

Jambai, Amara, and Carol MacCormack. 1996. "Maternal Health, War, and Religious Tradition: Authoritative Knowledge in Pujehun District, Sierra Leone" *Medical Anthropology Quarterly* 10 (2): 270–286.

Jenkins, Janis H. 1991. "The State Construction of Affect: Political Ethos and Mental Health among Salvadoran Refugees." *Culture, Medicine and Psychiatry* 15:139–165.

Jewson, N. D. 1976. "The Disappearance of the Sick Man from Medical Cosmology," *Sociology* 10:225–244.

Johns Hopkins Bloomberg School of Public Health. 2007. Updated Iraq Study Affirms Earlier Mortality Estimates. Available online at http://www.jhsph.edu/publichealthnews/press_releases/2006/burnham_iraq_2006.html.

Johnson, Lyman. 2004. "Why Dead Bodies Talk: An Introduction." In *Death, Dismemberment and Memory: Body Politics in Latin America*, ed. Lyman Johnson, 1–26. Albuquerque: University of New Mexico Press.

Jordan, Brigitte. 1993. *Birth in Four Cultures: A Crosscultural Investigation of Childbirth in Yucatan, Holland, Sweden, and the United States.* 4th ed. Prospect Heights, IL: Waveland Press.

Justice, Judith. 1986. *Policies, Plans & People: Foreign Aid and Health Development.* Berkeley and Los Angeles: University of California Press.

Kandel, Susan. 2002. "Migaciones, Medio Ambiente and Pobreza Rural en El Salvador." San Salvador: PRISMA (Programa Salvadoreño de Investigación Sobre Desarrolla y Medio Ambiente). Available online at http://prisma2.org.sv/web/publicaciones.php.

Kaufman, Robert R., and Joan M. Nelson, eds. 2004. *Crucial Needs, Weak Incentives: Social Sector Reform, Democratization, and Globalization in Latin America.* Baltimore: Johns Hopkins University Press.

Keune, Lou. 1995. *Sobrivimos la Guerra: Las Historia de las pobladores de Arcatao and San José de las Flores.* San Salvador: Adelina Editores.

Kiefer, Christie. 1992. "Militarism and World Health." *Social Science and Medicine* 347:719–724.

———. 2000. *Health Work with the Poor: A Practical Guide.* New Brunswick, NJ: Rutgers University Press.

Kim, Jim Yong, Joyce Millen, Alec Irwin, and John Gershman. 2000. *Dying for Growth: Global Inequality and the Health of the Poor.* Monroe, ME: Common Courage Press.

Kincaid, A. Douglas. 1987. "Peasants into Rebels: Community and Class in Rural El Salvador." *Comparative Studies in Society and History* 29 (3): 466–494.

Kirk, Robin. 2004. *More Terrible Than Death: Drugs, Violence, and America's War in Colombia.* New York: Public Affairs, Perseus Books.

Klare, Michael, and Peter Kornbluh. 1988. *Low-Intensity Warfare: Counterinsurgency, Proinsurgency and Antiterrorism in the Eighties.* New York: Pantheon.

Kleinman, Arthur. 1995. *Writing at the Margin: Discourse between Anthropology and Medicine.* Berkeley and Los Angeles: University of California Press.

Komter, A. E. 2005. *Social Solidarity and the Gift.* Cambridge: Cambridge University Press.

Krauss, Clifford. 1993. "How U.S. Actions Helped Hide Salvador Human Rights Abuses." *New York Times*, March 20.

Kuper, Leo. 1981. *Genocide: Its Political Use in the Twentieth Century.* New Haven, CT: Yale University Press.

Laclau, Ernest, and C. Mouffe. 1985. *Hegemony and Socialist Strategy: Towards a Radical Democratic Politics.* London: Verso.

LaFeber, Walter. 1993. *Inevitable Revolutions: The United States and Central America.* 2nd ed. New York: W. W. Norton.

Lan, David. 1985. *Guns & Rain: Guerrillas & Spirit Mediums in Zimbabwe.* London and Berkeley: University of California Press.

Lancaster, Roger N. 1988. *Thanks to God and the Revolution: Popular Religion and Class Consciousness in the New Nicaragua.* New York: Columbia University Press.

Langer, M. M. 1989. *Merleau-Ponty's Phenomenology of Perception: A Guide and Commentary.* Basingstoke, U.K.: Macmillan.

Laqueur, Thomas. 1989. "Bodies, Details and the Humanitarian Narrative." In *The New Cultural History*, ed. Lynn Hunt, 176–204. Berkeley and Los Angeles: University of California Press.

Leatherman, Thomas. 2005. "A Space of Vulnerability in Poverty and Health: Political-Ecology and Biocultural Analysis." *Ethos* 331:46–70.

Leonard, Stephen T. 1990. *Critical Theory in Political Practice*. Princeton, N.J.: Princeton University Press.

Lernoux, Penny. 1982. *Cry of the People: The Struggle for Human Rights in Latin America—The Catholic Church in Conflict with U.S. Policy*. New York: Penguin Books.

Levins, Richard. 1995. "Toward an Integrated Epidemiology." *TREE* 10 (7): 304.

Lewellen, Ted C. 2002. *The Anthropology of Globalization: Cultural Anthropology Enters the 21st Century*. Westport, CT: Bergin & Garvey.

———. 2003. *Political Anthropology: An Introduction*. Westport, CT: Praeger.

Lewis, Maureen, G. S. Eskeland, and X. Traa-Valerezo. 1999. "Challenging El Salvador's Rural Health Strategy" Policy Research Working Paper 2164. Human Development Sector Units and Development Research Group. Washington, DC: World Bank.

———. 2004. "Primary Health in Practice: Is It Effective?" *Health Policy* 70:303–325.

Linder, Fletcher. 2004. "Slave Ethics and Imagining Critically Applied Anthropology in Public Health Research." *Medical Anthropology* 23:329–358.

Lloyd-Sherlock, Peter. 2000. *Healthcare Reform and Poverty in Latin America*. London: Institute of Latin American Studies.

Lock, M. 2001. "The Tempering of Medical Anthropology: Troubling Natural Categories." *Medical Anthropology Quarterly* 15 (4):478–492.

López Vigil, María. 1987. *Don Lito de El Salvador: Habla Un Campesino*. San Salvador: UCA Editores.

Loveman, Brian, and Thomas M. Davies Jr. 1978. *The Politics of Antipolitics: The Military in Latin America*. Lincoln: University of Nebraska Press.

Low, Setha. 1994. Embodied Metaphors: Nerves as Lived Experience. In *Embodiment and Experience: The Existential Ground of Culture and Self*, ed. Thomas Csordas, 139–162. Cambridge: Cambridge University Press.

Lundgren, Rebeka I., and Robert Lang. 1989. "There Is No Sea, Only Fish": Effects of United States Policy on the Health of the Displaced in El Salvador." *Social Science & Medicine* 28 (7): 697–706.

Lungo Uclés, Mario. 1996. *El Salvador in the Eighties: Counterinsurgency and Revolution*. Philadelphia: Temple University Press.

Lutz, Catherine. 1988. *Unnatural Emotions: Everyday Sentiments on a Micronesian Atoll and Their Challenge to Western Theory*. Chicago: University of Chicago Press.

Lyon, Margot L. 1990. "Order and Healing: The Concept of Order and Its Importance in the Conceptualization of Healing." *Medical Anthropology* 12:249–268.

Lyon, Margot, and J. M. Barbalet. 1994. Society's Body: Emotion and the Somaticization of Social Theory. In *Embodiment and Experience: The Existential Ground of Culture and Self*, ed. Thomas Csordas, 48–66. Cambridge: Cambridge University Press.

MacLean, John. 1987. *Prolonging the Agony: The Human Cost of Low-Intensity Warfare*. London: El Salvador Committee for Human Rights.

Manwaring, Max. 1990. "Toward an Understanding of Insurgency Wars: The Paradigm." In *Uncomfortable Wars: Toward a New Paradigm of Low Intensity Conflict*, ed. Max Manwaring, 19–28. Boulder, CO: Westview Press.

Manwaring, Max, and Courtney Prisk. 1988. *El Salvador: An Oral History*. Washington, DC: National Defense University Press.

Martín-Baró, Ignacio. 1990. *Psicología Social de la Guerra*. San Salvador: UCA Editores.

———. 1998. *Ignacio Martín-Baró 1942–1989*: Psicología de la Liberación para América, comp. G. Pacheco and Bernardo Jiménez. Guadalajara: Instituto Tecnológico y de Estudios Superiores de Occidente Departamento de Extensión Universitaria Universidad de Guadalajara.

Matomora, M.K.S. 1989. "Mass Produced Village Health Workers and the Promise of Primary Health Care." *Social Science and Medicine* 28 (10):1081–1084.

Maupin, Jonathan. 2008. "Fruit of the Accords: Healthcare Reform and Civil Participation in Highland Guatemala." Unpublished manuscript, in author's possession.

Mazur, Laurie Ann. 1994. *Beyond the Numbers: A Reader on Population, Consumption, and the Environment*. Washington, DC: Island Press.

McClintock, Michael. 1985. *State Terror and Popular Resistance in El Salvador*. Vol. 1 of *The American Connection*. London: Zed Books.

McElroy, A., and P. K. Townsend. 2004. *Medical Anthropology in Ecological Perspective*. Boulder, CO: Westview Press.

McGuire, Meredith B. 1988. *Ritual Healing in Suburban America*. New Brunswick, NJ: Rutgers University Press.

Messer, Ellen. 1993. "Anthropology and Human Rights." *Annual Review of Anthropology* 22:221–249.

Metzi, Francisco. 1988. *The People's Remedy: Health Care in El Salvador's War of Liberation*. New York: Monthly Review Press.

Meyers, Alan, Adrienne Epstein, and Doris Burford, et al. 1989. "Community Health Assessment of a Repopulated Village in El Salvador." *Medical Anthropology Quarterly* 33:270–280.

Mittal, Anuradha. 2001. "Land Loss, Poverty and Hunger." *IFG Bulletin* 1 (3), International Forum on Globalization.

Montgomery, Tommie Sue. 1995. *Revolution in El Salvador: From Civil Strife to Civil Peace*. 2nd ed. San Francisco: Westview Press.

Moody, Ellen. 2005. "Public Death and Privatization in Post-War El Salvador." Paper delivered at the American Anthropological Association's annual meeting, December 2005.

Morgan, Lynn. 1989. " 'Political Will' and Community Participation in Costa Rican Primary Health Care." *Medical Anthropology Quarterly* 33:232–245.

———. 1993. *Community Participation in Health: The Politics of Primary Care in Costa Rica*. New York: Cambridge University Press.

Morgen, Sandra. 1990. "Two Faces of the State: Women, Social Control, and Empowerment." In *Uncertain Terms: Negotiating Gender in American Culture*, eds. Faye Ginsburg and Anna Lowenhaupt Tsing, 169–182. Boston: Beacon Press.

Muller, Frits. 1989. *Pobreza, Participacion y Salud: Casos Latinoamericanos*. Medellin: Editorial, Universidad de Antioquia.

Murray, Kevin, and T. Barry. 1995. *Inside El Salvador*. Albuquerque: Interhemispheric Resource Center.

Navarro, Vicente. 1977. *Medicine under Capitalism*. New York: Prodist.

———. 1988. "Professional Dominance or Proletarianization? Neither." *The Milbank Quarterly* 66 (2): 57–75.

NCAHRN. 1986. "Health Consequences of the War in Nicaragua, 1985–86." Joint publication of the National Central America Health Rights Network, New York, and the Committee for Health Rights in Central America, San Francisco.

Nelson, Anne. 1985. "Mercenary Marketers Cashing in on the Salvadoran Air War." *Multinational Monitor*, December/January: 6–7.

Nelson, Diane. 2002. "Relating to Terror: Gender, Anthropology, Law and Some September Elevenths" In *Duke Journal of Gender, Law and Policy*, Summer: 195–211.

Nelson, Joan M. 2004. "The Politics of Health Sector Reform: Cross-National Comparisons." In *Crucial Needs, Weak Incentives: Social Sector Reform, Democratization, and Globalization in Latin America*, ed. Robert R. Kaufman and Joan M. Nelson, 23–64. Baltimore: Johns Hopkins University Press.

Nelson-Pallmeyer, John. 1989. *War against the Poor: Low-intensity Conflict and Christian Faith.* Maryknoll, NY: Orbis Books.

Nichter, Mark. 1984. "Project Community Diagnosis: Participatory Research as a First Step toward Community Involvement in Primary Health Care." *Social Science and Medicine* 193:237–252.

———. 1986. "The Primary Health Center as a Social System: Primary Health Care, Social Status, and the Issue of Team-work in South Asia." *Social Science and Medicine* 234:347–355.

Nissenbaum, Dion, and Shashank Bengali. 2009. "Israeli Ground War Bisects Gaza, Deepens Humanitarian Crisis." *McClatchy Newspapers* (wire). Washington Bureau. January 4.

Nonini, Donald M. 2007. "Introduction: The Global Idea of 'the Commons.'" In *The Global Idea of "the Commons,"* ed. Donald M. Nonini, 1–25. New York: Berghahn Books.

Nordstrom, Carolyn. 1992. "The Backyard Front." In *The Paths to Domination, Resistance, and Terror*, eds. Carolyn Nordstrom and JoAnne Martin, 260–274. Berkeley and Los Angeles: University of California Press.

———. 1997. *A Different Kind of War Story.* Philadelphia: University of Pennsylvania Press.

———. 1998. "Terror Warfare and the Medicine of Peace" *Medical Anthropology Quarterly* 12 (1): 103–121.

O'Donnell, Guillermo. 1986. "Tensions in the Bureaucratic-Authoritarian State and the Question of Democracy." In *Promise of Development: Theories of Change in Latin America*, eds. P. Klarén, and T. Bossert, 239–275. Boulder, CO: Westview Press.

Ollman, Bertell. 1993. *Dialectical Investigations.* New York: Routledge.

O'Neill, John. 1985. *Five Bodies: The Human Shape of Modern Society.* Ithaca, NY: Cornell University Press.

———. 2004. *Five Bodies: Re-figuring Relationships.* Thousand Oaks, CA: Sage.

Ortner, Sherry B. 1984. "Theory in Anthropology since the Sixties." *Comparative Studies in Society and History* 261:126–166.

Paige, Jeffrey M. 1994. "History and Memory in El Salvador: Elite Ideology and the Insurrection and Massacre of 1932." Paper presented at the Annual Meeting of the Latin American Studies Association, Atlanta, March 11.

Palmer, Steven. 2003. *From Popular Medicine to Medical Populism: Doctors, Healers, and the Public Power in Costa Rica, 1800–1940.* Durham, NC: Duke University Press.

Pandolfi, Mariella. 2007. "Memory within the Body: Women's Narratives and Identity in a Southern Italian Village." In *Beyond the Body Proper: Reading the Anthropology of Material Life*, eds. Margaret Lock and Judith Farquhar, 451–458. Durham, NC: Duke University Press.

Pastor, Manuel, Jr., and Michael Conroy. 1995. "Distributional Implications of Macroeconomic Policy: Theory and Applications to El Salvador." *World Development* 23 (12): 2117–2131.

Paul, Benjamin D., and William J. Demarest. 1984. "Citizen Participation Overplanned: The Case of a Health Project in the Guatemalan Community of San Pedro la Laguna." *Social Science and Medicine* 193:185–192.

Pearce, Jenny. 1986. *Promised Land: Peasant Rebellion in Chalatenango, El Salvador.* New York: Monthly Review Press.

Pearce, Tola Olu. 1993. "Lay Medical Knowledge in an African Context." In *Knowledge, Power and Practice: The Anthropology of Medicine and Everyday Life*, eds. Shirley Lindenbaum and Margaret Lock, 150–165. Berkeley and Los Angeles: University of California Press.

Pedelty, Mark. 1995. *War Stories: The Culture of Foreign Correspondents.* New York: Routledge.

Petras, James, and Steve Vieux. 1992. "Myths and Realities: Latin America's Free Markets." *International Journal of Health Services* 224: 611–617.

Physicians for Human Rights. 1990. *El Salvador: Health Care under Siege: Violations of Medical Neutrality during the Civil Conflict.* Boston: Physicians for Human Rights.

Pinochet, Augusto. 1968. *Geopolitica.* Santiago, Chile: Editorial Gabriela Mistral.

Pion-Berlin, David. 1991. "The Ideological Governance of Perception in the Use of State Terror in Latin America: The Case of Argentina." In *State Organized Terror: The Case of Violent Internal Repression*, eds. P. T. Bushnell, Vladimir Shlapentokh, John Mccamant, Christopher Vanderpool, and Jeyaratnam Sundram, 135–152. Boulder, CO: Westview Press.

Porpora, Douglas V. 1990. *How Holocausts Happen: The United States in Central America.* Philadelphia: Temple University Press.

Poteliakhoff, A. 1987. The Arms Race and the Health Needs of the Developing Countries. *Medicine and War* 3:101.

PRODERE. 1992. "Propuesta de Plan de Trabajo en Salud en el Departamento de Chalatenango." Unpublished working paper. October.

Prokosch, M. 1997. "Fighting Phone Privatization in El Salvador." *Dollars & Sense.* July–August issue, 34–38.

Public Health Commission Report. 1983. "Report of the Second Public Health Commission to El Salvador." New York: Committee for Health Rights in El Salvador.

Puffer, R. R., and C. V. Serrano. 1973. *Patterns of Mortality in Childhood.* Washington DC: Pan American Health Organization (PAHO), Scientific Publication No. 262.

Quesada, J. 1998. "Suffering Child: An Embodiment of War and Its Aftermath in Post-Sandinista Nicaragua." *Medical Anthropology Quarterly* 12 (1):51–73.

Quinn, John R. 1981. "The Public Debate on Social Justice and Health Care: An Opportunity for Evangelization." In *The Ministry of Healing,* 79–82. St. Louis: The Catholic Health Association of the United States.

Rao, Mohan. 1999. *Disinvesting in Health: The World Bank's Prescriptions for Health.* London: Sage Publications.

Ratcliffe, John. 1978. "Social Justice and the Demographic Transition: Lessons from India's Kerala State." *International Journal of Health Services* 81:123–144.

Redfield, Peter. 2005. "Doctors, Borders and Life in Crisis." *Cultural Anthropology* 203:328–361.

Rifkin, Susan B. 1986. "Health Planning and Community Participation." *World Health Forum* 7:156–162.

Rifkin, Susan B., Frits Muller, and Wolfgang Bichmann. 1988. "Primary Health Care: On Measuring Participation." *Social Science and Medicine* 269:931–940.

Rifkin, Susan B., and Gill Walt. 1986. "Why Health Improves: Defining the Issues Concerning 'Comprehensive Primary Health Care' and 'Selective Primary Health Care.'" *Social Science and Medicine* 236:559–566.

Rodriguez, Claudia. 2009. "El Salvador's Presidential Elections." Latin American Working Group Web site. http://www.lawg.org/index.php?option=com_content&task=view&id=390&Itemid=68.

Rohter, Larry. 1994. "Remembering the Past, Repeating It Anyway." *New York Times*, July 24, sec. 4, p. 1.

Rosa, Herman. 1993. *AID y las Transformaciones Globales en El Salvador*. Managua: Coordinadora Regional de Investigaciones Economicas y Sociales CRIES.

Roseberry, William. 1994. "Hegemony and the Language of Contention." In *Everyday Forms of State Formation: Revolution and the Negotiation of Rule in Modern Mexico*, eds. G. M. Joseph, and D. Nugent, 355–366. Durham, NC: Duke University Press.

Rosenberg, Tina. 1992. *Children of Cain: Violence and the Violent in Latin America*. New York: Penguin.

Rubel, Arthur. 1990. "Compulsory Medical Service and Primary Health Care: A Mexican Case" In *Anthropology and Primary Health Care*, eds. Jeannine Coreil and J. Dennis Mull, 137–153. Boulder, CO: Westview Press.

Sabo, Lois, and Joachim Kibirige. 1989. "Political Violence and Eritrean Health Care." *Social Science and Medicine* 287:677–684.

Sarkesian, Sam C. 1993. *Unconventional Conflicts in a New Security Era: Lessons from Malaya and Vietnam*. Westport, CT: Greenwood Press.

Sauerborn, R. A., A. Nougtara, and H. J. Diesfeld. 1989. "Low Utilization of Community Health Workers: Results from a Household Interview Survey in Burkina Faso." *Social Science and Medicine* 29 (10): 1163–1174.

Sayer, Derek. 1994. "Everyday Forms of State Formation: Some Dissident Remarks on Hegemony." In *Everyday Forms of State Formation: Revolution and the Negotiation of Rule in Modern Mexico*, eds. G. M. Joseph and D. Nugent, 367–378. Durham, NC: Duke University Press.

Scarry, Elaine. 1985. *The Body in Pain: The Making and Unmaking of the World*. New York: Oxford University Press.

Schaull, Wendy. 1990. *Tortillas, Beans, and M-16s: A Year with the Guerrillas in El Salvador*. London: Pluto Press.

Scheper-Hughes, Nancy. 1992. *Death without Weeping: The Violence of Everyday Life in Brazil*. Berkeley and Los Angeles: University of California Press.

———. 1994. "Embodied Knowledge: Thinking with the Body in Critical Medical Anthropology" In *Assessing Cultural Anthropology*, ed. Robert Borofsky, 229–239. New York: McGraw-Hill.

Scheper-Hughes, Nancy, and Margaret Lock. 1987. "The Mindful Body: A Prolegomenon to Future Work in Medical Anthropology." *Medical Anthropology Quarterly* 1:6–41.

Scholl, E. A. 1985. "An Assessment of Community Health Workers in Nicaragua." *Social Science and Medicine* 203:207–214.

Schoultz, Lars. 1987. *National Security and United States Policy toward Latin America*. Princeton, NJ: Princeton University Press.

Schuld, Leslie. 2003. "El Salvador: Who Will Have the Hospitals?" *NACLA Report on the Americas*, 21 (January/February): 42–45.

Scott, James C. 1976. *The Moral Economy of the Peasant: Rebellion and Subsistence in Southeast Asia*. New Haven: Yale University Press.

———. 1985. *Weapons of the Weak: Everyday Forms of Peasant Resistance*. New Haven, CT: Yale University Press.

———. 1990. *Domination and the Arts of Resistance: Hidden Transcripts*. New Haven, CT: Yale University Press.

Second U.S. Public Health Commission. 1983. *Health and Human Rights in El Salvador*. New York, Boston: Committee for Health Rights in El Salvador.

Segall, M. 1983. "On the Concept of a Marxist Health System: A Question of Marxist Epistemology." *International Journal of Health Services* 13:221–225.

Selva-Sutter, Ernesto. 2000. "Historias prohibidas de la Reforma de Salud en El Salvador." March. Working paper. Universidad Centroamericana (UCA) Jose Simeon Canas, San Salvador.

Sen, Amartya K. 1999. *Development as Freedom.* New York: Knopf.

Silber, Irina Carlota. 2004. "Not Revolutionary Enough? Community Building in Postwar Chalatenango." In *Landscapes of Struggle: Politics, Society, and Community in El Salvador,* eds. A. Lauria-Santiago and L. Binford, 166–186. Pittsburgh: University of Pittsburgh Press.

Silverman, Marilyn, and P. H. Gulliver. 2006. " 'Common Sense' and 'Governmentality': Local Government in Southeastern Ireland, 1850–1922." *Journal of the Royal Anthropological Institute* 12:109–127.

Simpson, John, and Jana Bennett. 1985. *The Disappeared and the Mothers of the Plaza: The Story of the 11,000 Argentinians Who Vanished.* New York: St. Martin's Press.

Sinclair, Minor. 1995 .*New Politics of Survival: Grassroots Movements in Central America.* New York: Monthly Review Press.

Singer, Merrill, and Hans Baer. 1995. *Critical Medical Anthropology.* Amityville, NY: Baywood Press.

Singer, Merrill, and Scott Clair. 2003. "Syndemics and Public Health: Reconceptualizing Disease in Bio-Social Context." *Medical Anthropology Quarterly* 17 (4): 423–441.

Skalnick, Peter. 1989. *Outwitting the State.* New Brunswick, NJ: Transaction Publishers.

Sloan, John W. 1984. "State Repression and Enforcement Terrorism in Latin America." In *The State as Terrorist: The Dynamics of Governmental Violence and Repression,* eds. Michael Stohl and George A. Lopez, 83–98. Westport, CT: Greenwood Press.

Smith, Christian. 1991. *The Emergence of Liberation Theology: Radical Religion and Social Movement Theory.* Chicago: University of Chicago Press.

Smith, Sandy. 1985. "Rain of Terror: The Bombing of Civilians in El Salvador" *Health & Medicine,* Winter Issue, 21, 26–28.

———. 1987. "Nicaragua Schism: Clinics Often Destroyed in War; Contras Blamed." *American Medical News,* February 13: 1.

———. 1988. "Health Workers Fear Contra Attacks." *American Medical News,* January 15: 1.

———. 1989a. "MDs, Health Workers Caught in Crossfire in El Salvador War." *American Medical News,* March 15: 3, 17–18.

———. 1989b. "Health Care Battle in El Salvador." *San Francisco Chronicle,* May 10: Briefing Section, 5.

———. 1989c. "Health Workers Harassed in El Salvador War." *American Medical News,* September 1: 1, 13.

———. 1990. "Renewed Fighting Cripples El Salvador Health System." *American Medical News,* January 19.

———. 1997a. " 'Popular' Health and the State: Dialectics of the Peace Process in El Salvador." *Social Science & Medicine* 44 (5): 635–645.

———. 1997b. "Primary Health Care and Its Unfulfilled Promise of Community Participation: Lessons from a Salvadoran War Zone." *Human Organization* 56 (3): 364–374.

———. 1998. "Health 'Anti-Reform' in El Salvador: Community Health NGOs and the State in the Neoliberal Era." *Political and Legal Anthropology Review (PoLAR)* 21 (1): 99–111.

———. 2000. "The Smoke and Mirrors of Health Reform in El Salvador: Community Health NGOs and the Not-So-Neoliberal State." In *Dying for Growth: Global Restructuring and the Health of the Poor*, eds. Jim Yong Kim, Joyce V. Millen, Alec Irwin and John Gershman, 359–381. Monroe, ME: Common Courage Press.

Sollis, Peter. 1992. "Displaced Persons and Human Rights: The Crisis in El Salvador." *Bulletin of Latin American Research* III:49–67.

———. 1996. "Partners in Development? The State, NGOs and the UN in Central America." In *NGOs, the UN and Global Governance*, eds. Thomas Weiss and Leon Gordenker, 189–206. Boulder, CO: Lynne Rienner Publishers.

Solway, Jacqueline. 2006. " 'The Original Affluent Society': Four Decades On." In *The Politics of Egalitarianism*, ed. Jacqueline Solway, 65–78. New York: Berghann Books.

Stanley, William. 1996. *The Protection Racket State: Elite Politics, Military Extortion, and Civil War in El Salvador*. Philadelphia: Temple University Press.

Stark, Ruth. 1985. "Lay Workers in Primary Health Care: Victims in the Process of Social Transformation." *Social Science and Medicine* 203:269–275.

Starn, Orin. 1991. "Missing the Revolution: Anthropologists and the War in Peru." *Cultural Anthropology* 61:63–91.

———. 1992. " 'I Dreamed of Foxes and Hawks': Reflections on Peasant Protest, New Social Movements, and the Rondas Campesinas of Northern Peru." In *The Making of Social Movements in Latin America: Identity, Strategy, and Democracy*, eds. A. Escobar and S. Alvarez, 89–III. Boulder, CO: Westview Press.

Stephen, Lynn. 1994. *Hear My Testimony: Maria Teresa Tula, Human Rights Activist of El Salvador*. Boston: South End Press.

Stoll, D. 1999. *Rigoberta Menchú and the Story of All Poor Guatemalans*. Boulder, CO: Westview Press.

Strathern, Andrew. 1996. *Body Thoughts*. Ann Arbor: University of Michigan Press.

Stutzman, Ronald. 1980. "El Mestizaje: An All-Inclusive Ideology of Exclusion." In *Cultural Transformations and Ethnicity in Modern Ecuador*, ed. N. Whitten, 45–94. Chicago: University of Chicago Press.

Stycos, J. Mayone. 1984. "Sterilization in Latin America: Its Past and Future." *International Family Planning Perspectives* 102:58–64.

Suarez-Orozco, Marcelo. 1990. "Speaking of the Unspeakable: Toward a Psychosocial Understanding of Responses to Terror." *Ethos* 183:353–383.

———. 1992. "A Grammar of Terror: Psychocultural Responses to State Terrorism in Dirty War and Post–Dirty War Argentina." In *The Paths to Domination, Resistance, and Terror.*, ed. C. Nordstrom and J. A. Martin, 219–259. Berkeley and Los Angeles: University of California Press.

Sunkel, Osvaldo. 1995. "Uneven Globalization, Economic Reform, and Democracy: A View from Latin America." In *Whose World Order? Uneven Globilization and the end of the Cold War*, eds. Hans-Henrik Holm and Georg Sorensen, 43–67. Boulder, CO: Westview Press.

Tajer, Débora. 2003. "Latin American Social Medicine: Roots, Development during the 1990s, and Current Challenges." *American Journal of Public Health* 93 (12): 2023–2027.

Taussig, Michael T. 1978. "Nutrition, Development, and Foreign Aid: A Case Study of U.S.-Directed Health Care in a Colombian Plantation Zone." *International Journal of Health Services* 81:101–121.

———. 1986. *Shamanism, Colonialism, and the Wild Man: A Study in Terror and Healing*. Chicago: University of Chicago Press.

———. 1992. *The Nervous System*. New York: Routledge.

Third U.S. Public Health Commission to El Salvador. 1985. "El Salvador 1985: Health, Human Rights and the War." San Francisco: Committee for Health Rights in Central America.

Thornton, Lewis H., Peter Boddy, and M. Roy Brooks Jr. 1994. "Mid-Term Evaluation—Maternal Health and Child Survival Project PROSAMI," Project Number 519-0367. San Salvador: Report prepared for the U.S. Agency for International Development.

Tilley, Virginia. 2005. *Seeing Indians: A Study of Race, Nation, and Power in El Salvador*. Albuquerque: University of New Mexico Press.

Trinquier, Roger. 1964. *Modern Warfare: A French View of Counterinsurgency*. New York: Praeger.

Trostle, James. 1986. "Anthropology and Epidemiology in the Twentieth Century: A Selective History of Collaborative Projects and Theoretical Affinities, 1920–1970." In *Anthropology and Epidemiology*, eds. Craig R. Janes, Ron Stall, and Sandra M. Gifford, 59–94. Boston: Reidel Publishing.

Turner, Bryan S. 1992. *Regulating Bodies: Essays in Medical Sociology*. London: Routledge.

———. 1996. *The Body and Society: Explorations in Social Theory*. Thousand Oaks, CA: Sage Publications.

Turner, V. W. 1957. *Schism and Continuity in an African Society: A Study of Ndembu Village Life*. Manchester, U.K.: Rhodes-Livingstone Institute Northern Rhodesia/Manchester University Press.

Turner, Victor. 1974. *Dramas, Fields, and Metaphors: Symbolic Action in Human Society*. Ithaca, NY: Cornell University Press.

Ugalde, Antonio. 1985. "Ideological Dimensions of Community Participation in Latin American Health Programs." *Social Science and Medicine* 211:41–53.

Ugalde, Antonio, Ernesto Selva-Sutter, Carolina Castilla, Caroline Paz, and Sergio Cañas. 2000. "The Health Costs of War: Can They Be Measured? Lessons from El Salvador." *British Medical Journal* 321:169–172.

UN Truth Commission. 1992. *From Madness to Hope: The 12-Year War in El Salvador*. Report of the United Nations Truth Commission. New York: UN Security Council.

Unger, Jean-Pierre, and J. Killingsworth. 1986. "Selective Primary Care: A Critical Review of Methods and Results." *Social Science and Medicine* 22 (10):1001–1013.

Van der Geest, Sjaak, Johan D. Speckmann, and Pieter H. Streefland. 1990. "Primary Health Care in a Multi-level Perspective: Towards a Research Agenda." *Social Science and Medicine* 309:1025–1034.

Varela, F. J., E. Thompson, and Eleanor Rosch. 1991. *The Embodied Mind: Cognitive Science and Human Experience*. Cambridge, MA: MIT Press.

Vergara, Pilar. 1997. "In Pursuit of 'Growth with Equity': The Limits of Chile's Free-Market Social Reforms." *International Journal of Health Services* 272:207–215.

Vilas, Carlos M. 1995. *Between Earthquakes and Volcanos: Market, State, and the Revolutions in Central America*. New York: Monthly Review Press.

Virchow, Rudolf. 1985 (1848). *Collected Essays on Public Health and Epidemiology*, Vol. 2, ed. Lelland J. Rather, Canton, MA: Science History Publications, Watson Publishing International.

Wagelstein, John. 1985. "Post-Vietnam Counterinsurgency Doctrine," *Military Review* January: 42.

Waitzkin, H., and C. Iriart. 2001. "How the United States Exports Managed Care to Third World Countries." *International Journal of Health Services* 31:495–505.

Walsh, Julia A., and Kenneth Warren. 1979. "Selective Primary Health Care: An Interim Strategy for Disease Control in Developing Countries." *New England Journal of Medicine* 301 (18): 967–974.

Walt, Gill. 1994. *Health Policy: An Introduction to Process and Power*. Johannesburg, South Africa: Witwatersrand University Press.

Walt, Gill, Myrtle Perera, and Kris Heggenhougen. 1989. "Are Large-Scale Volunteer Community Health Worker Programmes Feasible? The Case of Sri Lanka." *Social Science and Medicine* 295:599–608.

Wartenberg, Thomas E. 1990. *The Forms of Power: From Domination to Transformation.* Philadelphia: Temple University Press.

Wayland, Coral, and Jerome Crowder. 2002. "Disparate Views of Community in Primary Health Care: Understanding How Perceptions Influence Success" *Medical Anthropology Quarterly* 16 (2): 230–247.

Weissman, Fabrice. 2004. *In the Shadow of 'Just Wars': Violence, Politics, and Humanitarian Action,* Ithaca, NY: Cornell University Press.

Wellin, Edward. 1955. "Water Boiling in a Peruvian Town" In *Health, Culture and Community: Case Studies of Public Reactions to Health Programs,* ed. Benjamin D. Paul, 71–103. New York: Russell Sage Foundation.

Werner, David. 1977. *Where There Is No Doctor.* Palo Alto, CA: Hesperian Foundation.

———. 1981. "The Village Health Worker: Lackey or Liberator?" *World Health Forum* 21:46–48.

Werner, David, and B. Bower. 1982. *Helping Health Workers Learn.* Palo Alto: Hesperian Foundation.

Weyland, Kurt. 1995. "Social Movements and the State: The Politics of Health Reform in Brazil." *World Development* 23 (10): 1699–1712.

White, Richard Alan. 1980. "El Salvador between Two Fires." *America,* November 1: 262–266. Published by the Council on Hemispheric Affairs.

Whitfield, Teresa. 1995. *Paying the Price: Ignacio Ellacuria and the Murdered Jesuits of El Salvador.* Philadelphia: Temple University Press.

Williams, Robert G. 1986. *Export Agriculture and the Crisis in Central America.* Chapel Hill: University of North Carolina Press.

Wisner, B. 1988. "Gobi Versus Primary Health Care: Some Dangers of Selective Primary Care" *Social Science and Medicine* 26 (9): 963–969.

Woelk, Godfrey B. 1992. "Cultural and Structural Influences in the Creation of and Participation in Community Health Programmes." *Social Science and Medicine* 354:419–424.

Woerner, Fred F. 1990. "The Strategic Imperatives for the United States in Latin America." In *Uncomfortable Wars: Toward a New Paradigm of Low Intensity Conflict,* ed. Max G. Manwaring, 57–67. Boulder, CO: Westview Press.

Wolf, Eric R. 1969. *Peasant Wars of the Twentieth Century.* New York: Harper & Row.

Wolfwood, Theresa. 2003. "Victory for Health Workers in El Salvador." *Island Net.* Available at www.islandnet.com/.

Wood, Elizabeth J. 2003. *Insurgent Collective Action and Civil War in El Salvador.* Cambridge, New York: Cambridge University Press.

World Bank. 1993. *Investing in Health.* World Development Report. New York: Oxford University Press.

Yarborough, William. 1989. "Counterinsurgency: The United States' Role—Past, Present, and Future." In *Guerrilla Warfare and Counterinsurgency,* eds. Richard Shultz, Robert Pfaltzgraff, Uri Ra'anan, and William Olson, 103–114. Toronto: Lexington Books.

Zola, Irving. 1972. "Medicine as an Institution of Social Control." *Sociological Review* 20:487–504.

Zwi, Anthony B. 1987. "The Political Abuse of Medicine and the Challenge of Opposing It." *Social Science and Medicine* 25 (6): 649–657.

Zwi, Anthony B., and Antonio Ugalde. 1989. "Towards an Epidemiology of Political Violence in the Third World." *Social Science and Medicine* 287:633–642.

INDEX

Italicized page numbers refer to figures and illustrations.

ABOUT THE AUTHOR

SANDY SMITH-NONINI, PhD, is a research assistant professor in the department of anthropology at the University of North Carolina, Chapel Hill. She previously taught on the sociology and anthropology faculty at Elon University from 2000 to 2005. Dr. Smith-Nonini received the Richard Carley Hunt Post-Doctoral Writing Fellowship in 2005 to complete this project, which draws on ethnographic research and human rights journalism in El Salvador dating to the late 1980s, when she lived in the country while reporting on the civil war for U.S. newspapers. She won the Peter K. New Award from the Society for Applied Anthropology for a 1995 article on primary health care in El Salvador. She has published on health, development, and immigrant labor in *Social Science & Medicine*, *Human Organization*, *Social Analysis*, *Medical Anthropology*, *Political and Legal Anthropology Review*, and numerous book collections.